Mosby's
E X P E R T
10-Minute
Physical Examinations

Mosby's
E X P E R T
10-Minute
Physical Examinations

Second Edition

ELSEVIER
MOSBY

ELSEVIER
MOSBY

11830 Westline Industrial Drive
St. Louis, Missouri 63146

MOSBY'S EXPERT 10-MINUTE PHYSICAL EXAMINATIONS   ISBN 0-323-02880-2
Copyright © 2005, Elsevier Inc.

NOTICE

Health and physical assessment is an ever-changing field. Standard safety precautions must be followed, but as new research and clinical experience broaden our knowledge, changes in treatment and drug therapy may become necessary or appropriate. Readers are advised to check the most current product information provided by the manufacturer of each drug to be administered to verify the recommended dose, the method and duration of administration, and contraindications. It is the responsibility of the licensed prescriber, relying on experience and knowledge of the patient, to determine dosages and the best treatment for each individual patient. Neither the publisher nor the author assumes any liability for any injury and/or damage to persons or property arising from this publication.

Previous edition copyrighted 1997

International Standard Book Number 0-323-02880-2

Executive Publisher: Barbara Nelson Cullen
Executive Editor: Cindy Tryniszewski, RN, MSN
Developmental Editors: Adrienne Simon, Laura Sieh Chu
Clinical Project Manager: Colleen P. Seeber-Combs, RN, MSN
Publishing Services Manager: John Rogers
Project Manager: Doug Turner
Designer: Amy Buxton

Printed in the United States of America

Last digit is the print number: 9   8   7   6   5   4   3   2   1

CONTENTS

CONTENTS

Appendixes

Cynthia Blank-Reid, RN, MSN, CEN
Trauma Clinical Nurse Specialist
Temple University Hospital
Philadelphia, Pennsylvania

Christopher J. Combs, PhD
Department of Psychiatry
Temple University School of Medicine
Philadelphia, Pennsylvania

Melissa M. Dikeman, MSN, CRNP
Nurse Practitioner, Primary Care
Philadelphia VA Hospital
Philadelphia, Pennsylvania

Ellie Z. Franzes, MSN, CRNP, CNRN
Nurse Practitioner, Neurosurgery
St. Luke's Hospital and Health Network
Bethlehem, Pennsylvania

Catherine Glynn-Milley, RN, CRND, CPHQ
Ophthalmic Coordinator
Veteran Affairs Palo Alto Health Care Systems
Palo Alto, California

Eva L. McCaully, RN, MSN
Independent Consultant
Collegeville, Pennsylvania

Kendra Menzies, RN, MS, CCRN, CNRN
Unit Educator
Neurological ICU
Harris Methodist Hospital
Fort Worth, Texas

Donna Perry, RN, MS, NP
Coordinator, The International Nurse Consultant
    Program
The Center for Clinical and Professional
    Development
Massachusetts General Hospital
Boston, Massachusetts

Teresa Regillo, RN, MSN
Independent Consultant
Philadelphia, Pennsylvania

Barbara A. Todd, MSN, CRNP
Director, Clinical Surgical Specialists and
    Practitioners (CSSP)
Hospital University of Pennsylvania
Adjunct Faculty
University of Pennsylvania School of Nursing
Philadelphia, Pennsylvania

SPECIAL THANKS TO

Villanova University
College of Nursing
Villanova, Pennsylvania
for use of their nursing laboratory and supplies.

Karen Fenstermacher, RN, MS, Certified FNP
Family Nurse Practitioner
Freeman Health Systems
Carthage, Missouri

Patricia Iyer, RN, MSN, LNCC
President
Medical League Support Services, Inc.
Flemington, New Jersey

Annabelle M. Keene, RN, MSN, BC
School Nurse
Bellevue Public Schools
Bellevue, Nebraska;
Former Associate Professor
College of Saint Mary
Omaha, Nebraska

Elizabeth Marci Rash, PhD, FNP-C
Adjunct Instructor
School of Nursing
College of Health and Public Affairs
University of Central Florida
Orlando, Florida

Dottie Roberts, RN, MSN, BC, MACI,
  CMSRN, ONC
Clinical Nurse Specialist
Rehabilitative & Medical Services
Palmetto Health Baptist
Columbia, South Carolina

Marianne Shaughnessy, PhD, CRNP
Associate Director of Education/Evaluation
Baltimore VA GRECC
Assistant Professor
School of Nursing
University of Maryland
Baltimore, Maryland

What can you accomplish in 10 minutes…Take a report?… Set up a tube feeding?…Irrigate and dress a wound? How about examine your patient from head to toe? That's exactly what the second edition of *Mosby's Expert 10-Minute Physical Examinations* will help you do. When you open this latest edition, you'll see a physical examination book like no other. Packed with time-saving tips, this book will help you to organize your physical examination so that you can move through the examination quickly—and without missing critical findings. The book's organization allows you to rapidly find what you need. The content is organized by body region—for example chest and back—rather than by body system, an approach that provides an excellent method for conducting a thorough examination. What's more, the book will help you realize when to shift gears and focus the examination on a critical sign or chief complaint.

How to use this book

There are two ways to use this book and approach the physical examination. Your choice of methods will depend on the condition and the most pressing problems of your patient. Let's say your patient is hospitalized for a specific condition, such as pneumonia, is resting comfortably, and is not in any distress. In this situation, you have the "luxury" of performing a head-to-toe examination, keeping in mind the admission diagnosis and reason for hospitalization. Working methodically, you can cover all areas of the body, picking up any abnormal findings. And you can pace yourself knowing you'll need to spend extra time examining the chest and back or other areas that reflect the patient's recovery from pneumonia. You'll find that Chapters 1 through 9 provide you with detailed knowledge of how to examine the major body regions. Chapter 10 then weaves together all aspects of a head-to-toe examination and helps you put it all together.

Now let's suppose your patient develops chest pain. After clarifying the chief complaint, you'll want to begin a focused, rapid assessment that addresses the most pressing problem. That's why throughout this book we've given you techniques for isolating your patient's chief complaint (such as chest pain, dyspnea, and nausea), performing a focused assessment, and pinpointing its probable cause.

Special features

Several special features, signaled by quick-reference symbols within the text, help speed you to important assessment information.

Disorder close-ups focus on the most common disorders encountered by nurses today, listing their characteristic findings as well as complications.

Disorders include angina pectoris, asthma, diabetes mellitus, hypertension, myocardial infarction, and many others.

◉ *Action STATs* tell you exactly what to do if, during your examination, you discover that your patient is in a potentially life-threatening situation.

▨ *Priority checklists* review the most important steps to cover when examining patients.

▐▌ *Anatomy reviews* present detailed illustrations of major body parts and organs.

▨ *Normal findings* summarize, at a glance, characteristic findings.

▨ *Interpreting abnormal findings* help you analyze abnormal findings and determine their causes.

▨ *Examination tips* feature time-saving pointers that make the examination faster and easier—and more accurate.

New to this edition

To keep you on the right track, we've packed even more information and features into the second edition of *Mosby's Expert 10-Minute Physical Examinations*. We've kept and improved all of the features you've told us you like, such as Chapter 2: *Examining Patients with Special Needs*. Chapter 11: *Documenting Your Findings Accurately* is a new chapter that highlights key information to document during the initial assessment and presents guidelines for documenting assessment findings for selected medical conditions. In addition, you'll find the following features that are new to this edition:

- *Updated content* throughout provides you with the latest information on assessment techniques, normal and abnormal findings, and the assessment of patients with specific diseases and disorders. Plus, we've added a section about examining the pregnant patient.
- ▨ *Lifespan Considerations* help you individualize the examination for patients of different ages, including children and older adults.
- ◉ *Cultural Considerations* provide you with information on variations in findings that may represent cultural anomalies.
- *Upgraded illustrations and photographs* better show you normal anatomy and assessment techniques.
- *Expansion of special features*, including Interpreting Abnormal Findings, Examination Tips, and Disorder Close-Ups, help you hone your skills.
- *Appendixes,* including assessment tools and normal laboratory values, serve as valuable quick references.

The added features have been selected, prepared, and reviewed by an expert team of nurses with your time constraints and patient-care needs in mind. The new and improved *Mosby's Expert 10-Minute Physical Examinations*, second edition, is a reference tool that no nurse should be without.

Barbara A. Todd, MSN, CRNP
Director, Clinical Surgical Specialists and Practitioners (CSSP)
Hospital University of Pennsylvania
Adjunct Faculty
University of Pennsylvania School of Nursing
Philadelphia, Pennsylvania

HEALTH HISTORY AND PHYSICAL EXAMINATION REVIEW

A complete head-to-toe examination must begin at the beginning, with a health history interview and a general physical examination. Because reliable patient health data lay the foundation for a thorough physical examination, Chapter 1 starts by describing how to build a rapport with your patient and promote cooperation. Then it details the components of the health history interview.

Next, the chapter reviews the four techniques you must master to conduct the physical examination and describes the equipment you may use. Finally, it explains how to document history and physical examination findings quickly, accurately, and completely.

Establishing a rapport with your patient

Establishing a trusting relationship with the patient will promote cooperation during the health history interview and physical examination. When you first meet the patient, introduce yourself and describe your role. If you're not sure how to pronounce the patient's name, ask. Then address him formally by his last name—for instance, "Mr. Wilson." Don't call him by his first name unless he gives you permission.

Providing a comfortable environment. A patient who's comfortable—both physically and psychologically—is more likely to offer complete history information and comply with the physical examination. As you

start the interview, help put the patient at ease by following these suggestions:
- Ensure privacy by drawing the curtains and closing the door.
- Make sure the room temperature is comfortable.
- Find out if the patient has any immediate needs—for example, for a glass of water or use of the bathroom. Address those needs before proceeding with the interview.

Using appropriate body language. Sit down when obtaining the history. Besides making you more comfortable, sitting shows the patient that you intend to spend some time with him. It also means you won't tower over him—a posture he could find intimidating.

Keep a *social distance*, staying several feet away from the patient. This distance—neither intimate nor remote—sets the proper tone for obtaining the interview.

CULTURAL CONSIDERATIONS

Keep in mind that certain cultural groups perceive space differently. A patient who's from a Hispanic or Middle Eastern background may feel more comfortable with a more personal distance, one that's less than 4 feet. If your patient moves closer to create a more intimate space, try not to move away—an act that could offend the patient. On the other hand, if your patient is of Native American, Vietnamese, Chinese, Korean, or West Indian heritage, he may prefer more distance during the interview.

Finally, maintain eye contact with the patient as much as possible. This means you should keep note-taking to a minimum. Why? Because you can't sustain eye contact with someone when taking notes. Excessive note-taking may also prevent you from detecting nonverbal clues to the patient's feelings and thoughts.

CULTURAL CONSIDERATIONS

Comfort with eye contact varies greatly among cultural groups. Patients who are of Asian, Arabic, Native American, or Hispanic heritage may avoid eye contact. Some cultural groups view steady eye contact as a form of aggression, while others avert their eyes as a sign of respect to authority.

Communicating effectively. As you interview your patient, word your questions wisely. Closed-ended questions are fine for obtaining basic information, such as name and age. But to elicit details—say, when exploring the chief complaint—switch to open-ended questions. For example, ask if the patient can describe the chest pain. (See *Avoiding Communication Pitfalls.*)

CULTURAL CONSIDERATIONS

If you and your patient speak different languages, enlist the help of an interpreter to get through the history and physical examination. While it's probably more convenient for a family member to translate, a professionally trained medical interpreter can offer added benefits because he knows medical terminology, understands patient's rights, and can provide culturally sensitive teaching and advice. If you use a family member to interpret, keep in mind that the patient might shield the family member from embarrassing or alarming information. Whomever you choose to translate, be sure to speak clearly and plainly (avoiding complicated terms), and pause every one or two sentences to allow for interpretation and responses.

OBTAINING A HEALTH HISTORY: A SYSTEMATIC APPROACH

Health history information provides a framework for an accurate physical examination, helping you focus your assessment on your patient's most important health problems. What's more, the health history interview provides an opportunity to assess your patient's understanding of his

AVOIDING COMMUNICATION PITFALLS

Poor communication can impede the health history interview and physical examination by alienating the patient and thwarting your efforts to build a rapport. The following guidelines can help you avoid common communication pitfalls.

- Make sure that you give your patient a chance to speak without interruption. If you interrupt the patient often or do most of the talking, you rob him of the chance to describe his symptoms and express his concerns. Instead, try to listen closely to what the patient is saying, interrupting only to ask for clarification.

- Steer clear of biased or leading questions, such as "You don't drink, do you?" Such questions give the impression that you're judging the patient. Instead, ask, "How many alcoholic drinks do you have a day?" Because this question is more precise and nonjudgmental, it will yield a more precise answer— without conveying disapproval.
- Avoid asking several consecutive questions that require "yes" or "no" responses. Your patient might become confused and answer incorrectly. Also, such questions tend to discourage the patient from elaborating on his answer.

PUTTING HIPAA INTO PRACTICE

The Health Insurance Portability and Accountability Act (HIPAA) national legislation was enacted to protect the patient's privacy by safeguarding disclosure of health care information, such as medical records and medical information collected by or communicated to health care providers by oral, electronic, or paper routes, as well as any information related to the patient's health, health care, or payment history. This act aims to provide the patient with better control over his personal health records and to give health care workers uniform standards of practice. Here's how you can comply with HIPAA standards when performing and documenting a health history and physical examination:
- When admitting a patient, provide him with a copy of his privacy rights.
- When taking a health history, keep your voice low and ask others to leave the room, if possible.
- Keep the results of the health history and physical examination, indeed all medical records, in a secure location. If charts are kept at the nurse's station, shield the names from the view of those passing by.
- If you're recording the health history and physical examination electronically, make sure the computer screen isn't visible to visitors and others.
- Request and distribute the results of the health history and physical examination—and all other private information—on a need-to-know basis. This rule applies to information given in writing, by phone or fax, or electronically.
- Check your institution's policies and procedures, or check with an administrator to determine if you need patient authorization before sharing information.
- Remove any patient identifiers, such as name and social security number, from documents that you transmit by fax or e-mail.

health problems or health maintenance needs and then guides you as you devise a plan of care.

If the patient's medical records are available, review these before starting the interview. Medical records can help you identify areas that need further exploration. But remember, reviewing a patient's medical records is never a substitute for obtaining a health history directly from the patient. Also, be sure to safeguard the privacy of all medical records and information obtained during the history and physical examination by keeping in mind the regulations put forth by the Health Insurance Portability and Accountability Act (HIPAA) of 1996. (See *Putting HIPAA into Practice.*)

Using a systematic approach to the health history will save you time and help you organize your thoughts and questions. Here are the main steps to follow:
- Collect basic patient information.
- Determine the chief complaint.
- Obtain a history of the present illness.
- Obtain a past medical and surgical history.
- Obtain a family history.
- Obtain a social history.
- Conduct a review of body systems.
- Conclude the health history.

Collecting basic patient information

Start the interview by gathering basic information, such as the source of the patient's referral, the source of patient information, and the reliability of the information provided.

The source of the referral may be another health care facility or provider. The source of patient information is usually the patient himself, along with his medical records. But for some patients, you may need to gather information from a friend, family member, caregiver, or combination.

To judge the reliability of the information provided, determine the patient's level of alertness and orientation. (You may not be able to judge reliability until later in the interview, when evaluating the patient's mental health status.) If you must gather information from a person other than the patient, find out how well that person knows the patient.

Determining the chief complaint

Next, determine the main reason your patient is seeking health care, called the *chief complaint*. Record the chief complaint in the patient's own words, using quotation marks—for instance, "I've had chest pain since early this morning." Then gather details about the symptom. (See *Investigating the Chief Complaint,* p. 6.)

If your patient has several complaints, ask him which one concerns him most. After investigating the primary complaint, explore the others.

Obtaining a history of the present illness

The history of the present illness usually provides additional information about the chief complaint. What's more, it may help you identify the underlying cause by placing the symptoms in the context of recent events.

Exploring previous treatment

Find out if the patient has ever been evaluated or treated for his symptoms. If so, determine the outcome of the treatment.

Ask the patient about his health status before symptoms began and before any treatment he received. Then find out how much time elapsed between the treatment and the recurrence or worsening of the symptoms. Also look for possible reasons for symptom recurrence: Did the patient discontinue prescribed medication? Did he recently change his diet or start exercising?

Next, try to determine if the patient has complied with his treatment. Ask if he has kept medical appointments and whether he has taken prescribed medication or maintained a restricted diet, if recommended, to treat his chief complaint.

Finally, once you've gathered the history of the present illness, review it and read the main points back to the patient. This gives him a chance to clarify any misconceptions or offer additional details and confirm your understanding. Then obtain the rest of his history.

INVESTIGATING THE CHIEF COMPLAINT

Ask your patient to describe the chief complaint—his main symptom or reason for seeking health care—as fully as possible. Further description may help you identify the underlying cause of his problem. If the problem is life-threatening, obtaining detailed information also promotes rapid intervention.

Dig for details

Obtain as many details as possible about the chief complaint. For instance, if the chief complaint is pain, ask whether the pain is sharp or dull, aching, burning, or shooting.

Find out what the patient was doing when his symptom began and how often the symptom occurs. Does he experience it during such activities as exercising, walking, doing housework, or showering? Does it occur during rest or awaken him from sleep?

Ask about onset, duration, and location

Determine the time of onset and the duration of the chief complaint. Ask when the patient first felt the symptom and how long it lasted. Then ask about its location. Find out if the symptom is confined to one area or affects other areas, too. To help identify symptom location, ask the patient to point to the affected area.

Use terms the patient is familiar with. For example, instead of asking if the pain radiates, ask if he feels pain in any other part of his body.

Evaluate symptom severity

Next, explore the severity or degree of the chief complaint by asking the patient to quantify the symptom. Suppose, for example, your patient reports he has been coughing up blood. You'll want to find out how often he coughs up blood and how much blood is involved. To elicit this information, ask such questions as:

- "How many times have you coughed up blood?"
- "Was the sputum merely streaked with blood or was there a larger amount of blood?"
- "How big was the bloody area? About the size of a nickel or more like the size of a half dollar?"
- "Did you cough into a tissue? If so, did the blood fill the tissue?"

Ask about aggravating and relieving factors

Aggravating and relieving factors can provide insight into the cause of the chief complaint. Ask the patient if the symptom seems to get worse at certain times—for instance, with a change in seasons or temperature, when he consumes certain foods or beverages, or when he takes part in certain activities.

Find out what measures, if any, bring relief. Does the symptom improve with rest? With medication? With heat or cold application?

Explore associated symptoms

Find out if the patient has other symptoms that could be associated with the chief complaint. These symptoms could provide clues to the underlying cause. For example, if chest pain is the chief complaint, ask if it's ever accompanied by nausea, shortness of breath, palpitations, or sweating.

Obtaining the medical-surgical history

A patient's past medical conditions and surgeries can affect his current health status. A patient with long-standing diabetes mellitus, for example, may experience delayed wound healing—important information to bear in mind if he has been admitted for surgery. Medical and surgical history data also may provide insight into the patient's perception of his health and health education needs.

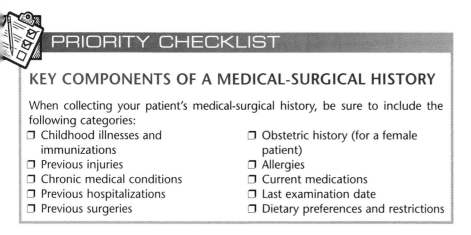

KEY COMPONENTS OF A MEDICAL-SURGICAL HISTORY

When collecting your patient's medical-surgical history, be sure to include the following categories:

- ❐ Childhood illnesses and immunizations
- ❐ Previous injuries
- ❐ Chronic medical conditions
- ❐ Previous hospitalizations
- ❐ Previous surgeries
- ❐ Obstetric history (for a female patient)
- ❐ Allergies
- ❐ Current medications
- ❐ Last examination date
- ❐ Dietary preferences and restrictions

When obtaining the medical-surgical history, be sure to cover the major categories. (See *Key Components of a Medical-Surgical History.*)

Childhood illnesses and immunizations

Ask your patient which common childhood illnesses he has had, such as measles, mumps, chicken pox, rubella, and whooping cough. This information may point to the possible cause of his chief complaint. It may also help you to fine-tune your physical examination.

Information about childhood immunizations may also help point to the cause of the chief complaint. Adults who didn't have the usual childhood diseases and haven't been vaccinated against them are at increased risk for contracting them.

Also ask about recent immunizations, such as hepatitis B, pneumococcal, and influenza vaccines. Hepatitis B status is particularly important if the patient is being admitted to the hospital and is likely to receive blood transfusions.

Previous injuries

Injuries and accidents may explain certain changes in a patient's physical condition and cognitive or motor function. They also may complicate a patient's current health problems and predispose him to certain secondary disorders. Therefore, be sure to note the circumstances surrounding any previous injuries. If an injury occurred during an alcohol-related accident, explore the patient's current alcohol consumption habits. If the patient injured himself in a fall, try to find out if the fall resulted from syncope—a possible indicator of an underlying illness.

Chronic medical conditions

Chronic medical conditions may affect the course of the present illness and help guide the physician's choice of treatments. Ask the patient if he has a chronic illness, such as diabetes mellitus, a thyroid disorder, anemia, hypertension, renal dysfunction, or heart disease.

Previous hospitalizations

Ask the patient if he has ever been hospitalized. If he has, find out the reason, the length of his stay, the treatment he received, any associated complications, and the names of the hospital and health care providers for each hospitalization. If the patient is now being admitted again, also explore his psychological responses to his previous hospitalizations.

Previous surgeries

Ask about all previous surgeries and medical procedures the patient has had. Document their dates, where they were performed, and the length of the patient's recovery. Find out if he experienced post-procedure complications; if he did, have him describe each complication. Also find out if he experienced excessive bleeding or adverse effects of anesthesia after the procedure and note whether or not he received blood transfusions.

Obstetric history

Obtain an obstetric history from all female patients. This history consists of the number of pregnancies (gravida), number of pregnancies carried to term (para), and number of abortions.

If the patient is of childbearing age, find out the date of her last menstrual period, and ask if she may be pregnant. Also inquire about her current use of birth control.

For females who are perimenopausal or postmenopausal, ask about symptoms such as hot flashes, and what methods, if any, she uses or has used to relieve them. Also, ask about whether or not she's using or has used hormone replacement therapy.

Sexual history

Although it might seem difficult to obtain a sexual history when time is of the essence or when you're not comfortable with the subject, try to weave in a few basic questions that could provide important information about your patient's health condition.
• Do you have more than one sexual partner?
• Do you ever have pain during intercourse?
• Do you have vaginal, anal, or oral sex?
• Have you ever had difficulty having sex because of physical or psychological problems?

Allergies

Ask your patient if he's allergic to any medications, foods, environmental substances, or other conditions. Have him describe his allergy symptoms in detail. Possible allergic responses include anaphylaxis, shortness of breath, rash, pruritus, rhinorrhea, and watery eyes.

Try to differentiate true allergies from medication side effects by asking if the patient was taking medication when the allergy symptoms arose. If he was, his symptoms may have resulted from the medication rather than an allergy. Clearly document reactions that you believe indicate true allergies and describe the patient's allergic reaction.

Current medications

Medications may cause or contribute to a patient's current health problem. Ask your patient which medications he currently takes—both prescription and over-the-counter. List the name of each medication, along with the dosage, administration route, frequency, and duration of use. Also ask if he uses home remedies or alternative treatments, such as herbs. (See *Exploring Your Patient's Medication Use*, p. 10.)

CULTURAL CONSIDERATIONS

Certain cultural groups, such as Chinese, Arab, and Hispanic cultures, view wellness in terms of balancing good and bad external forces. To maintain health and balance, these cultural groups often take a naturalistic approach to healing, using opposite forces to treat a condition. For example, hot conditions require cold foods, medications, and herbs. Not all cultural groups, however, use the same terms or define opposing forces in the same way. Chinese patients, for example, may use the terms *yin* for cold and *yang* for hot.

Last examination date

Ask the patient when he was last examined by a physician. This information provides insight into how often he receives health care and other aspects of his health maintenance habits. Also, ask him if he has ever received a chest X-ray, tuberculin test, or electrocardiogram (ECG) and whether he gets routine dental care. Ask female patients if they get regular Pap smears and breast examinations.

Dietary preferences and restrictions

Ask your patient to describe a typical day's meals and snacks. Then analyze his dietary report for nutritional value. Is he consuming too many high-fat foods or too few carbohydrates or proteins?

Also find out if he adheres to a special diet, such as vegetarian or kosher, or if his diet is restricted for health reasons, such as renal disease or celiac sprue. If he has been prescribed a restricted diet, determine his compliance.

EXPLORING YOUR PATIENT'S MEDICATION USE

When taking a patient's health history, ask to see any medication bottles he may have brought with him to the hospital. Besides allowing you to take a more accurate medication history, inspecting the bottles can help you detect and correct dangerous medication errors. For example, you may discover that the patient is doubling up on a particular medication—taking it under both a generic name and a trade name (such as propranolol and Inderal).

Verify medication names

Some patients may identify their medications only as "that blue pill" or "my water pill." If the bottles are available for inspection, note the exact drug name. Also check to see if any of the medications are outdated or show signs of improper storage.

Check for compliance

Find out if the patient complies with the prescribed drug regimen. Does he take the full dose as often as prescribed? Or does he sometimes skip doses or cut tablets in half in order to save money?

Other considerations

- Check for drug combinations that may lead to unwanted interactions.
- Ask the patient if he has had any undesirable effects from medication. If he has, ask what action, if any, he took. Did he call the doctor or did he simply stop taking the medication?

Obtaining the family history

A complete family history can reveal whether the patient is at risk for a disorder or disease with a genetic or familial tendency. To obtain the family history, ask your patient about the health of his parents, siblings, and grandparents (both maternal and paternal). Mention specific diseases by their names or symptoms to help him recall whether any family member has had them. Be sure to include such significant conditions as diabetes mellitus, hypertension, stroke, arthritis, pulmonary disease, cardiovascular disease, cancer, renal disease, mental illness, and alcoholism. To get a clearer picture of your patient's family history, you may want to make a genogram. (See *Constructing a Genogram*.)

Obtaining the social history

Social history data help place your patient within the context of his family and community. Because this part of the history requires you to ask about highly personal matters, be sure to convey a nonjudgmental attitude.

If you haven't already determined the patient's age and marital status, start the social history by obtaining this information. Then explore his

CONSTRUCTING A GENOGRAM

A genogram is a chart that shows a patient's family relationship and health history patterns. Health care professionals use genograms to help detect possible familial diseases and disorders.

When constructing a genogram, always provide a key that identifies important details about people in the patient's life. Identify male and female relatives and living and deceased relatives (as shown in the sample genogram). Be sure to fill in the ages of living family members, the age at which deceased family members died, and any diseases with a known or suspected familial or genetic tendency.

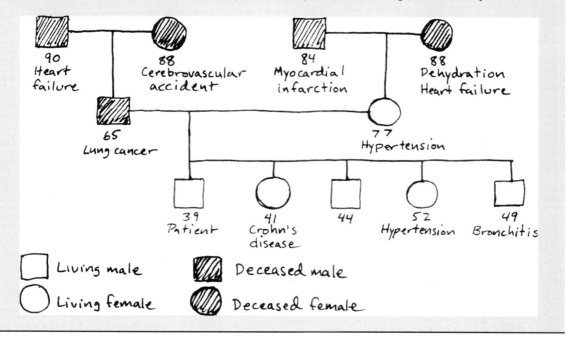

educational level, occupation, financial status, religious beliefs, leisure activities, sleep patterns, home environment, support systems, and personal habits.

Marital status and social support

A patient's marital status is a possible indicator of his support system. However, don't assume an unmarried patient lacks adequate support; investigate further by asking if the patient has a companion or close friend who should be contacted in case of an emergency. Also find out if the patient has children, either living at home or independently. This might be a good time to investigate possible abuse. You can start by asking the patient if he feels safe at home or in his relationships and progress to more direct questions as appropriate.

Educational level

Ask how many years of school the patient has completed, and find out if he can read and perform simple calculations. However, never make assumptions about a patient's intellectual abilities or understanding of his current condition based solely on his educational level.

Occupation

Occupational data may provide clues to work-related health hazards, such as asbestos exposure or chronic back pain caused by heavy lifting. Find out if the patient does manual labor or desk work, and determine if he works regularly, seasonally, or on a temporary or as-needed basis. Also ask if his employer provides health insurance. If the patient is unemployed, find out if he's able to pay for food, medication, and health care.

Religious, spiritual, and cultural beliefs

A patient's religious, spiritual, and cultural beliefs and customs may color his attitude toward health, illness, and medical treatment. For example, most Jehovah's Witnesses won't accept blood transfusions; consequently, major surgery may pose an increased risk for them.

The patient's belief system may also serve as a source of emotional support during illness. Ask if he belongs to a church, religious organization, or other spiritual group that could be a resource for him during or after illness or hospitalization.

Living conditions

Have the patient describe his home. Does it have heat, running water, electricity, and telephone service? Is there a smoke detector? A carbon monoxide detector? Does the home have more than one story? If so, is the patient able to negotiate the stairs easily?

If you haven't done so already, find out how many people the patient lives with. An overcrowded living environment may be responsible for the spread of certain infections.

Tobacco use

Ask the patient if he uses tobacco in any form—cigarettes, cigars, pipes, or chewing tobacco. If he does, find out how long he has used tobacco and how much he uses daily. Document cigarette use in terms of pack-years. (See *Determining Pack-Years.*)

Find out if the patient has ever quit smoking and, if so, when he quit and for how long. If he says he has quit smoking, ask when he last smoked. Some patients say they've quit when they've merely cut down on the number of cigarettes they smoke.

If the patient still smokes, ask if he'd like to stop. Later, you can help him explore options for smoking cessation.

DETERMINING PACK-YEARS

If your patient smokes cigarettes, be sure to document both the number of cigarettes he smokes a day and the length of time he has been smoking. A concise way to report this information is by describing his smoking history in terms of *pack-years*—the number of packs of cigarette the patient smokes per day multiplied by the number of years he has been smoking. Here's an example of how to perform the calculation:

Patient John Crane has smoked 2 packs of cigarettes per day for 20 years. To determine his pack-years, multiply 2 packs by 20 years; the result is 40 pack-years.

Alcohol use

Excessive alcohol use can cause or contribute to many medical conditions. Yet many health care providers hesitate to delve into this topic, perhaps fearing that questions about alcohol use might seem nosy or embarrassing. Nonetheless, your goal is to obtain a thorough health history—and that means you *must* investigate alcohol use. Keep in mind that the key to obtaining frank answers is to remain nonjudgmental.

First ask if the patient drinks alcohol. If he says he does, ask when he last had a drink. Find out what kind of liquor he drinks and how many drinks he has on a typical day. If his drinking seems excessive, ask if he thinks he has a drinking problem or if alcohol has ever interfered with his family life, occupation, or lifestyle.

Consider using the CAGE questionnaire to gather information about your patient's alcohol use. (See *Using the CAGE Questionnaire.*)

Recreational drug use

Like tobacco and alcohol use, recreational drug use may lead to or compound certain health problems. Ask the patient if he has ever used "street" drugs, such as cocaine, crack, amphetamines, LSD, or "downers." If so, find out how often and how they affected him. Also ask whether he has ever injected drugs; if he has, ask if he has been tested for HIV or hepatitis.

USING THE CAGE QUESTIONNAIRE

The CAGE questionnaire can help you get a better idea of your patient's history of alcohol use. If he answers "yes" to any of the following questions, suspect that he has a drinking problem:

C: Have you ever thought you should *cut* down your drinking?
A: Have you ever been *annoyed* by criticism of your drinking?
G: Have you ever felt *guilty* about your drinking?
E: Do you ever have an *eye*-opener (a drink) in the morning?

Conducting a review of body systems

After gathering the patient's social history, continue the health history interview by asking questions about each body system. The information you obtain from the review of systems may reinforce your initial impression of the patient's health problems. Also, exploring each system in detail may prompt your patient to mention additional signs and symptoms—not just the one that distresses him most. (See 📖 *Performing a Thorough Body-System Review.*)

As you conduct the review, maintain a systematic approach. Begin the review of systems by assessing your patient's overall health. Ask him to describe his present health status and how he feels overall. Be sure to note any general complaints, such as malaise, fatigue, or weakness, as well as problems with healing or unusual bleeding or bruising. Inquire about his weight and the presence of possible indicators of systemic diseases, such as lymphoma, tuberculosis, and AIDS. Then, focus on one body system at a time by asking questions relating to that system. (Later, when performing the physical examination, you'll proceed head-to-toe.)

Concluding the health history

After collecting health history data from your patient, take a few minutes to review your findings. Then, if necessary, ask more questions to clarify the patient's responses. For instance, if he gave conflicting or ambiguous information about a particular symptom, ask, "What do you think the problem is?" or "What concerns you most right now?"

Then, thank him for his time and cooperation and explain that you'll proceed with the physical examination.

PHYSICAL EXAMINATION TECHNIQUES

To obtain reliable findings from the physical examination, you must master the techniques of inspection, palpation, percussion, and auscultation. You must also gain proficiency in the use of examination equipment.

This section of the chapter provides the knowledge base you need to perform each examination technique and use essential equipment. In later chapters, you'll learn how to put these techniques and skills into practice as you examine your patient from head to toe.

Inspection

During inspection, the first step of the physical examination, observe your patient critically, evaluating what you see in light of your knowledge as a health care professional.

In an informal sense, inspection begins the moment you first encounter the patient. However, the formal inspection you conduct during the

PERFORMING A THOROUGH BODY-SYSTEM REVIEW

When performing a general review of body systems, be sure to ask the patient about the signs and symptoms listed below, noting anything unusual or abnormal, and addressing specific complaints.

Integumentary system
☐ Unusual hair loss or breakage
☐ Skin lesions or discoloration
☐ Unusual nail breakage or discoloration

Musculoskeletal system
☐ Joint pain or stiffness
☐ Tendon, ligament, or muscle pains or strains
☐ Bone aches or pains
☐ Muscle weakness

Head and neck
☐ Headaches
☐ Neck pain and stiffness
☐ Nasal discharge
☐ Nosebleeds
☐ Mouth lesions
☐ Sore throat
☐ Voice changes, such as hoarseness
☐ Dental problems

Eyes and ears
☐ Changes in vision, such as double or blurred vision
☐ Loss of vision
☐ Redness of eyes
☐ Eye drainage
☐ Eye pain
☐ Changes in hearing
☐ Loss of hearing
☐ Ear drainage
☐ Ear pain

Endocrine system
☐ Excessive thirst
☐ Excessive hunger
☐ Excessive urination
☐ Cold intolerance
☐ Heat intolerance
☐ Excessive sweating

Neurologic system
☐ Blackouts
☐ Seizures
☐ Loss of memory
☐ Mood swings
☐ Hallucinations
☐ Weakness
☐ Numbness
☐ Tremors
☐ Paralysis
☐ Loss of coordination

Cardiovascular system
☐ Chest pain
☐ Shortness of breath when lying flat
☐ Palpitations
☐ Edema
☐ Excessive urination at night
☐ Varicose veins
☐ Limb pain during exercise

Pulmonary system
☐ Shortness of breath
☐ Painful breathing
☐ Wheezing
☐ Sputum production
☐ Bloody sputum

Gastrointestinal system
☐ Changes in stool color, consistency, or frequency
☐ Heartburn
☐ Loss of appetite
☐ Food intolerances
☐ Painful swallowing
☐ Abdominal pain
☐ Blood in vomit or stool
☐ Nausea
☐ Constipation
☐ Diarrhea
☐ Fecal incontinence

Genitourinary system
☐ Painful urination
☐ Excessive urination
☐ Diminished urination
☐ Hesitancy
☐ Cloudy or darkened urine
☐ Pain in flank
☐ Pain above groin
☐ Urinary incontinence
☐ Blood in urine

Male reproductive
☐ Penile or testicular pain
☐ Penile lesions
☐ Penile discharge
☐ Impotence

Female reproductive
☐ Date of last menstrual period
☐ Possible pregnancy
☐ Breast lumps
☐ Vaginal discharge
☐ Vaginal itching
☐ Labial lesions
☐ Menstrual cramps
☐ Lack of menstruation
☐ Postmenopausal symptoms
☐ Premenstrual symptoms
☐ Sexual difficulties

Psychological status
☐ Anxiety
☐ Irritability
☐ Apathy
☐ Mood swings
☐ Depression
☐ Sleep disturbances
☐ Appetite disturbances
☐ Suicidal or homicidal thoughts
☐ Changes in libido

physical examination itself has two parts: the general inspection and the systematic inspection.

In the general inspection, you observe the patient from front to back and from each side, checking for symmetry of body parts, obvious injuries or abnormalities, and overall appearance. In the systematic inspection, you inspect each body region systematically from head to toe.

Accurate inspection requires adequate lighting and appropriate equipment, such as a penlight and possibly an ophthalmoscope and otoscope.

Palpation

Palpation involves using your hands to elicit information about skin temperature, bodily pulsations and vibrations, internal masses, and tenderness or rigidity of organs and structures. Certain parts of your hand are best used for palpating specific characteristics. For example, the finger pads are best used for palpating texture, shape, and pulsations, while the fingertips and nail tips are best for eliciting reflexes, such as the abdominal reflex. The forefinger and thumb are good for grasping tissue, hair, and nodules, while the ball of the hand is best for detecting vibrations and thrills. The back of the hand is best for assessing temperature and moisture, while the entire hand is used for testing strength and grip.

Palpation is usually the second step of the physical examination. However, when assessing the abdomen, always perform palpation after auscultation because palpation may increase the patient's intestinal activity, causing misleading auscultation findings, such as increased bowel sounds.

Palpation can be light or deep and may involve the use of one or both hands. In *light palpation,* you press on the skin gently. In *deep palpation,* you apply heavier pressure. In *bimanual palpation,* you palpate with both hands. (See *Palpation Techniques,* p. 18.)

Percussion

Perhaps the most challenging physical examination skill, percussion involves tapping or striking the patient's skin surface with your fingers or hands to elicit sounds, evaluate reflexes, uncover abnormal masses, and detect pain or tenderness. The tapping produces an audible vibration that helps to reveal the location, size, and density of the underlying structure. The three basic percussion techniques are direct, indirect, and blunt percussion. (See *Comparing Percussion Techniquesm,* p. 18.)

Because the body's organs, structures, and cavities differ in density, they produce sounds that differ in loudness, pitch, and duration. Percussion sounds are classified as dull, flat, tympanic, resonant, or hyperresonant and will vary depending on what part of the body or which organ you're percussing. What follows is a description of each percussion sound and where you may expect to hear it.

- Tympany, a high-pitched, drum-like sound, is usually heard over the stomach.

PALPATION TECHNIQUES

Depending on the part of the body you're examining or the particular characteristic you're assessing for, you may use light, deep, or bimanual palpation.

Light palpation

In this technique, you press gently on the patient's skin to a depth of no more than 1 cm, using one hand. Light palpation is best for assessing texture, temperature, moisture, pulsations, tenderness, vibrations, superficial masses, and papular lesions.

Deep palpation

In deep palpation, you press evenly on the patient's skin to a depth of approximately 4 cm. You may use one or both hands, keeping your fingers extended. Deep palpation is best for assessing abdominal structures, particularly the liver.

Bimanual palpation

This method involves the use of both hands to "trap" an organ and assess its texture and firmness. Expect to use this technique to assess the kidneys and female reproductive organs.

Photographs from Wilson, S. F., & Giddens, J. F. (2001). *Health Assessment for Nursing Practice* (2nd ed.). St. Louis: Mosby.

COMPARING PERCUSSION TECHNIQUES

To conduct a thorough physical examination, you must become proficient in the three percussion techniques: direct, indirect, and blunt percussion. No matter what technique you use, your nails should be trimmed so you won't scratch the patient.

Direct percussion

To perform direct percussion, tap directly on the patient's skin using short, sharp strokes of your fist or the fingertips of your dominant hand. Make sure the tapping movement originates from your wrist, not your elbow. After tapping, immediately lift your wrist from the skin surface so you don't muffle the sound. You can use this technique on any part of the body, including the back and the paranasal sinuses.

Indirect percussion

In this technique, used for most parts of the body, your nondominant hand serves as the striking surface. Place the middle finger of your nondominant hand firmly against the patient's skin surface; keep the other fingers of that hand fanned out slightly above the skin surface. Be sure to place only the *pad* of your finger against the skin. Then, with your dominant hand, strike the middle finger of your nondominant hand above or below the interphalangeal joint of your finger. Avoid striking directly on the joint because this can affect the sounds produced.

Blunt percussion

To perform blunt percussion, either strike the ulnar surface of your fist against the patient's skin surface or place your nondominant hand over the area and use it as a striking surface for your fist. Blunt percussion is useful for detecting pain or inflammation.

Before using this technique on a patient, practice it until you've learned to apply just enough force to elicit tenderness without hurting the patient.

Photographs from Wilson, S. F., & Giddens, J. F. (2001). *Health Assessment for Nursing Practice* (2nd ed.). St. Louis: Mosby.

- Resonance, a low-pitched, hollow sound, is usually heard over normal lung tissue.
- Hyperresonance, a loud, booming sound, is usually heard over a hyperinflated lung, as in patients with emphysema.
- Dullness, a soft, high-pitched, thudding sound, is usually heard over dense organs, such as the liver.
- Flatness, a soft, high-pitched sound, is usually heard over bones, muscles, and tumors.

Auscultation

Auscultation involves listening to sounds produced by internal body structures—usually the heart, lungs, blood vessels, and bowels. Typically, you'll use a stethoscope when you auscultate.

Generally, auscultation follows inspection, palpation, and percussion. However, when examining the abdomen, you should auscultate *after* inspection and *before* palpation and percussion, because auscultation findings may be influenced by the effects of palpation and percussion.

To master auscultation, you must have a thorough understanding of the physiologic changes that take place in the body. You must also be able to block out noises in the environment and sounds emanating from other organs. To help isolate sounds, close your eyes and concentrate on one auscultation sound at a time. For example, when listening to heart sounds, begin by concentrating on the first heart sound, and then move on to the second.

UNDERSTANDING PHYSICAL EXAMINATION EQUIPMENT

To gather certain types of information during the physical examination, you'll need to use special equipment, such as a stethoscope, thermometer, sphygmomanometer, automatic blood pressure cuff, penlight, reflex hammer, otoscope, and ophthalmoscope. In some situations, you may also need to use special cards to test for occult blood in stool or use a pulse oximeter to assess your patient's oxygenation status.

Stethoscope

The stethoscope is essential for auscultation. The acoustic stethoscope—the type most often used by nurses—consists of two earpieces, tubing, and an endpiece with a bell and a diaphragm.

Proper use of a high-quality stethoscope is crucial for auscultating sounds clearly. Following these guidelines can help you obtain accurate results:
- Use stethoscope tubing that's no more than 30 to 40 cm long and 4 mm in diameter. Longer and wider tubing may distort transmitted sounds.
- Make sure the earpieces fit comfortably and snugly in your ear canal. Angle them toward your nose so that sounds are directed toward the tympanic membrane.

- Hold the endpiece between your second and third fingers, and avoid holding or rubbing the tubing to minimize extraneous noise.
- Avoid placing the endpiece of the stethoscope on the patient's gown or clothing. Friction between the fabric and stethoscope could produce false sounds.
- Always use the correct component of the endpiece to auscultate. To detect high-pitched sounds, such as heart, lung, and bowel sounds, use the diaphragm, making sure you place it firmly on the skin surface. To detect soft, low-pitched sounds, such as heart murmurs and atrial and ventricular gallops, use the bell.

Thermometers

Thermometers measure the patient's body temperature. The most common types of thermometers currently in use are the electronic thermometer and the tympanic membrane thermometer. No matter which type you use, always wait 15 minutes after your patient has consumed a cold or hot beverage and 2 to 3 minutes after he has smoked a cigarette before measuring his temperature.

Electronic thermometer

The electronic thermometer measures body temperature within 30 seconds. Some models come with two color-coded probes: one for taking oral (and with some equipment, axillary) temperature and the other for taking rectal temperature. Disposable sheaths that fit over the temperature probe help to ensure hygiene. Faulty calibration may lead to false temperature readings, so be sure to check the thermometer's calibration often.

Tympanic membrane thermometer

This noninvasive device uses an infrared sensor to detect the temperature of blood flowing through the tympanic membrane, a semitransparent membrane in the middle ear. Highly accurate, the tympanic thermometer takes 2 to 3 seconds to obtain a measurement that's comparable to core body temperature.

Because it involves no contact with body fluids, the tympanic membrane thermometer is considered more sanitary than other thermometers. Nonetheless, like other thermometers, it comes with disposable covers that fit over the temperature probe. You should change the probe cover between patients and every time the thermometer is used so that cerumen, fingerprints, and dust won't interfere with the reading.

To use a tympanic membrane thermometer safely and accurately, follow these guidelines:

- Before taking the patient's temperature, remove cerumen from the ear canal by irrigation or use of a softening agent, such as carbamide peroxide. Otherwise, the cerumen may lower the temperature reading.

- Clean the probe window according to the manufacturer's instructions to ensure an accurate measurement.
- Straighten the adult patient's ear canal to insert the temperature probe, making sure to pull the external part of the ear—the pinna—upward and back.
- Insert the probe gently into the ear canal to avoid injuring or perforating the tympanic membrane. If you meet resistance, stop. Never force the probe into the canal.
- Make sure you advance the probe far enough into the ear canal to seal the opening. Otherwise, you may not get an accurate reading.

Sphygmomanometer

Used with a stethoscope to measure blood pressure, the sphygmomanometer consists of a blood pressure cuff, a pressure manometer, and a hand bulb with a pressure valve.

Usually, you'll measure blood pressure in the arm. Remember to avoid using an arm on the same side of the body on which a radical mastectomy has been performed or when an arteriovenous (AV) shunt is present. To ensure an accurate reading, make sure the inflatable rubber bladder on the blood pressure cuff is the correct size for your patient. The bladder should be about 40% as wide as the patient's arm circumference and about 80% as long as his arm circumference. For most adult patients expect to use a cuff that's 12 to 14 cm wide. Then follow these steps:

- Have the patient sit quietly with his arm relaxed.
- Wrap the cuff around his arm, approximately 2 cm above the inner aspect of the elbow (antecubital fossa). Support the patient's arm with your hand, keeping it level with his heart.
- Palpate the patient's brachial pulse, located slightly below and just medial to the antecubital area.
- Inflate the cuff until you no longer feel pulsations. Note the reading on the gauge.
- Deflate the cuff, put the stethoscope's earpieces in your ears, and position the stethoscope head over the brachial artery.
- Wait 30 seconds. Then reinflate the cuff by pumping the bulb until the aneroid gauge rises about 30 mm Hg above the reading that appeared when you felt the brachial pulse.
- Deflate the cuff slowly, about 3 mm Hg per second, until you start to hear pulse sounds (Korotkoff sounds). The reading you obtain at this point is the systolic pressure.
- Continue to deflate the cuff. When Korotkoff sounds start to grow faint or muffled, record this reading as the first diastolic sound.
- When Korotkoff sounds disappear, record this reading as the second diastolic pressure. (This technique decreases the chance of misinterpreting the systolic or diastolic pressure if an ausculatory gap exists—a silent period between Korotkoff sounds.)

- After you've measured blood pressure in one arm, measure it in the other. Be aware that blood pressure commonly differs by 5 to 10 mm Hg between arms.

Automatic blood pressure cuff

This blood pressure cuff inflates automatically, digitally displaying the systolic, diastolic, and mean arterial pressures. Convenient for taking multiple blood pressure readings over a short period of time, it's a good choice for critically ill patients who need frequent monitoring. Keep in mind, however, that if your patient has an irregular heart rhythm, such as that which occurs with atrial fibrillation, the automatic blood pressure cuff may not produce accurate results. When in doubt, compare your reading with one obtained manually.

When using the device, apply the cuff to the patient just as you'd apply a sphygmomanometer cuff. However, you don't need to auscultate to obtain a pressure measurement.

Otoscope

Used to visualize the ear canal and tympanic membrane, the otoscope consists of a base (or handle), a head, and an ear speculum. Several types of ear specula are available to accommodate ear canals of different sizes. Some otoscopes have a bulb attachment, called a pneumatic attachment, used to evaluate movement of the tympanic membrane.

When inspecting the ear of an adult:
- Tilt the patient's head slightly toward the side opposite the ear being examined to bring the eardrum into better view.
- Pull the pinna up and back to straighten out the ear canal.
- Hold the otoscope against the patient's head, handle end up.
- Keeping your hand alongside the patient's face to steady the otoscope, gently insert the speculum into the ear.
- View the tympanic membrane and its structures through the glass window.

Ophthalmoscope

Used to examine internal eye structures, the ophthalmoscope is a light source with lenses and mirrors. It has two major parts—a base (or handle) and a head. The base houses the batteries and serves as an appendage to grasp when inspecting the patient's eye. Parts of the head include a viewing window; apertures and an aperture selector dial, which changes the width of the light beam; a lens selector dial, which changes the lens to bring objects into focus; and a lens indicator, which displays lens magnification power as a number from 0 to +40 or from 0 to −20.

For reliable findings, follow these recommendations:
- Darken the room before beginning the ophthalmoscopic examination.

- Ask your patient to remove his eyeglasses. If you wear eyeglasses, remove them unless you're very nearsighted or astigmatic. (Contact lenses, on the other hand, can be worn during the examination.)
- Use your right hand and right eye to examine your patient's right eye. Use your left hand and left eye to examine his left eye.
- To help the patient hold his gaze steady, have him focus on a point on the opposite wall.
- Approach your patient from slightly off to one side, from a distance of about 15 inches. As you move toward him, place the thumb of your other hand on his eyebrow for guidance.

Pulse oximeter

A photoelectric device, the pulse oximeter noninvasively measures a patient's arterial oxygen saturation (SaO_2). A cutaneous sensor probe in the oximeter emits red and infrared light, which is then transmitted to the capillaries. When placed on the patient's finger or earlobe, the probe measures transmitted light passing through the vascular bed. It detects the relative amount of color absorbed by the arterial blood, then calculates the SaO_2 value. The pulse oximeter can be used either to obtain a single measurement or to provide continuous monitoring of a patient's oxygenation status.

For the most reliable pulse oximetry readings, follow these steps:
- Before placing the sensor probe, make sure the photodetectors in the probe are aligned.
- Place the probe at a site where capillaries are near the skin surface, such as a nail bed, an earlobe, or the bridge of the nose. If you choose the nail bed, remove any nail polish from the patient's finger to ensure the most accurate SaO_2 value. (To promote patient comfort, alternate probe sites periodically.)
- Instruct your patient to stay still during the measurement because movement can cause inaccuracies in the reading.
- Once the probe is in position, turn the pulse oximeter on and correlate your patient's radial pulse with the value on the digital display.
- Record the SaO_2 value shown on the digital display.

EXAMINING PATIENTS WITH SPECIAL NEEDS

A wide range of conditions—serious illness, sensory and cognitive impairments, anxiety, hostility, and more—can impede a thorough and accurate health history and physical examination. A patient with a cognitive impairment, for instance, may not understand your questions. An extremely anxious patient may be unable to focus on the interview.

In this chapter, you'll learn how to tailor your assessment approach and techniques for these patients, not only saving you time but producing reliable findings while preserving the patient's dignity.

SERIOUSLY ILL PATIENTS

Patients suffering from acute illnesses or serious injuries, such as cerebrovascular accident or head trauma, may be unable to communicate or respond fully because of their medical condition, mechanical ventilation, or heavy sedation. If your seriously ill patient can't supply a complete health history, obtain only the most important information—chief complaint, history of present illness, medications, and allergies. Then tell her that you'll ask more questions at a later time. That way, she won't feel rushed or taxed during the interview and will be more likely to answer your questions fully.

Establishing a communication system

A patient who is conscious but can't speak (for example, because of mechanical ventilation) may be able to respond nonverbally to simple questions. To obtain basic history information and assess the patient's level of pain and anxiety, establish gestures she can use to indicate her response to questions. For example, tell her to squeeze your hand once to indicate "no" and twice to indicate "yes." Before recording her answers, test her to make sure she understands and uses the gestures appropriately. For example, ask a simple question, such as "Is your name Mary?" Then make sure she responds correctly by squeezing your hand the proper number of times.

Providing comfort measures

Some seriously ill patients have trouble focusing on questions or instructions because of immobility, pain, discomfort, anxiety, or depression. So after establishing a communication system, evaluate your patient's ability to participate fully in the interview. Ask her how she's feeling. Is she able to talk at length despite immobility, pain, or discomfort? Or does she keep her responses short to get back to coping with the discomfort?

Before you can start the health history interview, you must address the immediate source of the patient's discomfort. Respond to her needs by helping her to a more comfortable position or offering her a cool beverage (if permitted). If she's in pain, give prescribed analgesics, then wait for the medication to take effect before proceeding with the interview.

You may also guide the patient through progressive muscle relaxation to ease pain and discomfort. For instance, you can instruct her to progressively tighten and then relax individual muscle groups until her whole body is relaxed. This exercise usually takes 10 to 30 minutes.

Some patients respond better to guided imagery. In this method, you gently instruct the patient to imagine she's in one of her favorite places. This should have a relaxing effect and enable you to proceed with the health history interview. (See *Interviewing a Seriously Ill Patient.*)

Performing an abbreviated assessment

With an acutely ill patient, expect to condense the health history interview and physical examination so that you can address her most immediate and life-threatening problem. For example, if you suspect your patient is experiencing a myocardial infarction, perform a brief but focused assessment of the cardiovascular system and other affected body systems so you can rapidly intervene. Later, when the patient's condition has stabilized, you can complete the history and physical examination at a more leisurely pace.

Modifying the physical examination

A bedridden or immobile patient may be unable to participate in some parts of the physical examination, such as evaluation of gait or active

INTERVIEWING A SERIOUSLY ILL PATIENT

You'll need to use your best interview skills when questioning a patient who's in marked pain or discomfort. To help the interview go more smoothly, follow these suggestions:

Get off to a good start
If your patient feels well enough to talk at length, start the history with open-ended questions. This will help her feel more comfortable with you. Then use natural pauses in the conversation to ask her closed-ended questions so that you can obtain more detailed information.

Maintain the flow of conversation so that the patient's attention stays focused on your questions, not on her discomfort or the surroundings. Also, nod your head or make a brief remark to show her that you're listening closely to her responses.

Deal with the patient's fears
What if your patient asks you if she's going to die or be permanently disabled or disfigured? Usually, your best response is to answer this type of question honestly. Remember, most patients don't ask such questions unless they're ready to hear the answer, whether it's good or bad.

However, before this situation arises, do some serious soul-searching. Before you can deal with the patient's fears, you need to examine your own fears and attitudes toward illness, disability, disfigurement, and death. Can you talk openly about these topics without getting lost in your anxieties?

If you don't think you're up to the task, ask the patient if she would like to speak with a counselor, religious leader, or some other person who feels comfortable discussing these difficult matters.

Accept the patient's crying
A patient who hears bad news about her health may respond by crying. Although this may make you uncomfortable, resist the urge to cut her crying short.

Usually, the best approach is to do nothing. Don't move away from the patient or rush to say something you hope will make her feel better. Instead, quietly offer a box of tissues or touch her on the arm to show that you're available for her and accept her feelings.

If you feel uncomfortable with her crying, resist the urge to talk just to fill the air. If you feel you must speak, offer a few sympathetic words about how hard it must be for her to go through such an ordeal. If you can accept her crying for what it is—coming to terms with painful emotions—you'll help her recognize that it's all right for her to feel the way she does.

---

range of motion. Also, you may need to alter the sequence or nature of the examination steps.

If the patient can't change her position easily, ask another nurse or caregiver to move her while you examine hard-to-reach areas. For instance, have a colleague hold the patient on her side so you can freely examine her posterior.

Examining a nonresponsive patient

If your patient is unconscious or comatose, don't assume she can't hear you. Instead, speak to her as you conduct the examination, providing explanations as if she were awake and conscious: "Now I'm going to listen to your heart." She may be able to hear what you're saying and find your words soothing.

ANXIOUS PATIENTS

Many people feel anxious and intimidated in a medical setting. Mild anxiety can be helpful during the assessment because it focuses the patient's attention on answering questions and following instructions and gives her the energy to carry through.

For most patients, a reassuring word is enough to reduce mild anxiety and promote cooperation. To convey empathy, tell the patient that you understand the stress she's feeling. For instance, you might say, "I know this experience can seem overwhelming. Take a deep breath and try to relax."

However, don't make reassuring statements just to calm the patient if the statement may not be true ("Everything will be all right"). False reassurance may jeopardize the patient's trust in you or other members of the health care team.

Dealing with moderately to severely anxious patients

A high anxiety level may interfere with a thorough history and physical examination. If your patient is moderately anxious, suggest breathing or relaxation exercises. Then, when she's calmer, start the interview with an open-ended question to invite her to begin talking, and proceed as appropriate.

If the patient is extremely anxious, consider discussing with the physician the need for a psychiatric consultation. The patient may need antianxiety medication to reduce her anxiety level before you can even begin to assess her.

Modifying the physical examination

An anxious patient may fear that the physical examination will cause pain or embarrassment, or worse, reveal a serious illness. Therefore, take special care to maintain privacy. Close the door and draw the curtain. Don't allow others to enter the room without the patient's permission.

During the examination, expose only the area of the body you're about to examine. Then promptly cover it when you're finished. As you examine the patient, state in advance what you're going to do so she knows what to expect. Before auscultating her lungs, for example, say: "Now I'm going to listen to your lungs. You'll feel the end of my stethoscope on your back. It might feel a little cold." That way, you'll avoid startling her and you'll keep her involved in the examination process.

If you need extra time to perform a certain part of the examination, such as auscultating heart sounds, tell the patient you're going to spend a few minutes listening to her heart. Otherwise, she might become anxious, fearing that the additional time you're spending listening to her heart means you've found something abnormal. After you've finished listening, say something reassuring like "Your heartbeat is regular and strong." (However, if this isn't true, don't give false reassurance.)

If you discover an abnormal finding, try to control your facial expressions and verbal response. Otherwise, the patient may become alarmed.

WITHDRAWN PATIENTS

Most withdrawn patients are anxious but will become more communicative with a little encouragement. For instance, you might try explaining to the patient that you need to ask some questions about her health. Then pose a few simple questions to elicit basic information, such as her full name, address, and telephone number. This gives her an idea of what to expect during the rest of the interview. Once she becomes more comfortable, you can follow up with open-ended questions.

If the patient remains uncommunicative during the interview, you may be able to draw her out of her shell simply by listening to her concerns, clearing up misconceptions, or providing assistance. Ask if she's troubled by something, and then offer assistance in dealing with her concern.

Suppose, for instance, the patient tells you she's concerned about a pet she had to leave unattended during her hospital stay. To relieve her of her worry—and establish a rapport—provide access to a telephone so that she can arrange for someone to look in on the pet, or offer to make the call yourself. She'll then be more likely to cooperate during the assessment.

You may also consider using touch to help draw a patient out. (See *Using Touch Appropriately.*)

Coping with silence

Expect frequent silences when interviewing a withdrawn patient. But remember, a silent period *doesn't* mean your interview skills are inadequate, so don't take these pauses personally. Instead, learn to become

USING TOUCH APPROPRIATELY

When used in a genuine way (rather than in a forced or scripted manner), touching can be helpful in dealing with a withdrawn patient. Holding the patient's hand or putting your hand on her arm or shoulder can send the message that you're in the moment with her. Touching also serves to help connect the patient's inner world with the outside world.

Try to exercise good judgment when you're about to touch a patient. Not all patients are comfortable being touched. And some patients may misinterpret your intentions and become upset.

A person's cultural background may also influence her views on when touching is acceptable and when it's an invasion of personal space.

comfortable with them so that you can resist the urge to jump in and "rescue" the patient.

When used appropriately, silent pauses can help elicit information. For instance, they can help the patient remember facts, organize thoughts, or think over important details. They also give the patient a chance to process painful emotions associated with her medical condition or personal life.

Modifying the physical examination

Remember that the withdrawn patient is usually anxious, so modify your physical examination as you would for an anxious patient—by ensuring privacy, telling the patient in advance what you're going to do, and controlling your facial expressions and verbal responses.

OVERLY TALKATIVE PATIENTS

Like withdrawn patients, many overly talkative patients are highly anxious. Typically, the overly talkative patient channels anxiety through speech, fearing that unless she relates every detail of her condition, she won't be diagnosed correctly. Your primary task with this type of patient is to maintain control while addressing her need to reduce her anxiety.

Allowing a "free speech" period

As the interview begins, give the patient an opportunity to talk without interruption. During this "free speech" period, make sure that every now and then you nod or say a few words to indicate that you're listening. As the patient talks, observe her and listen closely to what she's saying. By doing this, you can gain valuable insight into her thought processes, emotional state, coping mechanisms, and interaction style.

Note her speech pattern and characteristics. Is her speech pressured (rapid or urgent)? If so, this may indicate bipolar disorder. Is her speech incoherent, circumstantial, or tangential (veering off the subject)? These patterns suggest a possible thought disorder, such as schizophrenia. Does the content of her speech contradict her affect—that is, does she look sad but say she feels happy? Also observe nonverbal messages, such as body language and gestures. Are they consistent with what she's saying?

Taking control of the interview

After listening to the patient for a short time, wait for a natural break in the conversation. Then say you have some specific questions that will require short answers, and proceed with closed-ended questions to elicit the information you need to complete your assessment.

If the patient's answers veer from the topic, gently interrupt her to clarify information or steer the conversation back to the topic. For example, if your patient goes into excessive detail about events that occurred years ago, you might say: "It sounds like a lot happened to you in 1978. But before you go on, could you tell me about any other surgeries you've had?" Most overly talkative patients will tolerate interruptions if they believe the other party is truly listening to them.

You might also want to ask the overly talkative patient to fill out questionnaires and other forms. This can help channel her energy into something productive while giving her the sense that she's participating in her own care. It might also save you some time. Remember, though, that such forms aren't a substitute for formal history-taking.

Modifying the physical examination
During the examination, allow the patient to continue talking, provided it doesn't interfere with your ability to concentrate on findings or listen to sounds. If, for example, you need to listen to breath sounds, ask her not to speak because you don't want to miss important sounds—but emphasize that you'll gladly listen to her after you've finished.

HOSTILE PATIENTS

How you react to a hostile patient can be crucial to conducting a successful health history and physical examination. Many people use hostility and anger as a way to express fear. If this is true for your patient, expect her to watch you closely to observe how you handle her emotions. If she sees that you can deal with them effectively, she may realize that her emotions aren't so overwhelming that she can't handle them.

Don't take a patient's expression of anger personally. To a hostile patient, you may symbolize everything she's upset about at the moment—the health care facility, the medical profession, or even her illness. The patient may vent her anger at you because you're a convenient target.

Defusing anger
Before you start the interview, give the patient a chance to express her feelings. Simply by listening, you may be able to defuse her anger and frustration. Show her you can tolerate her feelings as long as the situation doesn't escalate into abuse.

Be genuine, acknowledging those things that you, too, would find frustrating if you were in her situation. Empathize with how difficult it must be for her to be hospitalized, to receive treatment for an acute illness, or to live with a chronic condition.

If the patient yells, don't yell back. Doing so could cause the situation to escalate into a confrontation. Instead, recognize that she's yelling because she feels the need to be heard. Hear her out in an uncritical manner, providing the sounding board she's seeking.

Avoid taking sides either for or against her. Arguing against her would probably prove pointless because most hostile patients aren't willing to listen to other people's arguments. Only after you've established rapport through supportive listening should you consider providing information that might change her mind.

As your patient calms down, redirect her attention to her primary goal: feeling better, getting well, or going home. Affirm your commitment to helping her reach this goal and to providing her with the best possible care. Help her use her determination and energy to focus on her recovery and will to live.

Dealing with abuse and violence

You should never tolerate abuse. If a patient becomes verbally abusive, firmly tell her that you'll continue the interview later, when she can express herself in a respectful manner. Set boundaries and be consistent in maintaining them.

Make sure you're familiar with your facility's policies and procedures regarding violent patients. And keep in mind that past behavior is the best predictor of future behavior. If you know a patient has a history of violent outbursts, take extra precautions when dealing with her. Notify another staff member that you'll be interviewing a potentially dangerous patient, and ask that staff member to check on you periodically. (See *Managing a Hostile Patient*.)

If you suspect a patient is about to become violent, position yourself between her and the door, making sure that the door stays open. If she does become violent, or you feel she poses a risk to herself or others, leave

MANAGING A HOSTILE PATIENT

When coping with a hostile patient, let the phrase *CALM DOWN* be your guide. Each letter of this mnemonic stands for one of the eight steps to follow when trying to keep the situation under control.

C: *Check* to see that everyone is safe.

A: *Agree* with the patient's affect, not her opinion. Let her know you understand her feelings without necessarily agreeing with her opinion.

L: *Listen* to the patient, hearing out her concerns.

M: Redirect the patient to your common goal: getting her the best ***medical*** care possible.

D: ***Don't debate*** with your patient.

O: *Old* (past) behavior is the best predictor of future behavior. If your patient has shown violence toward caregivers in the past, assume she may do so again.

W: *Walk away* from the patient if you feel threatened or abused.

N: Listen carefully and try to determine the patient's underlying ***need.*** What is she really trying to tell you?

the room and alert security. Ask the physician to order a sedative and restraints. After a violent episode, be sure to document your interventions and the patient's response.

Modifying the physical examination

You may need to provide the hostile patient with additional explanations and privacy measures before you can start the physical examination. Before you touch her, ask her permission so she won't react violently or accuse you of battery.

If you're afraid of being alone with her behind a closed door, enlist the help of a colleague who can be present during the examination. As you examine the patient, stay alert for clues that she's becoming more hostile or losing control—rapid breathing, gritting of the teeth, or avoiding eye contact. If you notice these signs, stop the examination and tell her that you'll resume later, when she's calmer. If necessary, ask for help from others for your protection.

COGNITIVELY IMPAIRED PATIENTS

Most patients with mild cognitive impairments can function adequately in daily life and can speak for themselves. This means you'll probably be able to obtain at least some health history information directly from the patient. However, some patients with mild cognitive impairments may not understand the complexities of their condition and may have emotional outbursts if they become confused or overstimulated. A few may even show psychotic symptoms.

Of course, patients with more severe cognitive impairments may be unable to provide any health history information. In that case, you'll need to interview a family member or other caregiver. (See *Taking a Patient History From a Family Member or Caregiver,* p. 34.)

Interviewing the patient with a mild impairment

Before starting the health history interview, eliminate distractions. The mildly impaired patient may not cope well with the stress or stimulation of being in an unfamiliar environment. Turn off any television or radio, and close the door to the interview room if there's a lot of activity in the hall.

Direct your questions at the patient even if a family member or caregiver is present. You may be tempted to bypass the patient and interview the third party because you'll spend more time and effort questioning the patient with a cognitive impairment. Resist this temptation—it could destroy any chance of building a rapport. If, after interviewing the patient, you need more information, ask her for permission to speak with the family or caregiver.

TAKING A PATIENT HISTORY FROM A FAMILY MEMBER OR CAREGIVER

If your patient can't speak for herself—for example, if she's severely ill or comatose or has a severe cognitive impairment—you'll probably need to obtain health history information from a family member or caregiver. Try to follow these important guidelines:

Ensure a conducive environment

Conduct the interview in a quiet, private, comfortable area away from the patient's room, if possible. Otherwise, the patient's presence may distract the family member or caregiver from concentrating on your questions.

After introducing yourself and explaining that you need to take the patient's health history, ask the family member or caregiver if she needs anything. Offer coffee, water, or another beverage, and ask how she's holding up. Reassure her that the patient is receiving proper attention, even though the two of you have left the patient's room. If the person is upset, allow her to express her thoughts and feelings. Offer reassurance and empathize with the difficulty of her circumstances.

Obtain basic information

Start the interview by asking simple, direct questions to obtain the patient's name, age, and telephone number. Find out what the relationship between the person you're interviewing and the patient is. If she's a family member, is she a close relative? If she's a friend or caregiver, how long has she known the patient? How often does she normally see the patient? Is the relationship informal or more distant? This will help you judge if the data the person provides are reliable, especially information about the patient's health habits and other sensitive areas.

Here are more suggestions to help you obtain a health history from a mildly impaired patient:

- Tailor your language to your patient's verbal abilities. Avoid jargon and technical terms, use concrete language whenever possible, and ask only one question at a time.
- Don't talk down to the patient. Doing so could work against your efforts to establish a rapport with her.
- If the patient reports a symptom, such as pain, ask her to rate its intensity on a scale of 1 to 10. This not only will help you assess the severity of her symptom but could prove useful for later comparison once treatment begins.

Interviewing the patient with a more severe impairment

Try to obtain this patient's health history from a family member or care-giver. Ask about the patient's ability to perform activities of daily living, such as dressing, toileting, personal hygiene, and managing money for small purchases. Besides indicating the patient's functioning level, the answers can give you a sense of the patient's ability to learn about her health care.

Modifying the physical examination

Like the health history interview, the physical examination of a patient with a cognitive impairment will proceed more smoothly if you've established a rapport. Here are some other suggestions that may promote a successful examination:

- Arrange for a family member or caregiver to be present, if possible, to help calm and reassure the patient.
- If necessary, change the sequence of examination steps so that you start with less intrusive areas, such as the hands, skin, and hair. Once you've shown the patient you're not going to hurt her, proceed to more intrusive areas.
- If you think a certain part of the examination will be painful or uncomfortable, tell the patient in advance—but choose your words carefully so as not to frighten her. "This might sting a little" is less frightening than "This might hurt."

HEARING-IMPAIRED PATIENTS

Dealing with hearing-impaired patients can present a number of challenges. If your patient communicates mainly in sign language, try to find an interpreter, or use sign language yourself if you know it. If you must rely on an interpreter, make sure the person does not summarize what is being communicated; otherwise, you might miss important details or clues about the patient's thought process.

If the patient can read lips, face her, speak slowly, and articulate your words clearly; where appropriate, add gestures or pantomime. If the patient relies largely on visual cues, make sure she's wearing eyeglasses, if she needs them, and that the room is adequately lit.

If the patient has some hearing, determine whether her hearing loss is unilateral or bilateral. If it's unilateral, position yourself near her good ear when speaking. If the patient has hearing aids, ask her to use them during the interview.

Communicating on paper

If the patient has adequate reading and writing skills, you can gather some health history information by having her fill out questionnaires and other preprinted forms during the interview or afterward. Or you can write down questions, and then have her write down her answers.

Remember, however, that if you leave preprinted forms for the patient to complete on her own, you won't be able to ask immediate follow-up questions to the responses she supplies. This could prevent you from obtaining a complete history.

Modifying the physical examination

You may need to give a hearing-impaired patient specific instructions during the examination—for example, you may have to ask her to change her position. If so, provide written instructions, pictures, or diagrams whenever possible.

VISUALLY IMPAIRED PATIENTS

Most visually impaired patients can respond to questions without difficulty. When you first approach the patient, introduce yourself and describe the purpose and format of the interview. Be sure to use a normal tone of voice, speak at a moderate speed, and enunciate words clearly. If the visually impaired patient also uses a hearing aid, ask her to wear it during the interview.

Orienting the patient

To reassure the patient and orient her to your location, use subtle gestures, such as resting your hand on her arm. If she hasn't been previously oriented to the room, take a few minutes to describe where everything is so she can get a sense of her surroundings. Whenever possible, use other aids to supplement oral instructions, such as materials on audio tape or in Braille.

Modifying the physical examination

Move slowly and deliberately during the examination, providing explanations and directions as you proceed. Tell the patient what you're about to do before you do it. Let her know where you'll be touching her and why.

OLDER ADULTS

From your first contact with an older adult, be sure to convey respect. For instance, address patient Jane Strayer as Ms. Strayer, not Jane. Never address an older adult by her first name unless she asks you to.

Early in the health history interview, determine if your patient has any sensory impairments. Some older adults with declining visual or hearing ability refuse to wear eyeglasses or hearing aids because they want to maintain a sense of independence and dignity. Unfortunately, this only compounds the sensory impairment. What's more, poor vision or hearing can lead to or worsen confusion when an older adult is in unfamiliar surroundings.

Keep in mind that older adults are likely to have a longer health history than are younger patients, so try to allot more time for the health history interview. That way, you won't need to rush through the interview or gloss over aspects of the patient's history that she feels are important.

Checking for memory deficits

Memory normally declines somewhat with age. Usually, age-related memory loss involves spontaneous recall of information about recent events. Thus, the older adult may have trouble recalling what she had for dinner the previous night but have no difficulty remembering the name of her high school.

Be sure to consider the possible impact of memory problems when assessing the patient's ability to perform activities of daily living. For example, does the patient sometimes forget she's cooking something on the stove? Does she occasionally forget where she is, even in her own neighborhood? To obtain such information, you may need to interview a close friend or family member. (See *Assessing a Patient's Psychosocial Status.*)

If, during the health history interview, you suspect that the patient has a significant memory problem, interrupt the interview to assess her mental status and level of consciousness. (For more information on assessing level of consciousness, see Chapter 3.) Later, you can interview a friend or family member to obtain complete health data.

Dealing with an incompetent patient

While competency is not an issue that arises exclusively with older adults, it may come into play if your patient has age-related dementia. Competency is a legal issue, and your facility will need to take certain steps to protect the patient's welfare and civil liberties. If you suspect

ASSESSING A PATIENT'S PSYCHOSOCIAL STATUS

Stay alert for signs that an older adult is experiencing personal or social difficulties. Such signs include poor hygiene and grooming and indications of abuse, neglect, or malnutrition. If you uncover these signs, you'll need to investigate the causes and be prepared to contact a social worker, if appropriate.

When assessing for depression and other psychological disorders, keep in mind that although depression is more common among older adults, its symptoms may be less severe in this age group. What's more, they may mimic normal signs of aging.

Therefore, make sure that you check for subtle indicators of depression, such as disruptions in a patient's sleep patterns (trouble falling asleep or waking up early in the morning), changes in her eating habits (eating too little or too much), and changes in her interests (loss of enjoyment derived from hobbies that the patient used to enjoy).

your patient is incompetent or unable to make decisions for herself, contact her physician and your nurse manager to determine who will make decisions about her care.

Consult with your nurse manager about the need to document specific patient deficits, such as lack of judgment, and how to involve your facility's risk-management team in the patient's care. Also, talk to the physician about obtaining a psychiatric consultation for the patient.

Modifying the physical examination

Proceed more slowly when conducting the examination to accommodate an older adult's slow response to your instructions or an increased number of symptoms to investigate. Also, keep in mind that the patient may be unable to assume certain positions because of decreased flexibility.

During the examination, don't confuse normal signs of aging with signs of disease. Age brings on many bodily alterations, including changes in fat distribution, skin elasticity, and posture. Age can also reduce a person's pain perception, so take special care to be gentle. This is especially important if you suspect the patient may have osteoporosis. Blunt percussion, for instance, may be contraindicated in this patient.

Also consider whether any medications the patient is taking could affect your physical findings. For example, if she's taking a beta-blocker, expect her heart rate to be slower than normal.

OBESE PATIENTS

When obtaining a health history from an obese patient, be sensitive to her feelings, especially when asking about her weight and eating habits. Most obese people are painfully aware that they're overweight; some have tried to lose weight numerous times. Also, many know of the health risks associated with obesity and feel guilty about endangering their health.

Checking for obesity-related health problems

Obesity in itself is good cause for a thorough investigation of the patient's health status. Ask about a history of obesity-related disorders such as diabetes mellitus and hypertension. Also, find out if the patient's serum cholesterol and triglyceride levels have been checked recently. If they have and the results were elevated, find out if she's currently being treated for these conditions.

Review the patient's dietary habits and discuss any past attempts at weight loss. Try to determine if her obesity is long-standing or more recent. If it's recent, ask if she knows what prompted the weight gain. For instance, did she recently start taking a medication that promotes weight gain, such as a corticosteroid?

Also investigate whether your patient is depressed, bored, or less mobile as a result of an injury or a disorder. Ask about recent pregnancies and changes in menstrual patterns.

Modifying the physical examination

Be sensitive to your patient's need for privacy and discretion. If the patient's gown isn't large enough to cover her fully, let her wear her own clothing, when appropriate.

Be sure to use the proper examination equipment, such as a large blood pressure cuff, to ensure accurate findings. In body areas that may be hard for the obese patient to reach, such as skinfolds, feet, and toenails, carefully examine the skin for signs of disease or poor hygiene.

Be aware that you may have difficulty performing certain examination steps with an obese patient, including eliciting deep tendon reflexes and palpating peripheral pulses and abdominal organs. To palpate, you may need to use both hands (bimanual palpation) to trap or hook an organ.

PREGNANT PATIENTS

You may care for a pregnant patient on your unit when she seeks health care for another problem. So you'll need to be prepared to alter the health history and physical examination for her special needs. Since her pregnancy may not be obvious, always ask a female patient of childbearing age if she's pregnant. When in doubt, check with the physician about ordering a pregnancy test.

Getting the details

In addition to other components of the health history, you'll need to ask specific questions about the progression of the patient's pregnancy, including duration of gestation, delivery due date, presence of contractions, and any complications, such as hypertension. Also, find out if this is her first pregnancy or if she has had previous pregnancies, abortions (spontaneous and induced), or deliveries.

While obtaining her nutritional history, ask the patient about her typical daily diet and any food intolerances, as you would ask any patient. But, also ask about food cravings. If she craves nonnutritive substances (pica), such as dirt, find out what she has eaten and how much. Also, ask if she's taking nutritional supplements, such as prenatal vitamins. If possible, determine her prenatal weight, and calculate her weight gain during pregnancy.

Be sure to ask about smoking, alcohol intake, and recreational drug use. If there's evidence of her use of any of these substances, warn her about the potential effects on the fetus, and consider a referral to a social worker or counselor.

Finally, try to get a handle on her social and emotional state. If you haven't asked earlier, find out if your patient is married or in a safe, stable relationship. If she's single and unattached, explore options for support during the pregnancy and after the delivery. Also try to gauge her reaction—positive or negative—to the pregnancy. Keep in mind that ambivalence and anxiety are common emotions—especially early in the pregnancy.

Modifying the physical examination

As you would with any patient, be sure to provide the pregnant patient with warmth, privacy, and comfort during the physical examination. Make sure that her gown is large enough to cover an advanced pregnancy, or allow her to wear her own clothing. If needed, bring a large-sized blood pressure cuff to the bedside, as well as an ultrasound stethoscope or fetoscope and measuring tape, if you perform a fetal examination.

Before starting the examination, ask your patient if she needs to void; increased glomerular blood flow and uterine pressure on the bladder can cause urinary frequency in the first and third trimester. As you proceed with the examination, pay special attention to her positioning. Whenever possible, keep her in the seated position or in the left-sided supine position with the head of the bed elevated. Avoid having her lie flat on her back for very long. Why? As the uterus expands in pregnancy, it can place pressure on the descending aorta and inferior vena cava, compromising blood flow to and from the lower extremities. If the blood flow is severely compromised, it can lead to supine hypotension, marked by a feeling of faintness. When she needs to lie on her back—for example when you're examining her abdomen,place a pillow beneath her bent knees to relax her abdominal muscles. Because the enlarged uterus can keep the diaphragm from descending fully and prevent complete lung expansion, keep her head elevated to help ease her breathing.

When you examine a pregnant patient, be prepared for unexpected findings related to the pregnancy and the hormonal changes it produces. Signs and symptoms present in a healthy, pregnant female might otherwise cause alarm if found in a nonpregnant patient. When performing a head-to-toe examination of the pregnant patient, consider the normal, physiological changes that pregnancy produces (See *How Pregnancy Affects the Result of the Physical Examination.*)

LIFESPAN CONSIDERATIONS

HOW PREGNANCY AFFECTS THE RESULT OF THE PHYSICAL EXAMINATION

Body region	Expected changes	Possible cause
Head and neck	• Irregularly shaped, brown patches on the face (chloasma), darkening of scars and moles, spider nevi	• Increased melanocyte activity
	• Increased facial hair, loss or thinning of scalp hair, oily scalp	• Increased androgen and corticotropic hormone formation
	• Gingival hyperplasia	• Increased gingival vascularity caused by hormonal changes
	• Symmetrically enlarged thyroid gland	• Increased thyroid gland vascularity, new thyroid follicle formation, hyperplasia of glandular tissue
	• Nasal congestion	• Increased vascularity and swelling of nasal mucosa
Eyes and ears	• Blurred vision when wearing contact lenses	• Increased lysozome content in tears
	• Darkening of eyelids	• Increased melanocyte activity
	• Feeling of fullness in ears	• Increased vascularity of auditory canal and tympanic membrane
Chest and back	• PMI displaced upward and to left, shallow respirations with increased rate, reduced respiratory excursion	• Upward displacement of diaphragm
	• Soft, blowing systolic murmurs, S$_3$ heart sound	• Increased blood volume and velocity
	• Darkening of areolae and nipples	• Increased melanocyte activity
	• Breast hypertrophy and tenderness, superficial venous pattern	• Increased breast glandular tissue and vascularity
Upper extremities Abdominal region	• Palmar erythema	• Cause unknown
	• Midline, brownish, black streak (linea nigra)	• Increased melanocyte activity
	• Purple or red straie	• Stretching of skin caused by uterine, fetal growth
	• Hypoactive bowel sounds, nausea, vomiting, dyspepsia, constipation	• Intestinal smooth muscle relaxation
	• Abdominal tenseness or firmness during palpation	• Uterine contractions caused by palpation (commonly third trimester)
	• Hemorrhoids	• Increased regional blood flow
Lower extremities	• Edema, varicosities	• Increased lower extremity venous pressure, caused by pressure of enlarged uterus

FIRST ENCOUNTERS:
A GENERAL SURVEY OF THE PATIENT

Physical examination begins the moment you meet your patient—during his admission to the hospital, upon your first encounter with him on your shift, or at the start of a clinic visit. Even before you begin a formal physical examination, you may be able to detect both obvious and subtle signs of a disease or disorder.

This chapter describes how to form a sound clinical impression of your patient's physical and psychological well-being from the first time you see him and then build on that impression step by step as you proceed with the examination. Your main tools for forming this impression are your senses of sight, hearing, smell, and touch.

The specific steps you'll take and the sequence you'll follow may vary with the patient's medical condition. Typically, however, you'll begin by observing facial expressions for clues to his emotional state, checking for obvious signs of distress. Then, proceeding with the initial portrait, you'll evaluate vital signs, body build, posture, body movements, gait, balance, coordination, position sense, level of consciousness, and nutritional status, as well as skin, hair, and nails. Of course, if the patient is seriously ill or bedridden, you may need to delay or omit certain parts of the initial assessment.

ASSESSING GENERAL PRESENTATION

A patient's general presentation can provide important clues to his health and well-being. To assess general presentation, observe the patient's facial expression, evaluate his self-care, and note any unusual odors.

Facial expression

A person's facial expression usually reveals the emotions he's experiencing at the time, such as fear, happiness, or anxiety. As you first enter a patient's room, check his expression for signs of distress. If present, these may affect the way you conduct the examination. For example, if he's grimacing in pain, you'll need to respond to his need for relief before proceeding. Throughout your first encounter, continue to assess his facial expression for clues to discomfort. As you perform each examination step, stay alert for grimacing, gritting teeth, or flushing. Also watch for pallor and diaphoresis, which suggest hypotension from severe discomfort that triggers a vasovagal reaction.

Try to determine if the patient's facial expression is consistent with what he's saying or appropriate for the conversation. For instance, does he look tense, even though he's telling you he feels fine? If so, this may mean he's reluctant to tell you that something's bothering him. On the other hand, if he complains of excruciating pain but has a relaxed or happy facial expression, he could be malingering.

CULTURAL CONSIDERATIONS

Keep in mind that cultural factors can play a role in facial expressiveness and the extent of eye contact a patient makes. A patient who comes from a culture that values stoicism may try to hide any sign of pain on his face. Also, be aware that in some cultures, avoiding eye contact does not indicate lack of interest or distrust. Rather, it's a sign of respect or deference to authority.

Self-care

Components of self-care include personal hygiene and grooming. Signs of poor hygiene and grooming may be obvious as you approach your patient. You can assess hygiene further by noting whether his hair, nails, and skin are clean. To assess grooming, check whether your patient has combed his hair and fastened his clothing properly, and whether he's dressed appropriately.

Poor hygiene and grooming may reflect illness or malaise, lack of social support or financial resources, or impaired thought processes (resulting from depression or a mental disorder).

CULTURAL CONSIDERATIONS

Also, consider whether cultural factors might be at play; different cultures have different customs and standards regarding hygiene. For example, the use of deodorant is unheard of and the shaving of a woman's axillary hair is rare in some cultures.

Unusual odors

Unusual body odors may result from a variety of physical illnesses. Fruity breath, for example, may indicate diabetic ketoacidosis. Other body odors may simply reflect variations in hygienic and grooming practices. If you detect an unusual odor, try to determine if the underlying cause calls for prompt attention. (See *Identifying Unusual Odors.*)

ASSESSING VITAL SIGNS

Vital signs include temperature, pulse, respirations, and blood pressure. Obtaining your patient's vital signs early in the assessment may enable you to immediately detect certain life-threatening problems, such as profound hypotension or tachycardia.

IDENTIFYING UNUSUAL ODORS

Stay alert for unusual body odors as you assess your patient's general presentation. The chart below presents possible causes of various odors.

Odor	Probable causes
Fruity breath	• Diabetic ketoacidosis
Halitosis	• Dental decay • Throat infection
Putrid breath or body odor	• Infection (such as lung abscess or wound infection) • Malignancy
Fishy vaginal odor	• Vaginal infection
Urine or ammonia-like odor	• Dehydration • Incontinence • Urinary tract infection
Fecal breath or body odor	• Bowel obstruction (with fecal breath odor) • Incontinence • Poor hygiene

Temperature

You can measure body temperature with a glass mercury thermometer, an electronic thermometer, or a tympanic thermometer. A tympanic thermometer measures core body temperature—the most reliable standard for temperature measurement. If your patient is in a critical care area and has a pulmonary artery catheter or an indwelling urinary catheter that records temperature, you can obtain his core body temperature using the thermistor port of the catheter.

Normal findings

- Body temperature ranging from 96.8° to 99.5° F (36° to 37.5° C). Normal temperatures may vary slightly with the measurement method used. (See 🧩 *Normal Temperature Variations.*)

Abnormal findings

- Oral temperature above 99.5° F (37.5° C), rectal temperature above 100.5° F (38° C), or tympanic temperature above 101.3° F (38.5° C). If your patient has any of these, investigate for possible causes of the fever, such as infection, tissue trauma, infarction, malignancy, a blood disorder, medication reaction, or immune disorder.
- Core body temperature exceeding 105° F (40.5° C), indicating a medical emergency called *hyperpyrexia,* which can lead to death unless the patient's temperature is promptly reduced. Clinical effects of hyperpyrexia include neurologic symptoms (such as seizures or changes in mental status) and direct thermal injury to muscle tissue.

NORMAL FINDINGS

NORMAL TEMPERATURE VARIATIONS

Many authorities refer to a range of normal body temperatures rather than a single number because temperature may vary slightly depending on how it's taken, as well as other factors. The following are normal ranges for oral, rectal, and tympanic temperatures:
- Oral temperature: 96.8° to 99.5° F (36° to 37.5° C)
- Rectal temperature: 97.3° to 100.2° F (36.3° to 37.9° C)
- Tympanic (core) temperature: 97.2° to 100° F (36.2° to 37.8° C)

Fluctuating temperatures

Body temperature tends to fluctuate throughout the day, peaking in the late afternoon and reaching its low point at about 3 to 4 A.M. Body temperature also varies over the life span, decreasing with age. That's why older adults are more vulnerable to hypothermia and less capable of mounting a febrile response.

Such injury may lead to rhabdomyolysis (breakdown of muscle tissue into myoglobin), which in turn may lead to renal failure. Other possible consequences of thermal tissue injury include disseminated intravascular coagulation, hypoxemia, and hypotension. In adults, hyperpyrexia rarely results from an infection. More often, it is caused by heatstroke or damage to the hypothalamus.

- Rapid and potentially fatal temperature elevation characterized by muscle rigidity, indicating a rare hereditary phenomenon called *malignant hyperthermia.* It may follow administration of inhaled anesthetic agents or muscle relaxants. Malignant hyperthermia may cause tachycardia, tachypnea, muscle rigidity, cyanosis, and skin mottling. To avert death, treat rapidly. Treatment may include a direct-acting muscle relaxant (such as dantrolene), discontinuation of the offending agent, and fever reduction through the use of cooling blankets.
- Core body temperature below 95° F (35° C), indicating hypothermia. This may result from prolonged exposure to cold, starvation, hypo-thyroidism, or hypoglycemia. Alcohol intoxication and sepsis worsen hypothermia by impairing vasoconstriction—the mechanism by which blood vessels constrict, reducing blood flow to peripheral organs and preserving body heat necessary for the vital organs. Hypothermia is life-threatening and calls for rapid intervention. (See *Assessing the Severity of Hypothermia.*)

ASSESSING THE SEVERITY OF HYPOTHERMIA

Hypothermia may be mild, moderate, or severe.

Mild hypothermia
Defined as a body temperature between 90° and 95° F (32.2° to 35° C), mild hypothermia causes shivering, piloerection (gooseflesh), cool skin, pallor, and cyanotic nail beds with slow capillary refill.

Moderate hypothermia
A body temperature between 82.4° and 90° F (28° and 32.2° C) causes loss of the ability to shiver, diminished deep tendon reflexes, and cardiac arrhythmias (such as atrial fibrillation). Although moderate hypothermia typically causes a decreased cardiac output and a slow heart rate, the person usually can maintain a normal blood pressure.

Severe hypothermia
A body temperature below 82.4° F (28° C) causes decreased blood pressure, ventricular arrhythmias, progressive bradycardia, and coma. If the temperature falls below 64° F (18° C), the heart may stop beating and brain wave activity may cease. Death ensues unless normal body temperature is restored.

Pulse

Assessing the pulse reveals the patient's heart rate, as well as certain aspects of his heart rhythm. For instance, the pulse amplitude and contour can tell you about the force of left ventricular ejection.

To assess the pulse, palpate the patient's radial artery by applying firm pressure with the distal pads of your index and middle fingers until you feel a pulsation. Don't press too hard because you may occlude the artery and make the pulse undetectable. If your patient has a thready pulse and low blood pressure, you might find it easier to palpate the carotid or femoral artery instead of the radial artery.

To obtain the heart rate, count the beats for 30 seconds. Then multiply by 2. If the pulse is irregular, determine if the irregularity has a regular pattern or no detectable pattern. Then confirm the pulse rate by auscultating an apical heart rate (in case some of the heart's impulses are not reaching the radial pulse). Record the difference between apical and radial pulse rates, known as the *pulse deficit.*

Also, note the pulse amplitude (weak, strong, or bounding) to get an idea of the circulating blood volume, strength of left ventricular contractions, and blood vessel tone. Finally, assess pulse contour or configuration, which reflects the amount and force of blood ejected into the aorta.

Normal findings

- Pulse rate between 60 and 100 beats per minute.
- Regular rhythm.
- Strong amplitude.
- Contour with a smooth upstroke and downstroke.
- Variations in pulse rate and amplitude within normal limits. For example, pulse rates below 60 beats per minute are common in athletes and in people taking beta-adrenergic blockers. Also, any condition that stimulates the sympathetic nervous system, such as exercise, stress, fear, caffeine ingestion, or medications like pseudoephedrine, may increase the pulse rate and amplitude.

Abnormal findings

- Weak, thready pulse, possibly indicating decreased pulse pressure, reduced stroke volume (for example, from heart failure, hypovolemia, or aortic stenosis), and increased peripheral vascular resistance (PVR).
- Bounding pulse, which is easy to palpate and typically has a sharp upstroke followed by a quick downstroke. The pulsations may seem to throb against your finger, then quickly collapse or retreat (called water-hammer or Corrigan's pulse). Conditions that may cause a bounding pulse include bradycardia; hypervolemia; severe hypertension; disorders that increase circulating catecholamines (such

IDENTIFYING PULSE ABNORMALITIES

Each pulsation you feel when palpating your patient's pulse corresponds to a heartbeat. Pulse rate, rhythm, and other characteristics reveal how well the patient's heart is handling its blood volume. The chart below describes some abnormal pulse patterns and their possible causes.

Pulse	Characteristics	Probable causes
Pulsus alternans	• Weak beats alternating with strong beats • Regular rhythm	• Left ventricular failure
Pulsus bigeminus (bigeminal pulse)	• Two beats occurring in rapid succession, followed by a pause during which no pulse is felt • Irregular rhythm • Premature beat with smaller amplitude than normal sinus contraction	• Cardiac arrhythmias, such as premature ventricular contractions
Pulsus paradoxus	• Pulse amplitude that decreases with inspiration and increases with expiration	• Conditions that impede left ventricular outflow during inspiration, such as constrictive pericarditis, cardiac tamponade, end-stage heart failure, and severe chronic obstructive pulmonary disease
Pulsus tardus	• Slow pulse rate • Gradual upstroke; prolonged, blunted downstroke	• Severe aortic stenosis

as pheochromocytoma and hyperthyroidism); disorders that increase stroke volume, reduce PVR, or do both (for instance, anemia, aortic regurgitation, hyperthyroidism, arteriovenous fistula, and patent ductus arteriosus); and decreased blood vessel compliance. (See *Identifying Pulse Abnormalities.*)

Respirations

Changes in the rate, depth, or character of a patient's respirations may suggest neurologic, respiratory, or cardiovascular compromise. If you discover such changes, be sure to investigate for associated symptoms to help uncover the underlying cause.

Consciously or not, some patients change their breathing when they're aware that a health care worker is assessing their respirations. To avoid this, measure the patient's respiratory rate right after taking his pulse, while your fingers are still on his wrist. Count respirations for one minute, noting their rhythm and depth.

Normal findings

- Breathing quiet and effortless.
- Rate between 12 and 20 breaths per minute.
- Regular rhythm.
- Slight thoracic movement and pronounced abdominal movement when the patient is supine. If he's sitting up, expect more obvious thoracic movement.

Abnormal findings

- Respiratory rate exceeding 20 breaths per minute (tachypnea), which may indicate restrictive lung disease, pleuritic chest pain, an elevated diaphragm, fever, metabolic acidosis, or salicylate poisoning. Breathing may be shallow as well. (For information on other abnormal respiratory patterns, see Chapter 6.)

Blood pressure

Blood pressure measurement provides insight into the patient's cardiac output, circulation, hydration, and arterial elasticity. Extremely high or low blood pressure may be life-threatening, requiring rapid assessment and quick intervention. (See ▨ *Hypertension.*)

Before taking a patient's blood pressure, check his arm for an arteriovenous shunt or fistula, lymphedema, an indwelling catheter, or evidence of a brachial artery incision in his arm. Inflating a blood pressure cuff could further impede the flow of blood and lymphatic fluid in this arm. (To use an automatic blood pressure cuff, follow the recommendations outlined in Chapter 1.)

To help detect *orthostatic hypotension*—a drop of 20 mm Hg or more in systolic pressure when the patient rises from a sitting or lying-down position—take blood pressure in three positions: with the patient lying down, sitting, and standing up. (See ▨ *Checking for Orthostatic Hypotension,* p. 52.)

Normal findings

- Systolic pressure between 90 and 119 mm Hg in an adult.
- Diastolic pressure between 60 and 80 mm Hg in an adult.
- Systolic pressure that drops only slightly (less than 20 mm Hg) when the patient rises from a sitting to a standing position).
- Diastolic pressure that rises only slightly when the patient rises from a sitting to a standing position.
- Pulse pressure (the difference between systolic and diastolic pressures) between 30 and 40 mm Hg.
- Pressure that follows a typical diurnal pattern, peaking at midmorning and falling progressively throughout the day to reach its lowest point at 3 to 4 A.M.

HYPERTENSION

A common disorder, usually of unknown cause, hypertension is marked by an intermittent or sustained rise in systolic or diastolic blood pressure. Most physicians diagnose and treat hypertension when a patient has three consecutive blood pressure readings of 140/90 mm Hg or higher. The threshold for treating a patient with diabetes mellitus or chronic renal failure is lower. For these patients, treatment begins when the blood pressure reaches 130/80 mm Hg. Patients with blood pressure readings of 120/80 to 139/89 mm Hg are considered prehypertensive.

Typically, hypertension causes no symptoms and is detected incidentally during routine screening or evaluation for another problem. If it seems to have no underlying cause, the disorder is called primary (or essential) hypertension. When the condition does have a detectable cause, as when the patient has an adrenal disorder, it's called secondary hypertension. If the patient's diastolic pressure rises when he stands up, he probably has primary hypertension. If it drops when he stands up, he probably has secondary hypertension.

Blood pressure rises in response to increased blood volume, heart rate, and stroke volume, or because of arteriolar vasoconstriction, which increases peripheral vascular resistance. Eventually, the result of hypertension can be seen in the patient's blood vessels. In the arterioles, alternating areas of dilation and constriction develop, leading to vascular injury and increased intra-arterial pressure.

Health history
- Family history of hypertension
- African-American race
- Stress
- Obesity or sedentary lifestyle
- Diet high in sodium or saturated fat
- Tobacco use
- Oral contraceptive use
- History of diabetes mellitus, arteriosclerotic disease, or renovascular disease
- Pheochromocytoma
- Cushing's syndrome
- Primary aldosteronism
- Renal failure
- Coarctation of the aorta
- Thyroid or parathyroid disease
- Sleep apnea

- Morning headache in the occipital region
- Fatigue, dizziness, or weakness
- Blurred vision
- Epistaxis
- Chest pain
- Dyspnea

Characteristic findings
Expect your physical examination findings to vary among patients with hypertension, depending on the extent and severity of the disorder. Use the information that follows to help distinguish between expected and unexpected findings.

Inspection
- Peripheral edema (in late stages, with heart failure)
- Retinal hemorrhages, exudates, and papilledema (in late stages, with hypertensive retinopathy)

Palpation
- Pulsating mass in the abdomen (suggests aneurysm, which can result from hypertension)
- Enlarged kidneys (suggests polycystic disease, which can cause hypertension)

Auscultation
- Abdominal bruit
- Femoral bruit
- Elevated systolic or diastolic pressure or both
- Prehypertension: Systolic pressure 120 to 139 mm Hg, diastolic 80 to 89 mm Hg
- Stage 1 hypertension: Systolic pressure 140 to 159 mm Hg, diastolic 90 to 99 mm Hg
- Stage 2 hypertension: Systolic pressure greater than or equal to 160 mm Hg, diastolic pressure greater than or equal to 100 mm Hg

Complications
- Cerebrovascular accident
- Coronary artery disease
- Angina
- Myocardial infarction
- Heart failure
- Arrhythmias
- Sudden cardiac death
- Renal failure
- Hypertensive encephalopathy
- Blindness

EXAMINATION TIP

CHECKING FOR ORTHOSTATIC HYPOTENSION

If your patient appears dehydrated, complains of light-headedness or fainting, or is taking antihypertensive medication, be sure to check for orthostatic hypotension—a decrease in blood pressure when he rises from a sitting or lying-down position.

Take three readings

First, measure blood pressure when the patient is lying down. Then, after waiting 1 to 5 minutes, have him sit up (with the blood pressure cuff still around his arm) and take his blood pressure again. Finally, after waiting 1 to 5 minutes, have him stand (with the cuff still in place) and obtain a third measurement. Also, auscultate his heart rate in these three positions.

Interpret the readings properly

Suspect orthostatic hypotension if the patient's sitting or standing systolic pressure is 20 mm Hg or more lower than his recumbent pressure, and his pulse rises by 10 to 20 beats per minute—especially if he says he feels light-headed when rising to a vertical position.

- Blood pressure rises slightly as the patient ages. Diastolic pressure increases up to about age 60; systolic pressure also increases (from stiffening of the arterial and aortic walls), as does pulse pressure.

Abnormal findings

- Below normal blood pressure, indicating hypotension. Generally, this involves a systolic pressure below 90 mm Hg or a diastolic pressure below 60 mm Hg. However, a patient with pressures above this range may still be hypotensive if his readings are considerably lower than his baseline. Possible causes include heart failure, dehydration, endocrine disorders (such as Addison's disease or hypothyroidism), neurogenic shock, vena cava obstruction, cardiac tamponade, adrenal hypofunction, and a vasovagal reaction.
- Pulse increase of 10 beats per minute and light-headedness or syncope when the patient is standing, indicating orthostatic hypotension. Possible causes include decreased autonomic tone (as seen in older adults and diabetics), decreased vasomotor tone, and medications such as diuretics, alpha-blockers, and tricyclic antidepressants.
- Blood pressure ranging from 120/80 to 139/89 mm Hg obtained on at least three occasions, indicating prehypertension. Although not always treated with medication (unless the patient has diabetes mellitus or renal disease), patients with prehypertension should be

instructed to implement lifestyle changes, such as weight loss and a low-sodium diet.

- Blood pressure 140/90 mm Hg or higher obtained on at least three occasions, indicating hypertension. Be aware that pain, emotional stress, and use of medications such as cyclosporine may cause blood pressure to rise. (For more information on hypertension, see Chapter 7.) If your older patient's systolic blood pressure is greater than 140 mm Hg, but the diastolic reading is less than 90 mm Hg, consider isolated systolic hypertension, a variation commonly seen with aging. (See ▨ *Recognizing Systolic Hypertension in an Older Adult.*)
- Widened pulse pressure, or a difference of more than 40 mm Hg between the systolic and diastolic pressures. It may result from aortic insufficiency or thyrotoxicosis.
- Narrowed pulse pressure, or a difference of less than 30 mm Hg between systolic and diastolic pressures. It may result from tachycardia, severe aortic stenosis, constrictive pericarditis, cardiac tamponade, pericardial effusion, or ascites.

LIFESPAN CONSIDERATIONS

RECOGNIZING SYSTOLIC HYPERTENSION IN AN OLDER ADULT

Approximately 54% of hypertension cases in patients aged 50 to 59 years and 87% of patients aged 60 years or older are attributed to isolated systolic hypertension—a systolic pressure greater than or equal to 140 mm Hg, with a diastolic pressure below 90 mm Hg.

Until he reaches the age of 50, both your hypertensive patient's systolic and diastolic pressures tend to rise. After this age his diastolic pressure tends to level off as his systolic pressure continues to rise, causing isolated systolic hypertension and a widening in pulse pressure. A loss of elasticity in the large arteries caused by atherosclerosis contributes to the development of isolated systolic hypertension.

Previously, isolated systolic hypertension wasn't treated because it was thought to be part of the normal aging process. But we now know, thanks to the Systolic Hypertension in the Elderly Program Study (SHEP), that isolated systolic hypertension increases the risk of stroke and cardiovascular disease in the elderly, even when the diastolic pressure is normal, and should be treated. Track your older patient's blood pressure with each visit to detect isolated systolic hypertension and monitor the effects of treatment. Include orthostatic blood pressure measurements, since impaired baroreceptor reflex mechanisms may occur in an older patient, especially if he has isolated systolic hypertension.

EVALUATING BODY BUILD AND POSTURE

Continue your initial assessment by evaluating your patient's body build and posture. Be sure to check the symmetry of the shoulder, scapulae, and iliac crests. Also, inspect the alignment and curvature of the spinal column. This part of the assessment also includes measuring his height and weight.

Height and weight

Measure your patient's height and weight (with his shoes off) using a standing platform scale with a height attachment. If the patient is hospitalized, try to weigh him every day on the same scale, at the same time, in the same clothing to ensure an accurate comparison. Record both English and metric values for each measurement.

If your patient is weak, immobile, or bedridden, you'll need to use a chair or bed scale to weigh him. Remember to subtract the weight of sheets, padding, and any other items with which he must be measured. Measuring this patient's height may be impractical or impossible; you'll probably have to rely on his report of his height.

Determining if a patient is overweight

Once you've obtained height and weight, determine if the patient's weight is appropriate for his age and height by calculating your patient's *body mass index* (BMI). (See *Assessing Your Patient's Body Mass Index*.) The BMI is weight in kilograms divided by height in meters squared. To save time and avoid calculation, refer to a BMI chart that shows BMIs for various heights and weights and determines whether the patient is a healthy weight, overweight, or obese. Individuals with a BMI greater than 25 are over their ideal body weights and considered at increased risk for obesity-related disorders. The BMI can be calculated using pounds and inches with this equation:

$$BMI = \frac{Weight\ in\ Pounds}{[(Height\ in\ inches) \times (Height\ in\ inches)]} \times 703.$$

For example, a person who weighs 220 pounds and is 6 feet 3 inches tall has a BMI of 27.5, based on the following calculation:

$$\frac{220}{[(75\ inches) \times (75\ inches)]} \times 703 = 27.5.$$

If your patient has gained or lost weight recently, determine the percentage of the weight change through the following steps. Consider any change exceeding 10% of the patient's usual weight significant, and be sure to document it.

- If the patient has lost weight, subtract his current body weight from his previous weight (say, from 6 months ago). If he has gained weight, subtract his previous weight from his current weight.

ASSESSING YOUR PATIENT'S BODY MASS INDEX

Body Mass Index (BMI) is a value that reflects body weight adjusted for height. You can calculate your patient's BMI using inches and pounds or meters and kilograms. For individuals 20 years or older, BMI is categorized as underweight (less than 18.5), normal (18.5 to 24.9) overweight (25 to 29.9), or obese (greater than 30). The following chart displays corresponding inches and pounds for individuals with BMIs ranging from 19-35.

Height (feet and inches)	Weight in pounds																
4'10" (58")	91	96	100	105	110	115	119	124	129	134	138	143	148	153	158	162	167
4'11" (59")	94	99	104	109	114	119	124	128	133	138	143	148	153	158	163	168	173
5' (60")	97	102	107	112	118	123	128	133	138	143	148	153	158	163	168	174	179
5'1" (61")	100	106	111	116	122	127	132	137	143	148	153	158	164	169	174	180	185
5'2" (62")	104	109	115	120	126	131	136	142	147	153	158	164	169	175	180	186	191
5'3" (63")	107	113	118	124	130	135	141	146	152	158	163	169	175	180	186	192	197
5'4" (64")	110	116	122	128	134	140	145	151	157	163	169	174	180	186	192	197	204
5'5" (65")	114	120	126	132	138	144	150	156	162	168	174	180	186	192	198	204	210
5'6" (66")	118	124	130	136	142	148	155	161	167	173	179	186	192	198	204	210	216
5'7" (67")	121	127	134	140	146	153	159	166	172	178	185	191	198	204	211	217	223
5'8" (68")	125	131	138	144	151	158	164	171	177	184	190	197	203	210	216	223	230
5'9" (69")	128	135	142	149	155	162	169	176	182	189	196	203	209	216	223	230	236
5'10" (70")	132	139	146	153	160	167	174	181	188	195	202	209	216	222	229	236	243
5'11" (71")	136	143	150	157	165	172	179	186	193	200	208	215	222	229	236	243	250
6'(72")	140	147	154	162	169	177	184	191	199	206	213	221	228	235	242	250	258
6'1" (73")	144	151	159	166	174	182	189	197	204	212	219	227	235	242	250	257	265
6'2" (74")	148	155	163	171	179	186	194	202	210	218	225	233	241	249	256	264	272
6'3" (75")	152	160	168	176	184	192	200	208	216	224	232	240	248	256	264	272	279
BMI	19	20	21	22	23	24	25	26	27	28	29	30	31	32	33	34	35

Source: Evidence Report of Clinical Guidelines on the Identification, Evaluation, and Treatment of Overweight and Obesity in Adults, 1998. NIH/National Heart, Lung, and Blood Institute (NHLBI).

- Multiply the result by 100.
- Divide the result you obtained in the previous step by the patient's previous weight. This is the percentage of recent weight change.

The following example is calculated for a patient now weighing 185 pounds who weighed 162 pounds 6 months ago. As the result shows, his recent weight gain represents 14.2% of his previous weight.

$$\text{Percentage of recent weight change} = \frac{(185 - 162) \times 100}{162} = \frac{2300}{162} = 14.2$$

Normal findings

- Shoulders, scapulae, and iliac crests symmetrical bilaterally.
- Spinal column midline, with aligned spinal processes, when patient is bent forward. Lumbar spinal curvature is convex.
- Spinal curvature concave in the lumbar region and convex in the thoracic region with the patient standing.

LIFESPAN CONSIDERATIONS

AGE-RELATED CHANGES WITHIN NORMAL LIMITS

With age, a person's posture changes and height decreases as the intervertebral disks shrink, the bony structures between the disks become shorter, and full knee and hip extension becomes more difficult. Also, the lower abdomen typically protrudes from weakened abdominal muscles and redistribution of fat to the hips and lower abdomen. Spinal column alterations may lead to kyphosis.

Abnormal findings

- Accentuated lateral curvature of the spine when the patient bends forward, indicating structural scoliosis. The shoulders appear uneven and the rib cage seems to bulge to one side. This form of scoliosis is associated with thoracic deformity and vertebral rotation.

ASSESSING BODY MOVEMENTS AND GAIT

A patient's body movements and gait may provide clues to such disorders as Parkinson's disease and other neuromuscular or neurologic conditions. Assessing these features can help you gauge your patient's functional status and progress, as well as alert you to the need for possible intervention. For example, a patient with a gait disturbance that predisposes him to falls may require safety interventions or physical therapy for gait or balance retraining.

Observe your patient's body movements both at rest and in motion, paying special attention to movements of the arms, legs, and head. Check for involuntary movements, such as tremors (trembling movements in the hands or head) or tics (spasmodic muscle contractions).

Testing for involuntary movements

You may be able to detect involuntary movements simply by observing your patient as he moves about the room or performs simple activities. Alternatively, you can ask him to hold his arms in front of him and flex his wrists upward with fingers spread as you watch for abnormal involuntary movements.

Another way to check for involuntary movements is to perform *point-to-point testing*. Used mainly to assess coordination, this test also may reveal tremors. Ask the patient to place his index finger on his nose and then touch your finger as you hold it 12 inches to 14 inches directly in front of his nose. Have him continue to alternately touch his nose and your finger several times, watching him closely for tremors.

Normal findings
- Body movements smooth, easily controlled, and coordinated.
- Patient able to hold his arms in front of him with little difficulty or extraneous movement.
- Point-to-point testing smooth, with reasonably accurate movements. The patient should touch his nose and your finger without missing the target or trembling.

Abnormal findings
- Tremors, tics, and dystonic movements, possibly indicating neurologic, neuromuscular, endocrine, or psychological disorder. If you note tremors, tics, or other involuntary movements, document their location, rate, rhythm, and amplitude. And note whether they're related to particular postures, activities, or emotions.

Observing a person's gait
Analyzing a patient's manner or style of walking may help you detect various neurologic disorders. Observing the gait of a patient who's suffered a neurologic or musculoskeletal injury or amputation can also help you assess recovery and rehabilitation.

To analyze a patient's gait, ask him to walk a straight line for several feet and then turn and walk back toward you. Observe his walking rhythm, cadence, and speed, as well as his posture, balance, leg movements, and arm swing. (See ▨ *Identifying Ataxic Gaits,* p. 58.)

Be sure to observe his gait during both the stance and swing phases of walking. The stance phase occurs when one leg and one foot bear most of the patient's weight; it includes double stance, when both feet are in contact with the ground. Most gait abnormalities occur during the stance phase. The swing phase occurs when one foot is raised above the walking surface and the opposite leg and foot bear all of the patient's weight.

During a complete two-step cycle, the stance phase accounts for 60% of total gait time (a quarter of this time in double stance, when both feet are in contact with the ground); the swing phase accounts for the remaining 40%.

When assessing a person's gait, be sure to rule out painful or restrictive foot conditions, such as corns and calluses, which can affect the way someone walks.

EXAMINATION TIP

IDENTIFYING ATAXIC GAITS

When evaluating your patient's gait, check for signs of ataxia—a condition marked by impaired ability to coordinate body movements. Depending on the cause of ataxia, the patient may display either a sensory ataxic gait or a cerebellar ataxic gait.

Sensory ataxic gait
In this uncoordinated gait, the patient may watch the ground for guidance as he walks and may throw his feet forward and outward, toes and heels striking the ground in tandem. This gait is usually caused by loss of position sense resulting from such conditions as peripheral neuropathy (possibly caused by diabetes mellitus) or posterior spinal column damage.

Cerebellar ataxic gait
This wide-based, staggering gait is characterized by difficulty turning. The patient seems to waver and has difficulty standing steadily with eyes open or closed. Possible causes include cerebellar disease, vestibular disease, and alcohol intoxication.

Illustrations from Seidel, H. M., Ball, J. W., Dains, J. E., & Benedict, G. W. (2003). *Mosby's Guide to Physical Examination* (5th ed.). St Louis: Mosby.

Normal findings

- Patient holding his body and head erect, maintaining balance easily, swinging his arms at his sides, and turning smoothly, with shoulders and hips remaining level with each stride. His center of gravity moves up and down about 2 inches, and his pelvis and trunk shift laterally about 1 inch. His left and right feet are held about 2 to 4 inches apart and his step averages 15 inches.

LIFESPAN CONSIDERATIONS

AGE-RELATED CHANGES WITHIN NORMAL LIMITS

A person's gait slows and his balance and grace diminish with age. Reduced muscle strength, especially in the quadriceps, results in short, shuffling steps. Elderly males typically have a wide-based, short-stepped gait; elderly females typically have a narrow-based, waddling gait.

Abnormal findings

- Short-stanced, limping gait, indicating antalgic gait, which is often associated with pain originating from the feet or knees.
- Waddling gait characterized by exaggerated alternation of lateral trunk movements and increased hip elevation, indicating gluteal gait. Possible causes include gluteal medius paralysis, progressive muscular dystrophy, bilateral hip dislocations from joint infections, spastic paralysis, and polio.
- Wide-based, unsteady, uncoordinated gait, indicating ataxic gait.
- Slow, stiff gait in which the thighs cross each other at each step, and the patient looks as if he's walking through water, indicating scissors gait. It may result from bilateral spastic paresis of the legs.
- Slow gait, with the patient taking short accelerating steps, possibly indicating festinating gait (generally associated with Parkinson's disease). Other features include a decreased arm swing, stiff turning, stooped posture, forward lurching of the head and neck, slight flexion of the hips and knees, and arm flexion at the elbows and wrists.

ASSESSING BALANCE, COORDINATION, AND POSITION SENSE

Balance is the ability to maintain the body's equilibrium. Coordination refers to the harmonious functioning of various muscle groups to perform purposeful actions. Position sense is the ability to perceive head, arm, and leg movements and orient oneself without visual cues.

Balance, coordination, and position sense require the smooth integration of the various parts of the nervous system. Use your clinical judgment to determine whether your patient is able to perform tests that involve standing, walking, or performing other maneuvers that require him to leave his bed or expend energy. For example, you would defer most of these tests for a patient who's recovering from surgery or a myocardial infarction until he is stable or no longer in an acute care setting.

Testing balance and coordination

To test balance, have the patient perform the *Romberg test* by standing with his feet together and eyes closed. Observe him for 45 to 60 seconds, watching for signs he's losing his balance. (See ▧ *Evaluating Balance and Coordination.*)

Normal findings

- Romberg test showing patient can stand with his feet together without losing his balance. Although he may sway slightly when his eyes are closed, he shouldn't fall.

Abnormal findings

- Marked swaying or loss of balance during the Romberg test, possibly indicating a cerebellar or vestibular (inner ear) problem.

Evaluating position sense

You can assess your patient's position sense by performing tests that evaluate symmetrical positioning, his ability to identify toe direction, and pronator drift.

Symmetrical positioning. Have your patient close his eyes. Then move his arm or leg into a specific position and ask him to place his other arm or leg in the same position. Determine how closely he duplicates the position in which you placed his arm or leg.

Identifying toe direction. Grasp the patient's great toe by the sides. Ask him to close his eyes. Then move his toe up or down. Ask him to identify which direction you've moved it in. (Before performing this test, clarify which direction you are calling up and which you are calling down.)

Pronator drift. Have the patient stand and extend his arms in front of him, palms up. Then instruct him to close his eyes and maintain this position for 20 to 30 seconds.

Nylen-Bárány test. To assess vestibular function, ask your patient to sit on the side of the bed and then recline to a lying position. As he reclines, have him turn his head toward you while keeping his eyes open.

EXAMINATION TIP

EVALUATING BALANCE AND COORDINATION

To assess your patient's balance and coordination, ask him to perform the maneuvers shown. Throughout these tests, stand nearby to support him in case he starts to lose his balance. (Note: An elderly, weak, or disabled patient may be unable to perform some of these maneuvers.)

Romberg test

In this test of balance, the patient stands with his feet together and then closes his eyes. Watch for swaying or loss of balance.

Walking on heels and toes

To evaluate balance and strength of the foot extensor and flexor muscles, instruct your patient to walk several feet on his heels and then turn around and walk toward you on his toes.

Hopping in place

To test proximal and distal muscle strength in the legs, instruct the patient to hop in place for 10 seconds on each foot. Ask a weak, frail, or older adult to stand up from a sitting position without using his arms. This also tests proximal muscles and hip extensors.

Normal findings
- Symmetrical positioning test showing that the patient can duplicate the position in which you moved his leg or arm.
- Toe direction test showing that the patient can accurately identify the position of his toe after you have moved it.
- Pronator drift test showing that the patient can keep his arms extended without one of them drifting.
- Nylen-Bárány's maneuver showing that the patient doesn't feel dizzy or make extraneous eye movements while moving into a reclining position.

Abnormal findings
- Inability to accurately duplicate the position of the arm or leg, indicating poor position sense, possibly stemming from such conditions as posterior spinal column disease or a peripheral nerve root lesion.
- Inability to identify the direction of toe movement, indicating poor position sense, possibly stemming from such conditions as posterior spinal column disease or a peripheral nerve root lesion.
- Slow downward drift of the arm and supination of the hand during the pronator drift test, possibly indicating mild hemiparesis (paralysis of one side of the body). The patient may rely on visual cues to maintain correct arm position. Hemiparesis may result from a lesion in the contralateral cerebral hemisphere or the corticospinal tract.
- Reporting a sensation of revolving in space or of the surroundings revolving (vertigo) during Nylen-Bárány test, possibly indicating an inner ear problem.
- Involuntary, rhythmic eye movements (nystagmus) when moving from a seated to a recumbent position, possibly indicating an inner ear problem.

ASSESSING LEVEL OF CONSCIOUSNESS

From the first exchange, you should be able to assess your patient's level of consciousness (LOC) simply by calling him by name in a normal tone of voice and then observing his response. The patient should turn his head when he hears your voice and should respond appropriately, indicating alertness.

If he doesn't respond, call his name again while gently touching him or shaking his shoulder. If he still doesn't respond, you may need to apply strong stimulation, such as nail bed pressure. (Keep in mind, though, that a simple hearing impairment may explain a patient's lack of response to verbal stimulation.)

If you must use stimulation, be sure to document the amount and type of stimulation used, as well as your patient's response. That way, other caregivers can use the same type of pressure to reliably assess changes in the patient's LOC.

To document LOC, you can use the Glasgow Coma Scale, especially if the patient has been critically injured. (See *Using the Glasgow Coma Scale.*) Or you may prefer to document your patient's state of arousal using one of the following terms:

- *Alert.* The patient is awake and responds appropriately when addressed in a normal tone of voice.
- *Lethargic.* The patient awakens and responds briefly to a loud voice or gentle shaking but then falls back to sleep.
- *Obtunded.* The patient opens his eyes only when vigorously shaken or stimulated but does not fully awaken. His response may be slow and confused.
- *Stuporous.* The patient can be aroused only with strong stimulation (such as nail bed pressure) and lapses quickly back into an unresponsive state.

USING THE GLASGOW COMA SCALE

Once used mainly to evaluate patients' prognoses and recovery from head injuries, the Glasgow Coma Scale (GCS) is now widely used to evaluate level of consciousness (LOC). To use the GCS, score your patient's response to motor, verbal, and eye stimulation according to the numbers and responses listed. Then total his score. When reporting the results, break down the total score into its components, such as M5, V3, E3 = GCS 11. A patient who scores 15 points, the maximum, is fully awake, alert, and oriented. A patient who scores 3 points is deeply comatose.

Motor response		
	6	Follows commands
	5	Localizes pain on stimulus
	4	Withdraws from painful stimulus
	3	Shows abnormal flexion in response to pain
	2	Shows abnormal extension in response to pain
	1	No responses
Verbal response		
	5	Oriented
	4	Confused
	3	Inappropriate words
	2	Unintelligible sounds
	1	No responses
Eye-opening		
	4	Spontaneous
	3	Opens eyes on verbal command
	2	Opens eyes on painful stimulus
	1	No responses
Total:		

- *Comatose.* The patient can't be aroused even with strong stimulation.

Remember that different facilities may define these terms differently. To avoid confusion, check your facility's policy on documenting LOC.

ASSESSING SKIN, HAIR, AND NAILS

Careful assessment of the skin, hair, and nails (known as the integumentary system) usually provides a clear sense of a patient's overall health. Similarly, changes in the skin, hair, and nails are typically the first indications of a person's declining health. Therefore, when assessing the skin, hair, and nails, you need to look for subtle changes in color, texture, moisture, and temperature, as well as unusual markings or areas of injury.

Skin
The body's largest organ, the skin often serves as a mirror reflecting underlying illnesses, such as those of the liver, kidney, or heart. (See *Structures of the Skin, Hair, and Nails.*)

A thorough skin assessment requires removal of some or all of the patient's clothing. So before you start the examination, make sure the room is well lit, comfortably warm, and private. For greater efficiency, you may reserve much of the skin examination for later, when you assess the different parts of the patient's body. For example, you can assess the skin on the legs when examining the lower extremities.

Inspection
Start the examination by inspecting all exposed areas of the patient's skin. Pay particular attention to areas associated with the patient's chief complaint and other symptoms. Check skin pigmentation and complexion and note areas of skin breakdown, lesions, and bruising.

Inspect the pigmentation and general color of the patient's skin, checking for mottling, cyanosis, or jaundice.

CULTURAL CONSIDERATIONS

To check for cyanosis in a dark-skinned patient, look for an ashen color in the conjunctivae, oral mucosa, or nail beds. Jaundice, on the other hand, is best observed in the soles of the feet and palmar surface of the hands. However, remember that color irregularities may be difficult to determine in a dark-skinned patient.

ANATOMY REVIEW

STRUCTURES OF THE SKIN, HAIR, AND NAILS

The illustration on the left shows a cross-section of skin and hair structures. The one on the right shows the structures of the nail and surrounding tissue.

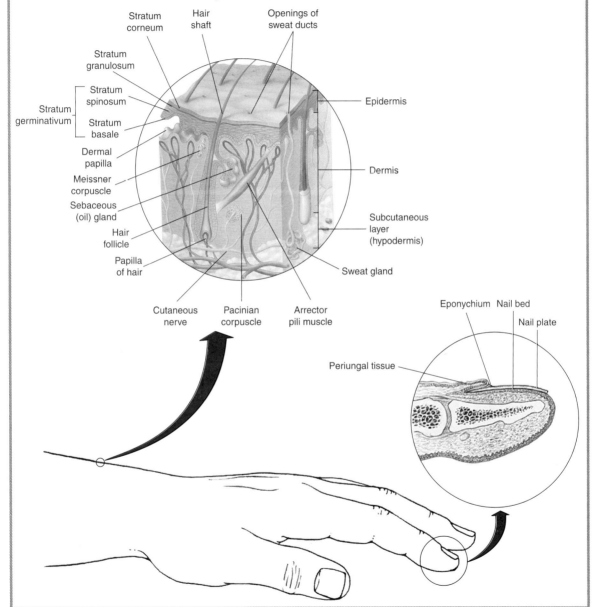

A, from Thibodeau, G. & Patton, K. (2003). *Anatomy and Physiology* (5th ed.) St. Louis: Mosby.
B, modified from Thompson, J. M., McFarland, G. K., Hirsch, J. E., and Tucker, S. M. (2002). *Mosby's Clinical Nursing* (5th ed). St. Louis: Mosby.

Also note pigment abnormalities, freckles, birthmarks, and moles. Ask the patient if he has noticed any changes in the color, shape, or size of a mole.

If the patient appears sunburned or tan, ask if he uses sunscreen—especially if he's taking a medication that makes his skin photosensitive, such as ciprofloxacin, methoxsalen, or a tetracycline.

If the patient is chronically ill or hospitalized, look closely for signs of skin breakdown.

CULTURAL CONSIDERATIONS

Be aware that a patient with dark skin may reveal pressure changes differently than a patient with lighter skin. In a darker-skinned patient, look for gray or yellowish-brown discoloration at the site of pressure, which can turn purple before returning to its baseline color.

In areas that have served as recent insertion sites for intravenous (IV) lines or catheters, look for signs of infiltration of medication or IV fluid, infection (manifested by pus or erythema), phlebitis, and tape burns. Also check for skin breakdown at all pressure points, such as the ears, scalp, scapulae, shoulders, iliac crests, sacrum, malleoli, and heels. Be sure to look beneath dressings, prostheses, and restraints.

Inspect any area that may be excoriated or infected from incontinence, heavy perspiration, lack of exposure to air, or obesity. Typically, these areas include the skin beneath the breasts, in the axillae, between the thighs, and in the gluteal folds.

Finally, check the skin for lesions, rashes, wounds, and bruising.

LIFESPAN CONSIDERATIONS

In an older adult, normal changes that occur with aging include wrinkled, thickened, pale, or translucent skin. You might also observe purple macular lesions that resemble bruises, called actinic purpura, bright red lesions called cherry angiomas, or brownish-gray macular lesions (known as liver spots) called actinic lentigines.

Palpation

For optimal patient comfort, warm your hands before beginning palpation. If you suspect the patient may have an infection that can be transmitted through the skin, don gloves before touching lesions.

Palpate skin temperature using the back of your hand, which is more sensitive to temperature. To help detect a temperature abnormality, simultaneously compare the patient's skin temperature to your own, using both hands. To uncover localized temperature changes, compare body parts on both sides of the body. For example, move your hand rapidly from the left leg to the right leg to compare their temperatures.

To check skin turgor (resiliency or elasticity), gently pinch the patient's skin between your thumb and forefinger. Then release it. In an elderly or dehydrated patient, test skin turgor on the forehead, sternal area, or beneath the clavicle—areas where the skin normally is more taut.

LIFESPAN CONSIDERATIONS

Expect skin turgor changes in the older adult that reveal loosened, thinning skin on the back of the hands, forearms, and other areas.

Using the tips and pads of your fingers, palpate for areas of increased roughness or smoothness. Also check the skin for suppleness or tautness, thickness, and strength.

Palpate for dry areas. To avoid confusing the patient's skin moisture with your own, use the backs of your hands and fingers. If you are wearing gloves, you can defer this part of the examination because gloves will interfere with moisture assessment.

If inspection reveals a skin lesion, gently palpate the borders of the lesion to see if the area is raised (papular) or flat (macular). Because the lesion may be infectious, either wear gloves or avoid direct palpation.

Normal findings
- Skin color varying with race but appearing even over the entire body.

CULTURAL CONSIDERATIONS

Dark-skinned people have lighter skin on their palms, the soles of their feet, and their nail beds. Also, in areas that get regular sun exposure, expect darker skin and greater pigmentation.

Abnormal findings
- Skin abnormalities reflecting a wide range of conditions. (See ▓ *Recognizing Skin Abnormalities*, p. 68.)

Hair
Like changes in the skin, changes in a patient's hair may reflect underlying illness, so you'll need to examine it carefully. Be sure to assess both types of hair—terminal and vellus. Terminal hair, long and coarse, is found

INTERPRETING ABNORMAL FINDINGS

RECOGNIZING SKIN ABNORMALITIES

An abnormal skin finding may suggest that the patient has a particular disease or disorder. Use the following table to correlate skin abnormalities with possible causes.

Abnormality	Probable causes
Patchy pigmentation	• Vitiligo • Tinea versicolor
Absence of pigmentation	• Albinism
Jaundice	• Hepatic disease
Cyanosis	• Hypoxemia
Mottling	• Blood flow disturbance (for example, from hypotension, if generalized, or a blood clot, if localized)
Flushing	• Fever • Embarrassment • Too-rapid infusion of certain drugs (such as vancomycin) • Medications or supplemental vitamins (such as niacin)
Pallor	• Anemia • Hypotension
Erythema	• Polycythemia • If localized: infection, burn, or infiltration of IV medication
Skin breakdown	• Pressure ulcer • Infection
Macule (flat lesion)	• Allergic reaction • Pigmentation change • Systemic lupus erythematosus (butterfly rash)
Papule (raised lesion)	• Hives • Acne
Scaling patches	• Psoriasis • Seborrheic dermatitis
Bruising	• Clotting disorder • Anticoagulant therapy • Trauma
Change in appearance of mole	• Melanoma
Hot, dry skin	• Fever
Cool, moist skin	• Circulatory compromise • Hypotension
Decreased turgor	• Dehydration
Oily skin	• Hyperthyroidism
Dry, thin skin	• Hypothyroidism

on the scalp, eyebrows, axillae, and pubic areas. Vellus hair is short, fine in texture, and lighter than terminal hair; it covers most areas of the skin except the palms and soles.

For efficiency, you can assess the patient's hair at the same time you assess his skin. To prevent piloerection (gooseflesh), ensure adequate lighting and warmth. If you suspect the patient's hair and scalp are infested with lice, wear protective gear, such as gloves.

Begin your assessment of the hair by inspecting the terminal hair on the patient's scalp, noting its color, distribution, and quantity. If you see areas of hair loss or thinning, determine if the hair shafts are broken or burned off or if the hair is completely absent.

LIFESPAN CONSIDERATIONS

Hair quantity and thickness tends to diminish with age. Fewer functioning melanocytes in the hair shafts result in loss of hair color.

Grasp the hair between your thumb and forefinger, noting its moisture and texture, and whether the hair falls out as you gently grasp it. Next, part the hair and inspect the scalp, noting any wounds, lesions, dryness or oiliness, scaling, infection, or signs of infestation.

Then inspect the fine vellus hairs on the patient's face, chest, back, arms, legs, and abdomen. Note the color, distribution, and quantity. Check for areas of hair loss or unusually dense or coarse hair, especially on the face of a female patient.

Finally, inspect the coarse, terminal hairs in the axillae and pubic areas, noting color, texture, and distribution. Remember, the pubic hair normally forms an upright triangle in the male and an inverted triangle in the female.

Normal findings
- Hair distributed evenly over the scalp and body, except in males with male-pattern thinning or baldness. Thin, fine, lighter-colored (vellus) hair covers all areas of the body except the palms and soles. Terminal hair is coarser, darker, and thicker than vellus hair.
- Hair color usually ranging from light blond to black. Hair color is consistent throughout the scalp, except in patients who use hair coloring or have graying hair.
- Hair fine or coarse, straight or curly.
- Scalp free of injuries, lesions, excessive dryness or oiliness, scaling, infection, or signs of infestation.

Abnormal findings
- Decreased hair growth, possibly indicating hypopituitarism. Patchy baldness with breakage of the hair shaft at the scalp surface indicates

alopecia areata, a disease of unknown origin. Hair loss associated with scalp scarring and destroyed hair follicles typifies scarring alopecia. Incomplete hair loss or thinning may result from wearing tightly bound hairstyles (traction alopecia), or from habitual hair pulling (trichotillomania). These disorders also cause scalp inflammation. Hirsutism (excessive body hair) may result from hormonal dysfunction (such as Cushing's syndrome), hereditary factors, porphyria, or certain medications.

- Altered hair color, possibly indicating malnutrition. Sometimes graying is associated with pernicious anemia. Nerve injury may cause patchy graying.
- Dry, brittle hair, possibly indicating malnutrition or hypothyroidism. Increased silkiness and fineness of the hair may be associated with hyperthyroidism.
- Scaling eruptions of the scalp, possibly indicating psoriasis or seborrheic dermatitis. Excoriation of the scalp, eyelids, and pubic area with small, nitlike flakes along the hair shaft indicates infestation with *Pediculus humanus corporis* (lice). Infection of one or more hair follicles results in folliculitis or carbuncles (clusters of staphylococcal boils or abscesses beneath the skin).

Nails

Because nails are extensions of the epidermis, their shape, color, texture, and condition may be affected by disease. Also, capillaries visible under the nail plate may reflect color changes associated with altered circulation and oxygenation.

For efficiency, you can assess the patient's nails when examining his upper and lower extremities. Before examining the nails, make sure the room temperature is comfortable; extremes in temperature can affect nail bed color. Also check for nail polish, artificial nails, and nail wraps, which can interfere with your assessment. If you must check the nail bed for signs of circulatory or oxygenation problems, have the patient immerse artificial nails or nail wraps in an acetone solution to loosen or dissolve them.

You can inspect and palpate the nails simultaneously. To begin, inspect the nail surface, noting its shape, color, and opacity. Feel the nail surface to determine smoothness and areas of unevenness. Check for horizontal or longitudinal ridges, opaque white spots, and small, splinter hemorrhages visible through the nail bed. Inspect the curvature to detect clubbing or spooning. (See 🖾 *Assessing for Finger Clubbing.*)

Next, gently squeeze the nail between your thumb and forefinger to determine how well the nail plate adheres to the nail bed and to assess the firmness of the nail bed. Also note how long the nail bed takes to recover from blanching (capillary refill).

Finally, inspect and palpate the periungual tissue. Note any erythema, edema, induration, or tenderness.

EXAMINATION TIP

ASSESSING FOR FINGER CLUBBING

You can use the Schamroth technique to identify clubbing of the fingers and nail beds—an abnormality resulting from chronic hypoxemia. Ask your patient to place the first phalanges of both index fingers together, as shown. Check the space between the two nail tips; normally, it's small and diamond-shaped. With clubbed fingers, there's no space between the two nail tips and the transverse diameter of the nail is wider than the distal phalanx. That's because the angle between the nail and the point where the nail enters the skin is convex, exceeding 180 degrees.

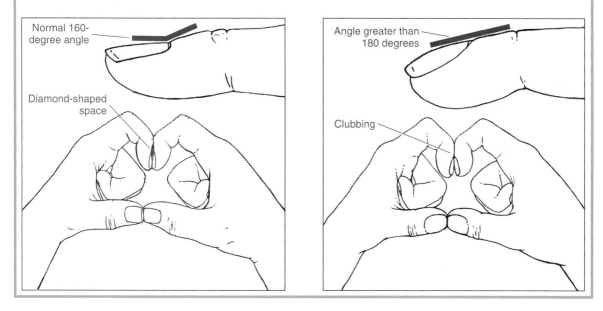

Normal findings

- Nail plate smooth, round, fairly translucent, and firmly attached to the nail bed. The nails should have slightly convex curvature, with an angle of about 160 degrees between the nail and the skin at the nail base. The nail surface should feel smooth, even, and hard, with smooth, rounded edges.

CULTURAL CONSIDERATIONS

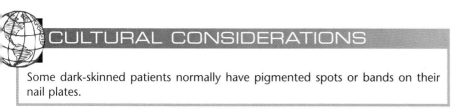

Some dark-skinned patients normally have pigmented spots or bands on their nail plates.

LIFESPAN CONSIDERATIONS

Older adults often have thickened, yellowish nails, with longitudinal furrows, especially on the toes.

- Nail bed pinkish and firm upon palpation. Capillary refill should take less than 4 seconds
- Cuticles smooth, flat, and unbroken.

Abnormal findings

- Brittle, thinning, or peeling nail plates, suggesting nutritional or circulatory deficiencies. Occasionally the nail plate is congenitally absent.
- Cracks or fissures in the nails, possibly indicating undernutrition.
- Thickened nails, which may result from trauma, decreased circulation, or fungal infection.
- White nail plates, suggesting hypoalbuminemia.
- Pale nail plates, possibly indicating anemia.
- Greenish-black nail plates, suggesting a fungal or bacterial infection (such as *Pseudomonas*).
- Yellow nail plates, suggesting psoriasis or respiratory disease, although yellowing can also stem from cigarette smoking or use of nail polish.
- Spoon-shaped nails, possibly reflecting iron deficiency.
- Poor adhesion of the nail plate to the nail bed, suggesting psoriasis—as does pitting of the nail plates.
- Rough, jagged, or bitten nails, possibly indicating poor hygiene or habits
- An abnormal curvature or a nail base angle of 180 degrees or greater, indicating clubbing, a sign of cardiopulmonary disease.
- Splinter hemorrhages of the nail bed, possibly resulting from endocarditis, psoriasis, or trauma.
- A white band suddenly appearing in the nail bed of a light-skinned person, suggesting melanoma.
- Transverse white lines (Mees' lines) or grooves (Beau's lines), possibly following certain systemic illnesses. However, white lines occasionally result from clinically insignificant nail trauma as well.
- Pallor of the nail bed, suggesting anemia.
- Bluish mottling or cyanosis, indicating hypoxemia or compromised peripheral circulation.
- Capillary refill greater than 4 seconds, indicating compromised circulation.
- Broken, bitten, erythemic, or swollen cuticles, possibly indicating paronychia, an acute or chronic infection of the tissue around the nails.

EVALUATING NUTRITIONAL STATUS

Nutritional status can affect a person's growth and development, wound healing, resistance to infection, and recovery from illness or surgery. Many facilities employ registered dietitians to identify and correct patients' nutritional deficiencies. Nonetheless, the nurse is often the first staff member to suspect a nutritional problem or to recognize that a patient's nutritional needs have changed. This means you're in a position to rapidly intervene to correct actual or potential nutritional deficiencies.

Before formally evaluating your patient's nutritional status, review his health history for possible risk factors for nutritional deficiencies. Pay special attention to recent weight changes, special dietary needs, changes in bowel elimination patterns (such as diarrhea), a history of chronic illness (such as chronic obstructive pulmonary disease), or a history of poor wound healing. Also review any prescription medications he's taking; some drugs can cause appetite changes. Note the presence of psychosocial factors that can affect nutritional status, such as low income, depression, alcoholism, or a history of anorexia or bulimia.

If possible, review the patient's 24-hour dietary recall and determine if he's consuming the proper number of servings from each of the six food groups: breads and grains, fruits, vegetables, dairy, meat or meat substitutes, and fats.

Nutritional imbalances

Nutritional imbalances fall into one of two general categories—undernutrition and overnutrition. If your patient has an actual or potential nutritional imbalance, he'll need to undergo a thorough examination, including anthropometric assessment. Anthropometric assessment includes height, weight, and skinfold measurement.

Undernutrition

If your patient is undernourished or at risk for undernutrition, try to identify the cause. Usually, undernutrition is associated with poor nutritional intake, altered nutrient digestion or absorption, increased nutrient excretion, inability to process nutrients, or increased nutritional demand.

Conditions that cause poor nutritional intake include appetite loss from nausea, dysphagia, and psychosocial problems such as depression, anorexia nervosa, bulimia, and alcoholism. Altered nutrient digestion or absorption can result from conditions such as diarrhea and pancreatitis, and procedures such as gastrectomy and small bowel resection.

Increased nutrient excretion can be caused by dialysis, diarrhea, and hemorrhage. Conditions that impair nutrient processing include alcoholism, congenital metabolic disorders (such as celiac sprue), and liver disease. Nutritional demands may increase from fever, sepsis, and surgery.

Overnutrition and obesity

One of the largest health concerns facing the United States, obesity is defined as a BMI that's greater than 30 (a BMI between 25 and 29.9 ranks as overweight). An obese, or overnourished, person typically consumes more calories than he expends, but that doesn't necessarily mean he's getting adequate nutrition. For example, a patient who takes corticosteroids may be overweight and yet experience protein breakdown—a condition that may call for protein supplementation.

Sometimes, obesity stems from a medical condition, such as Cushing's syndrome (cortisol overproduction) or Klinefelter's syndrome (a chromosomal disorder). Also, certain medications—for instance, tricyclic antidepressants (amitriptyline) and corticosteroids (prednisone)—can predispose a person to weight gain. What's more, an obese patient is prone to related health problems, such as diabetes mellitus, cardiovascular disease, and osteoarthritis.

What to do

If your assessment reveals that your patient is at risk for undernutrition or overnutrition, plan to refer him to a registered dietitian who can develop a diet plan that will address his nutritional needs.

EXAMINING THE HEAD AND NECK

After taking your patient's complete health history and performing a general assessment, you're now ready to move on to the head-to-toe physical examination. Throughout your physical examination of all parts of the body, be sure to keep pertinent points of your patient's health history and chief complaints foremost in your mind.

The physical examination starts with the patient's head and neck. This region includes the skull, nose, mouth, throat, and neck to the clavicle. The examination also covers assessment of several cranial nerves that control various sensory functions, including taste and smell. Assessment of the eyes and ears, although mentioned occasionally in this chapter, appears in detail in Chapter 5.

The head is the part of the human body that interacts most, and at the highest level of complexity, with the environment. Partly because of this, the head is the site of a number of common ailments, including headaches, sinus congestion, neck pain, nosebleeds, sore throats, and injuries.

In general, the chief complaints discussed in this chapter can and often do result from simple, temporary medical problems. However, virtually all of these complaints can also stem from serious, even life-threatening disorders. That's why assessing this area of the body completely and accurately is so important. Before beginning, be sure you're familiar with the important structures and functions you'll be assessing. (See █ *Structures of the Head and Neck,* pp. 76-79.)

(Text continued on p. 80.)

ANATOMY REVIEW

STRUCTURES OF THE HEAD AND NECK

The skull

Composed of flat, irregular bones tightly joined by sutures, the skull houses and protects the brain. It also positions and protects the eyes, ears, and teeth. The skull's major bony structures are shown as follows:

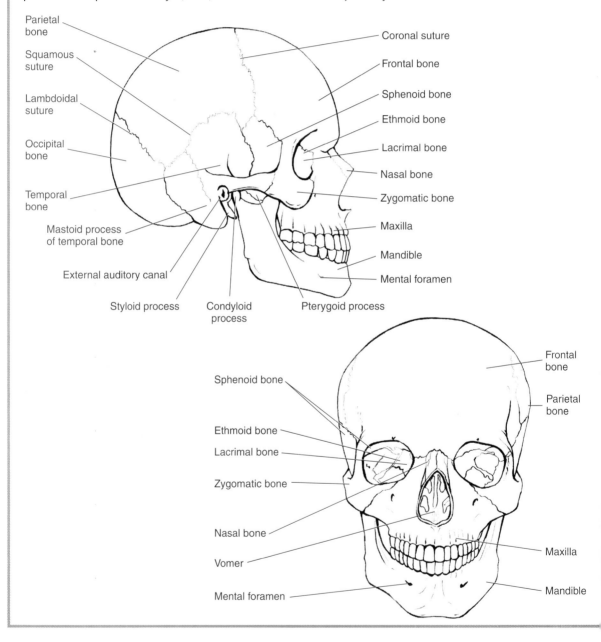

Muscles

The neck is divided into two triangles by the sternocleidomastoid muscle. The anterior triangle is bounded by the mandible and the sternocleidomastoid muscle, which meet at the body's midline. Midline structures of the neck are located in the anterior triangle. The posterior triangle is bounded by the trapezius muscle, the sternocleidomastoid muscle, and the clavicle. Major muscles of the head and neck are shown as follows:

(Continued)

ANATOMY REVIEW

STRUCTURES OF THE HEAD AND NECK—cont'd

Internal structures

A wide variety of internal structures support the functions of the senses, respiratory system, digestive system, endocrine system, and lymphatic system.

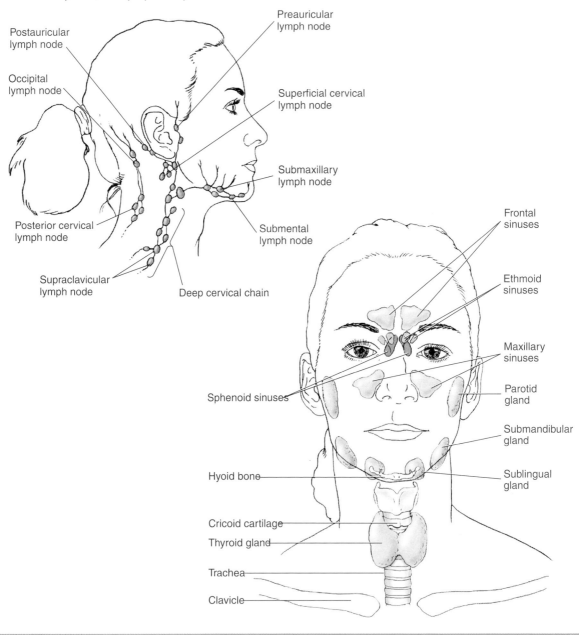

The mouth

Bordered superiorly by the hard and soft palates, inferiorly by the tongue, laterally by the pillars of the soft palate and tonsils, and anteriorly by the lips, the mouth serves as entryway to the digestive and respiratory systems. Major oral structures are shown as follows:

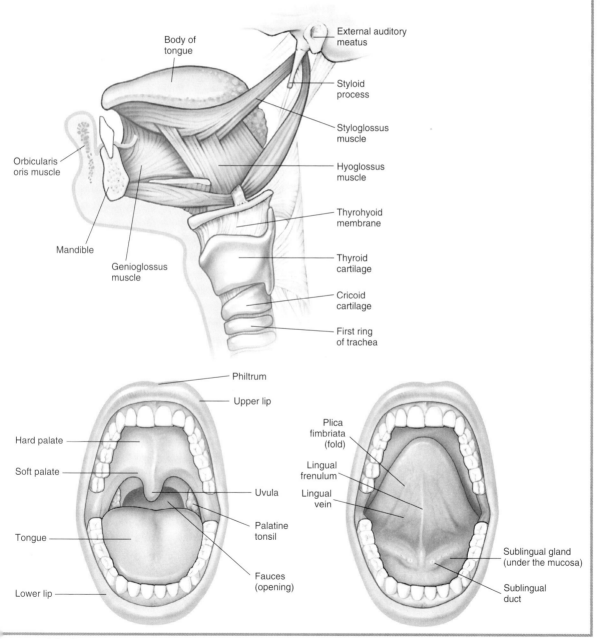

From Thibodeau, G., & Patton, K. (2003). *Anatomy and Physiology* (5th ed.). St. Louis, Mosby.

Keep in mind that the brain exerts fine control over many of the characteristics you'll be assessing. That makes the brain another structure with which you should be familiar if you want to bring your best talents to bear in the assessment. (See ▯ *Parts of the Brain.*)

Clearly, assessing the head and neck is a complex assignment. But with thorough preparation, careful attention to detail, and sound clinical judgments, you can meet this challenge successfully.

EXAMINATION STEPS AND FINDINGS

Before beginning your examination, be sure to assemble the necessary equipment, including examination gloves, a bright light source (such as a penlight), an otoscope with a wide speculum (if available), a cotton-tipped applicator, a tongue blade, a pin or other sharp object, several samples of familiar scents and tastes, and a stethoscope.

For best results when assessing the head and neck, make sure the room is well lit and the temperature is comfortable.

Inspection

In most cases, you'll start your examination at the top of the patient's head and proceed systematically downward toward the neck, performing inspection and palpation simultaneously to maximize your efficiency. (See ▯ *Key Examination Steps for the Head and Neck,* p. 84.)

Skull and scalp

Begin by asking your patient to sit comfortably upright so you can easily examine the top of her head. Working step by step, inspect the patient's hair, noting its quantity, distribution, texture, and any evidence of hair loss. If the patient has hair loss, describe its pattern.

Part the patient's hair and inspect the scalp. Look for scales, redness, open lesions, scabbed areas, or nits (lice eggs). Also look for lumps. Observe the general size and shape of the patient's skull. Make note of any deformities, swelling, or masses. Also perform a general assessment of the ears, noting their position and size in relation to the patient's head.

Face

Observe the patient's face for symmetry. Watch for any involuntary movements or tics. Then test cranial nerve (CN) VII, the facial nerve, by asking the patient to perform a series of movements to demonstrate her use of facial muscles. (See *Understanding Cranial Nerves,* p. 85.)

Begin by asking the patient to raise her eyebrows, frown, smile, show her teeth, puff her cheeks, and close her eyes tightly. Later, when you're examining the patient's mouth, you can test her sense of taste.

ANATOMY REVIEW

PARTS OF THE BRAIN

Seat of the central nervous system, the brain is composed of three major parts: cerebrum, cerebellum, and brain stem. Beneath the cerebrum and on top of the brain stem lie the structures of the diencephalon, including the thalamus and hypothalamus. The brain stem controls vital involuntary functions, such as breathing.

(Continued)

ANATOMY REVIEW

PARTS OF THE BRAIN—cont'd

Locating the cranial nerves

Twelve pairs of cranial nerves carry impulses between the brain stem and structures of the head and neck, including the eyes, mouth, face, pharynx, larynx, and tongue. These peripheral nerves control both motor and sensory functions, as follows:

Nerve		Function
I	Olfactory	Sensory
II	Optic	Sensory
III	Oculomotor	Motor
IV	Trochlear	Motor
V	Trigeminal	Mixed
VI	Abducens	Motor
VII	Facial	Mixed
VIII	Acoustic	Sensory
IX	Glossopharyngeal	Mixed
X	Vagus	Mixed
XI	Spinal accessory	Motor
XII	Hypoglossal	Motor

Complete your examination of the patient's face by observing her facial skin. Note its color, pigmentation, texture, and the distribution of any hair. Document the size, shape, and configuration of any lesions.

Eyes

Perform a general inspection of the eyes, eyelids, eyebrows, and eyelashes. Note any asymmetry or obvious abnormalities. Inspect the skin beneath and around the eyebrows and eyelashes for erythema, scaling, or drainage. Note the distribution of the eyelashes and whether they're thick or sparse. Check the eyebrows as well. Keep in mind that many females and some males remove all or part of their eyebrows for cosmetic reasons. Inspect the patient's periorbital area for edema, erythema, and lesions. (See Chapter 5 for a full assessment of the eyes and ears.)

Nose

Inspect the patient's nose for symmetry, deformity, and inflammation. If the patient currently has or recently has had a nasogastric tube or nasal oxygen therapy, inspect the skin around the nares for signs of breakdown.

Ask the patient to tip her head back. Using an otoscope with a wide speculum, gently insert the speculum through one nostril and into the vestibule. Observe the mucosa for erythema, swelling, and drainage. Then inspect the nasal septum for bleeding, perforation, and deviation. Now repeat the process for the other nostril.

If you notice any nasal drainage, be sure to document its color, amount, and consistency. If your patient has a basilar skull fracture and you notice a clear, thin, nasal discharge, use a glucose testing strip to see if it contains high levels of glucose, possibly indicating the presence of cerebrospinal fluid (CSF). Blood-tinged drainage that forms droplets with bloody centers and clear halos may also indicate the presence of CSF.

To assess the function of CN I (the olfactory nerve), ask your patient to identify familiar scents, such as soap, coffee, chocolate, and vanilla. However, you should avoid this test if you've already observed inflamed nasal mucosa or nasal discharge because it could worsen the irritation.

Before performing this part of the examination, however, first confirm the patency of the patient's nasal passages by obstructing one nostril and asking her to inhale through the other. If one side is obstructed, be sure to use the other nostril to complete the test. Then, with the patient's eyes closed, pass a fragrance under one nostril and ask your patient to identify the scent. Repeat this process with the other nostril and the remaining scents. Note the patient's responses.

Mouth

Inspect the patient's lips for color, moisture, and lesions. To examine the inside of her mouth, ask your patient to remove her dentures (if she's wearing them). Then use a penlight to examine the condition of the oral mucosa, noting any lesions or infected areas. Ask her to open her mouth wide. Then use a tongue blade to expose the mucosa on both sides of the mouth. Note the color, pigmentation, and overall condition of the interior structures. Inspect the color and shape of the hard palate. Look at the gingiva and teeth for swelling, bleeding, retraction, and discoloration. Identify any abnormalities in the position or shape of the teeth.

Next, observe the patient's tongue for symmetry, position, size, color, and texture. Ask her to touch her tongue to the roof of her mouth while you inspect its underside for lesions or other abnormalities. Inspect the lingual frenulum at the floor of the mouth. Look for the submandibular ducts, located on either side of the base of the frenulum.

Use your penlight and tongue blade to inspect the floor of the mouth and the underside of the tongue (where malignancies may occur) for white or red spots. If you find any ulcerations or nodules, palpate them with a gloved hand for tenderness and consistency. Inspect the soft palate, uvula, tonsils, and posterior pharynx. Look for symmetry of structures, color, and signs of exudate, edema, or ulceration. Note whether the patient still has her tonsils and whether they are enlarged.

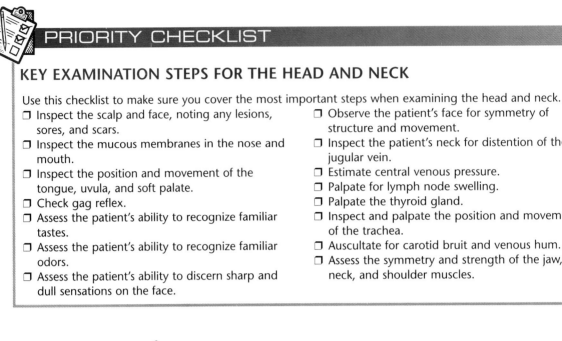

PRIORITY CHECKLIST

KEY EXAMINATION STEPS FOR THE HEAD AND NECK

Use this checklist to make sure you cover the most important steps when examining the head and neck.

- ❏ Inspect the scalp and face, noting any lesions, sores, and scars.
- ❏ Inspect the mucous membranes in the nose and mouth.
- ❏ Inspect the position and movement of the tongue, uvula, and soft palate.
- ❏ Check gag reflex.
- ❏ Assess the patient's ability to recognize familiar tastes.
- ❏ Assess the patient's ability to recognize familiar odors.
- ❏ Assess the patient's ability to discern sharp and dull sensations on the face.

- ❏ Observe the patient's face for symmetry of structure and movement.
- ❏ Inspect the patient's neck for distention of the jugular vein.
- ❏ Estimate central venous pressure.
- ❏ Palpate for lymph node swelling.
- ❏ Palpate the thyroid gland.
- ❏ Inspect and palpate the position and movement of the trachea.
- ❏ Auscultate for carotid bruit and venous hum.
- ❏ Assess the symmetry and strength of the jaw, neck, and shoulder muscles.

LIFESPAN CONSIDERATIONS

Keep in mind that tonsils generally shrink after the age of 5. In some adults, the tonsils aren't visible because they shrink back into the folds of the palatine arches.

Now test the function of CNs IX, X, and XII (glossopharyngeal, vagus, and hypoglossal). These nerves work together to control movements of the pharynx, larynx, soft palate, and tongue. If you've heard your patient speak and cough, you've already partially assessed these cranial nerves. First, ask your patient to stick her tongue out and move it up, down, and sideways. Watch for awkward movements or deviations to one side or the other. To test the sensory function of CN VII, place sugar, salt, and lemon solutions on the anterior two-thirds of the tongue and ask your patient to identify the tastes. To test the sensory function of CN IX, place those same recognizable tastes on the posterior third of the patient's tongue and ask her to identify them.

Then, using the tongue blade to depress your patient's tongue and a penlight to illuminate her oral cavity, ask your patient to yawn or say "ah" and observe the movement of her soft palate, uvula, and posterior pharynx for symmetry. Next, with the tongue still depressed with a tongue blade, use a clean cotton-tipped swab to touch either side of the pharynx to stimulate the gag reflex.

UNDERSTANDING CRANIAL NERVES

Use this table to assess cranial nerves and their functions and to help identify abnormalities.

Cranial nerve	Function	Origin	Structures innervated	Assessment
I Olfactory	Sensory	Olfactory bulbs below frontal lobes	• Olfactory mucous membranes	• Ability to identify familiar odors
II Optic	Sensory	Diencephalon	• Retina of the eye	• Visual acuity • Visual fields
III Oculomotor	Motor	Midbrain	• Medial, superior, and inferior rectus muscles of the eye • Inferior oblique eye muscles • Sphincter of the iris	• Extraocular movement • Pupillary reaction to light and accommodation
IV Trochlear	Motor	Midbrain	• Superior oblique muscle of the eye	• Extraocular movement
V Trigeminal	Mixed	Pons	• Sensory: pain, touch, and temperature sensations in the forehead, cheeks, jaw and chin, corneal reflex • Motor: muscles of mastication	• Sensation in the fore head, cheeks, jaw, and chin • Mastication
VI Abducens	Motor	Pons	• Lateral rectus muscle of the eye	• Extraocular movements
VII Facial	Mixed	Pons	• Sensory: anterior two-thirds of the tongue • Motor: muscles of the face, forehead, and eye	• Taste for anterior two-thirds of the tongue • Movement of the facial muscles
VIII Acoustic	Sensory	Pons	• Cochlear organ of Corti • Vestibule and semicircular canals	• Hearing acuity • Balance
IX Glosso- pharyngeal	Mixed	Medulla	• Sensory: posterior third of the tongue • Motor: muscles of the pharynx	• Taste for posterior third of the tongue • Movement of the pharynx • Gag reflex
X Vagus	Mixed	Medulla	• Sensory: skin of external ear and mucous membranes • Motor: muscles of larynx, pharynx, esophagus, and thoracic and abdominal viscera	• Swallowing • Movement of the pharynx • Gag reflex
XI Spinal accessory	Motor	Medulla	• Sternocleidomastoid and trapezius muscles	• Movement and strength of neck and shoulder
XII Hypoglossal	Motor	Medulla	• Tongue	• Movement and strength of tongue

Neck

Inspect the neck for symmetry, masses, scars, pulsations, or swelling. If the patient has no history of neck or spine trauma, ask her to drop her chin to her chest and then slowly roll her head in a full circle. Observe any limitations in movement or discomfort with movement. Note the position of the patient's trachea and whether it's deviated to one side or the other. Identify the thyroid gland. If your patient is thin, the thyroid's isthmus (the part that joins the two lobes) may be visible. But the isthmus may be difficult or impossible to find if her neck is short and thick.

Normal findings

- Head round and symmetrical. The scalp appears clean, with unbroken skin. The ears should be symmetrically shaped, in proportion to the face, and vertically positioned to line up with the eyes.
- Facial expressions, such as smiles and frowns, leaving symmetrical wrinkles on the forehead. The cheeks should appear symmetrical when puffed with air.
- Facial skin smooth, unbroken, and clean.
- Eyes clear, bright, and symmetrical. The eyelids close completely. The eyebrows and eyelashes should be evenly distributed, with unbroken skin at the base.
- Nasal mucosa moist, pink, and slightly darker than the oral mucosa. The nasal septum should be midline and intact.
- Nasal passages patent bilaterally. The patient should be able to identify scents correctly in both nostrils, indicating normal function of CN I.
- Lips soft, pink, and intact.
- Oral mucosa smooth, moist, pink, and intact, without inflammation or lesions. Fordyce's spots (sebaceous glands), characterized by small yellowish spots on the buccal mucosa, are normal in adults.
- Gingiva smooth and shiny. In Caucasians the gingiva is pale red. In dark-skinned people, it's commonly a patchy brown.
- Margins around teeth sharp and crevices between the gingiva and teeth shallow. The patient should have 32 teeth, each seated firmly in a bony socket.
- Tongue pink and slightly rough, with a midline depression. Its underside should be smoother and pinker than the top; the sublingual fold should be pink and moist. The tongue should be midline, fill the floor of the mouth, and move freely from side to side.
- Patient able to distinguish between sweet, sour, salty, and bitter tastes, indicating normal function for CN VII and CN IX.
- Soft palate rising, uvula moving forward, and posterior pharynx moving inward (like a curtain closing) when your patient says "ah."
- Gag reflex when your patient's posterior pharynx touched.
- Trachea at midline of patient's neck.

Abnormal findings

- Scaling skin and erythema around the eyelashes and eyebrows from seborrheic dermatitis.
- Red and swollen nasal mucosa, indicating rhinitis. With allergic rhinitis, the mucosa is swollen, but color varies from gray to dull red or blue.
- Nasal polyps, characterized by mobile, gelatinous, gray lesions in the middle meatus of the septum.
- Septal deviation, causing nasal obstruction, possibly congenital or caused by injury.
- Reduction or loss of sense of smell (anosmia), possibly caused by frontal bone or sinus trauma, disorders of the base of the frontal lobe (such as tumors), or decreased blood flow from atherosclerosis. It can also result from sinus infection, nasal congestion, smoking, or cocaine use, and can alter a patient's ability to recognize tastes.
- Blisters caused by the herpes simplex virus. Clusters of vesicular blisters develop around the lips and mucous membranes. As the blisters break, a crust forms.
- A thickened plaque, ulcer, or warty growth of the lower lip that doesn't heal, possibly indicating a carcinoma.
- Painful, small, round or oval white ulcers surrounded by a halo of reddened mucosa. Known as aphthous ulcers or canker sores, these ulcers usually recur. Their cause is unknown.
- White plaquelike exudate on the tongue and oral mucosa, resulting from moniliasis or thrush.
- Gingival hypertrophy (swelling of the gingiva), possibly caused by pregnancy, leukemia, or medications such as phenytoin and cyclosporine.
- Gingivitis (inflamed gingiva), characterized by erythema and swelling of the margins of the gingiva. The gingiva becomes fragile and bleeds easily. This condition typically results from poor oral or dental hygiene. If the disease progresses, gum margins recede and erode, causing teeth to loosen—a condition known as periodontitis.
- A smooth, red tongue with loss of papillae, suggesting a deficiency of cyanocobalamin (vitamin B_{12}), niacin (vitamin B_3), or iron.
- A swollen tongue, swollen face, rhinitis, and urticaria, possibly indicating anaphylaxis, a life-threatening allergic reaction. (See ⊚ *Responding to Anaphylaxis,* pp. 88-89.)
- Mildly red, slightly swollen pillars, and prominent lymphoid patches on the posterior wall of the pharynx, caused by viral pharyngitis. Severe redness, swelling, and patchy exudate may result from strep-tococcal pharyngitis.
- Loss of gag reflex and a hoarse or nasal-sounding voice from dysfunction of CN X. Because CN X also controls involuntary functions, the patient's heart rate and respiratory patterns also may be affected. Loss of the gag reflex and dysphagia reveal dysfunction of CN IX.

RESPONDING TO ANAPHYLAXIS

A life-threatening allergic reaction, anaphylaxis results from the body's overwhelming immunologic response to an allergen found in food, medication, blood products, insect venom, or chemicals (such as contrast medium used in medical testing).

On first exposure to the antigen, the body becomes sensitized to it. Then, on second exposure, the allergic person's humoral immune system activates immunoglobulins IgE, IgG, and IgM, prompting the release of chemical mediators, including histamine and complement, from mast cells.

Once released, these chemical mediators cause a massive systemic reaction marked by laryngeal edema and vasodilation. If allowed to progress, anaphylaxis leads rapidly to respiratory arrest, profound hypotension, and death. For any patient experiencing anaphylaxis, your response must be swift and sure. It could easily mean the difference between life and death.

What to look for
Signs and symptoms of an anaphylactic reaction can appear within seconds. Look for the following:
- Flushing of the skin
- Urticaria
- Pruritus
- Hoarseness and stridor
- Coughing and wheezing
- Extreme shortness of breath
- Angioedema, or swelling of the eyelids, lips, tongue, hands, and feet
- Copious watery nasal secretions
- Nasal congestion and sneezing
- Nausea, vomiting, and abdominal pain from edema of the gastrointestinal tract
- Signs of shock, including hypotension, tachycardia, and a weak, thready pulse

What to do immediately
Anaphylaxis requires rapid intervention. Have someone notify a physician immediately, then:
- If the anaphylactic reaction is caused by a blood transfusion or intravenous medication, stop the infusion immediately and change the intravenous (IV) tubing down to the hub of the catheter. Then start an infusion of normal saline through new IV tubing.
- Ensure a patent airway by positioning the patient's head and neck in slight hyperextension.
- Administer supplemental oxygen.
- Insert an oral or nasal airway if the patient is unconscious.
- Prepare for endotracheal intubation or tracheotomy if the airway can't be restored.
- Administer epinephrine (1:1,000 aqueous solution) immediately, as prescribed, to counteract the effects of chemical mediators and reduce bronchospasm. The usual dose is 0.1 to 0.5 ml every 10 to 15 minutes subcutaneously (SC) or intramuscularly (IM) until your patient responds. Or you can give 1 to 2.5 ml IV (1:10,000 concentration) every 5 to 15 minutes.
- When giving epinephrine SC or IM, massage the injection site to promote faster absorption.
- After giving epinephrine, expect to give the histamine$_1$ (H$_1$) antagonist diphenhydramine 1-2 mg/kg IV or IM. Also plan to give a histamine$_2$ (H$_2$) antagonist, such as ranitidine, 1 to 1.5 mg/kg IV or IM (to a maximum dose of 150 mg). These drugs prevent further release of histamine from mast cells.
- Maintain circulatory volume and blood pressure with intravenous fluids.

What to do next
Once your patient has been stabilized, identify and remove the allergen to prevent further reaction and respond as follows:
- If the allergen was administered by IV line, remove the bag and change the tubing down to the catheter hub.
- Plan to give a corticosteroid, such as methylprednisolone 1 to 2 mg/kg to prevent a late-phase reaction.
- To treat bronchospasm or wheezing, administer an inhaled beta$_2$ agonist, such as albuterol, as prescribed.

ACTION STAT

RESPONDING TO ANAPHYLAXIS—cont'd

- If the reaction was to an insect bite, remove the stinger by gently scraping it out.
- If the reaction was caused by food, induce vomiting to prevent further absorption.
- Administer other medications, as prescribed, such as corticosteroids and aminophylline.
- Monitor vital signs carefully after the event.
- Monitor respiratory effort and oxygenation.
- Comfort and reassure your patient.
- Teach your patient to avoid the suspected allergen.
- Instruct your patient to carry an anaphylaxis kit, and demonstrate how to use it.
- Encourage your patient to wear a medical information alert that lists the allergy.

- Facial weakness. If the weakness affects the entire side of your patient's face, the problem most likely stems from damage to CN VII, as seen in Bell's palsy. If, however, your patient can wrinkle her forehead while one side of the lower part of her face remains weak or immobile, the problem most likely stems from upper motor neuron damage from a cerebrovascular accident (CVA) or tumor.
- Impaired sense of taste from damage to CN VII and CN IX, caused by chemotherapy, radiation of the head and neck, or aging. It may be a sign of myasthenia gravis or amyotrophic lateral sclerosis (ALS) if accompanied by anesthesia of the tongue and palate, difficulty swallowing, increased salivation, and difficulty speaking.
- Soft palate that fails to rise, along with deviation of the uvula to one side. This may occur with paralysis of CN X.

Palpation

To maximize efficiency, perform palpation during your inspection of the structures. But be sure to protect yourself from infection by wearing examination gloves when examining the mouth or other areas where transmission of microorganisms may occur.

Head and neck

Begin by palpating the head and neck. Feel for the contour, symmetry, and size of the skull. Use your gloved hands to palpate lumps or lesions that you've observed, testing for tenderness, mobility, and consistency. Note their size and shape.

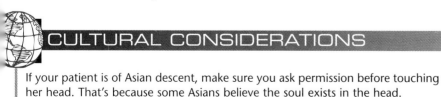

CULTURAL CONSIDERATIONS

If your patient is of Asian descent, make sure you ask permission before touching her head. That's because some Asians believe the soul exists in the head.

You'll also want to test your patient's muscle strength in the neck and shoulders by asking her to shrug her shoulders against the resistance of your hands. Then have her turn her head side to side, also against the resistance of your hands.

Face

CN V (the trigeminal nerve) controls the strength of the temporal and masseter muscles and sensations around the face. To assess its function, first palpate the temporal muscle by placing your middle and index fingers on your patient's temples and asking her to clench her teeth, comparing the strength of contraction of each side. Then move your middle and index finger to the mastoid process and again ask your patient to clench her teeth.

To assess the sensory component of CN V, ask your patient to close her eyes. Using the stick end of a clean cotton-tipped swab, press the patient's forehead, cheeks, and jaw (but make sure you don't press too hard). Ask the patient to identify whether the stimulus is sharp or dull. Occasionally, substitute the soft, cotton-covered end of the swab to test your patient's reliability.

Palpate the temporal pulses, located near the temples on either side of the face. Be sure to compare sides. Note the strength, amplitude, and rhythm of the pulsations.

When palpating the frontal and maxillary sinuses for tenderness, avoid placing pressure directly on the eyes to prevent injury. To palpate the frontal sinus, place your thumb on the upper inner aspect of the orbit and press gently but firmly upward, noting any increase in pain or tenderness. To assess the maxillary sinus, place your thumb under the zygomatic bone and gently press upward, also noting any increase in pain or tenderness.

Mouth

Palpate the upper and lower lips with a gloved hand to evaluate muscle tone, lumps, or areas of tenderness. To palpate the tongue, grasp it with a 4-inch by 4-inch gauze pad and move it from side to side to inspect and palpate the lateral borders for lesions or tenderness.

Trachea

In addition to inspecting the trachea's position, you can also palpate it to see if it's displaced or moving. Place your thumbs on either side of the trachea and feel the space between it and the sternocleidomastoid muscle. Is it equal? Then, with your patient's neck extended, place your index finger and thumb on each side of the trachea, below the thyroid's isthmus. Feel for the presence of tracheal movement or tugging.

Thyroid gland

Examine the thyroid gland for size, texture, and pulsation. (See *Palpating the Thyroid Gland*.)

PALPATING THE THYROID GLAND

The thyroid gland has two lobes connected by a central isthmus, giving it a butterfly appearance. In most people, a normal or slightly enlarged thyroid can't be palpated, although you can feel the isthmus rise as the patient swallows.

Palpating the thyroid gland is an advanced procedure you should perform with caution. It can release thyroid hormone into the circulation, possibly sparking a thyroid storm if the patient has hyperthyroidism. Do not palpate the thyroid if it is visibly enlarged.

The thyroid gland can be palpated by posterior or anterior approach. Many nurses find the posterior approach to be the easier of the two.

Midline structures of the neck

- Sternocleidomastoid muscle
- Hyoid bone
- Thyroid cartilage
- Thyroid gland
- Cricoid cartilage
- Thyroid isthmus
- Clavicle

Posterior approach

With your patient sitting upright, approach her from behind. Ask her to lower her chin slightly and relax her neck muscles. Then start by locating the thyroid isthmus, placing your thumbs against the back of her neck and resting the tips of your forefingers over the lower half of the trachea. You'll feel the isthmus rise in the patient's neck as she swallows.

To palpate the right lobe, have your patient keep her chin down and flex her neck slightly to the right. Use your left hand to displace her trachea to the right. Palpate the right lobe with your right hand as your patient swallows. Then assess the left lobe with your left hand while using your right hand to displace the trachea to the left.

Palpating the right lobe by posterior approach

Anterior approach

Approach your patient from the front and slightly to one side. Ask her to relax her neck muscles. To palpate the thyroid isthmus, use your index and middle fingers to palpate the cricoid cartilage as your patient swallows.

To palpate the lobes, grasp and palpate each one by placing your fingers on either side of the sternocleidomastoid muscles. Alternatively, you can displace the trachea toward your examining hand as with a posterior approach, thus moving the thyroid lobe to your fingertips.

Palpating the right lobe by anterior approach

Lymph nodes

For best results when examining the lymph nodes of the head and neck, ask your patient to relax her muscles and bend her neck slightly forward or toward the side that you're palpating. Use the pads of your index and middle fingers to gently move the skin over the tissue where the nodes are located. If you palpate an enlarged gland, note its size, consistency (hard or soft), mobility, tenderness, temperature, and location. Ask the patient if the enlarged node is tender. Also assess the areas adjacent to the lymph node for signs of infection or malignancy.

Systematically palpate the lymph nodes on both sides of the patient's neck. Be sure to include the following:

- Preauricular (in front of the ear)
- Postauricular (at the mastoid process)
- Occipital (at the base of the skull)
- Tonsillar (at the base of the mandible)
- Submaxillary (halfway between the angle and tip of the mandible)
- Submental (in the midline behind the tip of the mandible)
- Superficial cervical (just over the sternomastoid)
- Posterior cervical chain (just at the anterior edge of the trapezius)
- Deep cervical chain (deep in the sternomastoid)
- Supraclavicular (deep in the angle formed by the clavicle and sternomastoid)

As you palpate the lymph nodes, compare sides for symmetry, taking note of their size, shape, borders, mobility, consistency, and tenderness.

Vascular structures

When examining the neck, you'll want to palpate the carotid artery's pulsations and evaluate the jugular veins for distention, which is a possible sign of overhydration or heart failure. For best results, ask your patient to lie down with her head elevated on a pillow. Elevate the head of the bed slightly to maximize visibility of the jugular veins. Keep the patient's neck in a neutral position, neither flexed nor extended. Use tangential lighting, and be sure to remove any clothing that might interfere with your examination. If your patient has difficulty changing positions at this point in the examination, you can delay evaluating vascular structures until she's supine.

First, feel the carotid pulsations on either side of the neck. Use the pads of your fingertips and feel along the side of the trachea, midway between the angle of the jaw and the clavicles. Apply gentle pressure, and note the contour, rate, and rhythm of the pulsations. If you feel a thrill, be sure to note it. Also auscultate the carotid artery for bruits.

Distinguish between the internal and external jugular veins, which usually aren't visible unless your patient is reclining at an angle of at least 45 degrees. The external jugular veins lie posterior to the internal jugular veins and appear just above the clavicles. The internal ones will pulsate in response to pressure changes in the right atrium as your patient reclines.

You can distinguish internal jugular pulsations from those of the carotid artery because internal jugular pulsations are rarely palpable (only visible), and the level of pulsation usually diminishes with inspiration. Also, when your patient is upright, the pulsations disappear.

To measure jugular venous pressure, follow these steps:
- Identify the highest point at which you can see the internal jugular vein's pulsations. Also identify the sternal angle.
- Hold a centimeter rule in a vertical position with the bottom placed at the patient's sternal angle.
- Hold another ruler in a horizontal position so that one end rests at the highest jugular vein pulsation and the other intersects with the vertical ruler.
- The vertical distance on the centimeter ruler where it intersects with the horizontal ruler equals the patient's jugular venous pressure. Normally, it does not exceed 4 cm.
- Document the angle at which the head of the patient's bed is elevated.
- Estimate central venous pressure (right atrial pressure) by adding 4 cm to the patient's jugular venous pressure reading because the right atrium lies about 4 cm below the sternal angle.

Normal findings
- Skull contour smooth and symmetrical.
- Patient able to distinguish between sharp and dull stimuli bilaterally in all three distributions of CN V.
- Temporomandibular joint (TMJ) smooth. Joint movement produces no pain or crepitation.
- Frontal and maxillary sinuses nontender when palpated.
- Lips smooth and nontender, with good muscle tone. The tongue surface should be nontender and without palpable lesions.
- Trachea straight and midline, without movement or tugging.
- Thyroid thin, smooth, and mobile. The isthmus is the only portion of the thyroid that's usually palpable, although you may feel one or both lobes in some patients.
- Lymph nodes nonpalpable or small, soft, round, and mobile. They should not be tender.
- Carotid pulse regular, full, and smooth.
- Jugular venous pressure 3 cm or less above the sternal angle (at 45 degrees), reflecting a central venous pressure of approximately 7 cm. The pulsations of the internal jugular vein should be barely visible above the clavicles.
- Neck and shoulders overcome resistance equally well, indicating intact function of CN XI (the spinal accessory nerve).

Abnormal findings
- Asymmetrical skull, with bulging or protrusions, possibly indicating injury or tumor.

- Patient unable to distinguish sharp stimuli in one or all distributions of CN V, possibly indicating injury.
- Sharp, bullet-like facial pain in the distribution of CN V, from trigeminal neuralgia. This pain is more common in females than in males and usually affects the right side of the face.
- Limited jaw movement, crepitation or clicking heard on jaw movement, or pain on jaw movement, possibly indicating TMJ dysfunction.
- Tender frontal and maxillary sinuses, indicating fluid pressure, inflammation, or infection.
- Lesions or tenderness involving the lips or tongue, indicating injury, infection, or malignancy.
- Tracheal deviation, indicating a mediastinal shift.
- Tracheal tugging in a downward direction in synchrony with the pulse, indicating an abdominal aortic aneurysm.
- Diffusely enlarged thyroid gland. The surface may feel lobulated (bumpy or lumpy), but no discrete nodules are palpable. Thyroid enlargement can be associated with hyperthyroidism, hypothyroidism, endemic goiter (normal levels of thyroid hormones), or thyroiditis. (See *Hyperthyroidism,* pp. 96-97.)
- Enlarged thyroid with two or more identifiable nodules, known as multinodular goiter, suggesting metabolic disease, such as thyrotoxicosis.
- Tender, palpable lymph nodes, indicating a recent infection. In an acute infection, the nodes feel large and well defined. In a chronic infection, node borders are less defined. Firmly enlarged, nontender, immobile lymph nodes may indicate malignancy. If three or more node groups are involved, the patient has generalized lymphadenopathy, possibly indicating an autoimmune disease or neoplasm.

LIFESPAN CONSIDERATIONS

Keep in mind that palpable, nontender submandibular glands can be normal in an older patient. Also, cervical lymph nodes are often palpable in late childhood and throughout adolescence.

- Jugular vein distention related to elevated central venous pressure. The internal jugular pulsations may be visible well above the clavicles, as high as the mandible or the tragus. It may indicate heart failure, fluid overload, constrictive pericarditis, or obstruction of the superior vena cava.
- Bounding carotid pulse related to a hyperdynamic state, such as fever or thyroid storm.
- Weak carotid pulse from decreased stroke volume, indicating left ventricular heart failure or profound hypotension.

- Unilateral weakness or paralysis of muscles in the neck and shoulders, indicating a disorder of CN XI.

Percussion

When examining the head and neck, you'll percuss only the frontal and maxillary paranasal sinuses. Using your index or middle finger as the plexor, gently tap the area above the eyebrow (frontal sinuses). To percuss the maxillary sinuses, tap your middle or index finger on both sides of the nose in line with the pupil.

LIFESPAN CONSIDERATIONS

If you suspect increased intracranial pressure (ICP) in a child, percuss her skull with one finger behind the junction of the frontal, temporal, and parietal bones to try to elicit Macewen's sign. If you hear a sound that is more resonant than normal and resembles a cracking pot, suspect increased ICP after fontanel closure.

Normal findings
- Resonance on percussion, indicating sinuses are filled with air.
- No discomfort or tenderness on percussion.

Abnormal findings
- Dullness or flatness on percussion of the maxillary and frontal sinuses, indicating fluid.
- Pain and pressure on percussion in the maxillary and frontal sinuses, possibly indicating bacterial, viral, or allergic sinusitis.

Auscultation

When auscultating blood vessels in the head and neck for abnormal sounds, be sure to include the temporal and carotid arteries, as well as the jugular vein. First, place the bell of the stethoscope over the temporal artery just lateral to the outer canthus of the eye. Listen for several seconds. Repeat this procedure on the opposite temporal artery.

To listen to the carotid arteries, gently place the bell of your stethoscope over each artery and ask your patient to hold her breath so that the sound of her respirations doesn't interfere with the examination. Don't press too hard or you'll occlude the artery.

Bruits are most readily heard at the lateral end of the clavicle and the posterior margin of the sternocleidomastoid muscle. If you need extra time to listen, let your patient take deep breaths between listening. And be sure to listen to both sides of the neck.

To listen for venous hums, move the bell of your stethoscope to the medial end of the clavicle and the anterior border of the sternocleidomastoid

DISORDER CLOSE-UP

HYPERTHYROIDISM

A hypermetabolic disorder, hyperthyroidism results from an excess of circulating free thyroxin, triiodothyronine, or both. Hyperthyroidism is considered a multisystem disorder. Of its many forms, the most common is Graves' disease.

Pathophysiology

As secretion of thyroid hormones increases, the thyroid gland enlarges and becomes more vascular, and thyroid function increases. As excessive thyroid hormones are secreted, systemic adrenergic activity magnifies, causing epinephrine overproduction and hypermetabolism. The result is a sustained hypermetabolic state with increased oxygen consumption, along with heightened sensitivity and stimulation of the sympathetic nervous system.

Hyperthyroidism also causes fluid accumulation in the fat pads behind the eyeball and inflammatory edema of the extraocular muscles. As a result, the eyeballs protrude and the extraocular muscles may become inflamed and fibrotic (See illustration). The skin may take on an orange-peel texture from hyperpigmentation and nonpitting edema of the pretibial area, ankles, and feet.

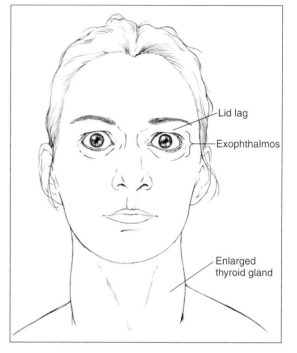

Health history
- Family history of Graves' disease
- Heat intolerance accompanied by excessive sweating
- Weight loss despite increased appetite
- Diarrhea
- Tremors
- Palpitations
- Dyspnea on exertion and possibly at rest
- Pruritus
- Menstrual irregularities (in females); impotence (in males)
- Emotional lability and nervousness
- Difficulty concentrating
- Insomnia

muscle. With your patient's head turned away from the area of auscultation, press firmly on the endpiece and listen for a continuous low-pitched sound during ventricular diastole. If you ask your patient to bear down, the sound will soften.

If the thyroid gland feels enlarged, auscultate it for a bruit as well. Using the bell of your stethoscope, listen over the lateral lobes of the thyroid gland while your patient holds her breath. To differentiate a bruit from a venous hum, gently occlude the jugular vein on the side

Characteristic findings

Expect physical findings to vary among patients with hyperthyroidism, depending on the extent and severity of the disease. Use the information that follows to help distinguish between typical findings and complications.

Inspection
- Anxious and restless appearance
- Tremors of the fingers and tongue
- Shaky handwriting
- Clumsiness
- Emotional instability
- Mood swings
- Flushed skin
- Soft, fine hair with premature graying and hair loss
- Fragile nails with distal nail separating from nail bed
- Raised, hyperpigmented, and well-demarcated pretibial edema on dorsa of legs and feet
- Plaquelike or nodular lesions
- Generalized or localized muscle atrophy
- Soft-tissue swelling, with underlying bone changes in areas of new bone formation
- Periorbital edema
- Infrequent blinking
- Staring and eyelid lag
- Exophthalmos
- Ocular muscle weakness, with impaired upward gaze, convergence, and strabismus

Palpation
- Asymmetrical, enlarged, and smooth or lobular thyroid gland
- Rubbery, soft or firm thyroid gland
- Thrill over thyroid gland
- Moist, warm, smooth skin
- Bounding pulse
- Hyperreflexia

Auscultation
- Bruit over thyroid gland
- Supraventricular tachycardia and atrial fibrillation (especially in elderly patients)
- Systolic murmur at left sternal border (occasionally)
- Increased bowel sounds

Vital signs
- Tachycardia
- Bounding pulse
- Widened pulse pressure

Complications
- Thyrotoxicosis
- Arrhythmias, especially atrial fibrillation
- Cardiac insufficiency and decompensation
- Muscle weakness and atrophy
- Paralysis
- Osteoporosis
- Skin hyperpigmentation
- Corneal ulcers
- Impaired fertility
- Gynecomastia

you're auscultating. A venous hum will disappear when you compress the vein.

Normal findings
- No audible sounds when auscultating the temporal and carotid arteries (other than normal heart sounds commonly heard in the neck).
- Venous hum in pregnant females.
- No audible sounds when auscultating the thyroid.

Abnormal findings

- Soft, low-pitched, rushing sound heard during the cardiac cycle, indicating a bruit in the temporal or carotid artery. The bruit may signify narrowing of the artery or radiation of a systolic murmur from the aortic valve area, as heard in aortic stenosis.
- Venous hum heard in the presence of anemia, thyrotoxicosis, or intracranial arteriovenous malformation.
- Bruit in the thyroid gland caused by accelerated blood flow through an enlarged gland and found with hyperthyroidism.

To close your examination of the head and neck, take a few minutes to summarize your findings. (See 🖼 *What to Expect When Examining the Head and Neck.*)

EXPLORING CHIEF COMPLAINTS

To be sure, most of your head and neck examinations will revolve around a chief complaint brought to you by a patient seeking medical care. In the section that follows, you'll find a number of common chief complaints, instructions on how to focus your assessments when examining patients with those complaints, and possible causes.

Headaches

If your patient complains of headaches, investigate further by asking her the following questions:

- Is the pain on one side of your head or on both sides? Is it diffuse or localized?
- Is the pain so severe that it interrupts your activities of daily living, or can you carry on despite the pain?
- Would you describe the headache as viselike or stabbing? Are you nauseated and vomiting? Are you dizzy or experiencing visual changes or weakness?
- Do the headaches begin suddenly or gradually? Are they preceded by an aura or characteristic sensation, such as flashing lights?
- When did you first notice the headaches? How often do they occur? How long do they last? Have they become more severe over time?
- What seems to bring the headaches on (noise, lights, coughing or sneezing, sexual intercourse, fatigue, certain foods, or menstruation)?
- What relieves them (sleep, analgesics, or avoiding certain foods, alcohol, or cigarettes)?
- Have you experienced any changes in your sleep pattern? Do you awaken early without cause?

NORMAL FINDINGS

WHAT TO EXPECT WHEN EXAMINING THE HEAD AND NECK

Use this review to confirm normal findings when examining the head and neck.
- Head round and symmetrical.
- Scalp pink in color, without scales, and covered with hair. Hair distributed evenly, without excess oils.
- Facial features symmetrical. Eyes open evenly and are equally displaced from the midline of the face.
- Nasolabial folds symmetrical.
- Skin of the face and neck pink, smooth, and firm in tone.
- Nasal mucosa flat and somewhat redder than oral mucosa. Nasal septum lies at the midline of the nose.
- Lips moist, without cracks or fissures.
- Gums with a red stippled surface. Margins around the teeth are sharp, and the teeth are firm in the sockets.
- Internal jugular vein pulsations regular and varying with inspiration and expiration. They aren't visible when the patient sits upright. Patient has no jugular distention.
- Skin of the head and neck warm and dry, without masses or tenderness.
- Frontal and maxillary sinuses free of pain.
- Trachea straight and at the midline of the neck. Thyroid gland moves freely when patient swallows; isthmus is free of nodes.
- Lymph nodes in the neck nonpalpable, nontender, and not swollen. If nodes are palpable, they're soft, round, and freely mobile.
- Carotid artery pulsation regular, full, and smooth.
- Resonance on percussion of the sinuses.
- No audible sounds over carotid and temporal arteries, other than normal heart sounds generally heard in the neck.
- Venous hum over jugular vein in pregnancy.

Cranial nerve function
- Patient can identify various odors (CN I).
- Temporal and masseter muscles equal in strength bilaterally. Patient can differentiate between sharp versus dull in all three distributions of the nerve (CN V).
- Facial movements symmetrical (CN VII).
- Movements of the pharynx, larynx, and palate symmetrical; gag reflex intact; patient's voice clear and easily audible (CN IX and X).
- Shoulder and neck muscles equal in strength and contraction bilaterally (CN XI).
- Tongue at the midline of the mouth, with full, rounded appearance and smooth movement (CN XII).

Focusing your assessment
When examining a patient who complains of headaches, focus your assessment as follows:
- Check the patient's vital signs because fever and hypertension can cause headache.
- Palpate the head and neck for tenderness or muscle tightness, signs of tension headaches.

- Assess for bruising, swelling, neck stiffness, otorrhea, and rhinorrhea, signs of trauma.
- Assess level of consciousness. Check for photophobia and pupil reaction to assess for migraines or hemorrhage.
- Auscultate for bruits in the temporal and carotid arteries, signs of temporal arteritis and carotid stenosis.
- If the headache is acute and very painful, check for nuchal rigidity and positive Kernig's sign or Brudzinski's sign, signs of meningeal irritation. (See *Assessing for Signs of Meningeal Irritation.*)
- Check muscle strength and reflexes for symmetry. Paresthesias may occur with migraines, hemorrhage, or tumors.
- Palpate and percuss the sinuses for tenderness.

Possible causes

- *Muscular pain or tension.* This benign headache is characterized by aching, bandlike pain around the head and neck. Often, tension headaches can be relieved by mild analgesics or muscle relaxants. (See 🔖 *Determining Causes of Headache,* pp. 102-103.)
- *Migraine.* This headache is severe and commonly preceded by an aura or characteristic sensation. Nausea and vomiting may ensue, and the migraine may last for several minutes, hours, or even days. The pain occurs in clusters in several parts of the head and face. It may be triggered by stress, menstruation, or eating certain foods.
- *Cluster headache.* This headache is associated with release of histamine, which causes the carotid arteries to dilate. Cluster headaches are marked by sudden, severe pain on one side of the head and excessive tearing of the eye on the same side as the pain.
- *Temporal arteritis.* This headache results from an inflammatory process that affects the cranial vessels, especially the temporal arteries. The headache is typically intractable and usually accompanied by swelling and tenderness in the temporal region, weakness, difficulty chewing, and visual changes.
- *Sinusitis.* This headache is characterized by pain and tenderness in the sinuses and worsens when the patient bends down. It may be relieved by decongestants.
- *Hypertension.* Headaches caused by hypertension are characterized by occipital pain in the morning.
- *Infection, as in meningitis or encephalitis.* This headache is accompanied by high fever, decreased level of consciousness, and neck pain. Your patient may also have seizures.
- *Malignancy.* Brain tumors cause headaches that are dull, localized, and worsen with changes in head position.

(Text continued on p. 104.)

ASSESSING FOR SIGNS OF MENINGEAL IRRITATION

If your patient with fever also complains of a stiff neck, check for signs of meningeal irritation, which can point to meningitis. Check for these cardinal signs of meningeal irritation: Kernig's and Brudzinski's signs, and nuchal rigidity.

Kernig's sign

With the patient supine, flex his leg at the hip to a 90-degree angle. With his leg in this position try to straighten his knee. If you feel resistance or the patient has severe lower back pain, Kernig's sign is present.

Nuchal rigidity and Brudzinski's sign

With the patient relaxed and supine, place your hand under the patient's head at the base of the skull and gently try to bend the head forward so his chin touches his chest. If nuchal rigidity is present, look for neck stiffness and reduced forward flexion. If he flexes his hips and knees or experiences neck and back pain, Brudzinski's sign is present.

From Chipps, E. M., Clanin, N. J., and Campbell, V. G. (1992). *Neurologic Disorders.* St. Louis: Mosby.

INTERPRETING ABNORMAL FINDINGS

DETERMINING CAUSES OF HEADACHE

Headaches are common and usually harmless. Most result from stress and muscle tension. Sometimes, however, a headache can warn of a serious, even life-threatening, medical condition. The following table lists possible causes of headaches and their characteristic signs and symptoms. By assessing your patient carefully and reviewing symptoms and examination findings closely, you can help your patient obtain an accurate diagnosis and appropriate treatment.

Characteristics	Location	Possible findings	Probable causes
• Gradual onset • Steady ache • Progressive pain that waxes and wanes and can last for days	Usually bilateral; occipital and upper neck region; may also occur in the frontal and temporal area	• Patient may report specific triggers, such as anxiety or stress • Findings usually normal, although muscles around the face and neck may be tense or tight	• Tension • Stress • Depression • Sleep disturbance • Fatigue
• Severe, throbbing pain, typically occurring in the morning • Commonly triggered by stress, menstruation, or certain foods • Peaks in about 1 hour and may last 1 to 2 days • Commonly ends with sleep	Usually, pain is unilateral and occurs in characteristic, localized regions of the head	• Photophobia • Unusual sensitivity to noise • Aura, usually visual, that precedes headache • Nausea and vomiting • Fatigue • Occasional unilateral sensory loss, hemiplegia, aphasia, or third nerve palsy	• Migraine
• Episodes of steady, excruciating pain • Onset sudden • Lasts 30 minutes to a few hours • Occurs repeatedly (6 to 8 a day) for a few weeksor months, commonly followed by a headache-free period • Typically seasonal • Occurs most commonly at night, awakening the patient from sleep	Unilateral, usually orbital or behind the eye	• Unilateral rhinorrhea • Miosis • Ptosis • Flushing of the cheek on the affected side • Conjunctival redness and tearing on the affected side	• Cluster headache
• Severe pain • Worsens with stooping or bending over • Lasts for hours or days • Sudden, severe onset • Described as the worst headache ever experienced	Periorbital, frontal, or maxillary None specific	• Pain or tenderness over the involved sinus • Fever • General malaise • Nuchal rigidity • Photophobia • Nausea and vomiting • Focal neurologic deficits	• Sinusitis • Cerebrovascular hemorrhage (subarachnoid)

Characteristics	Location	Possible findings	Probable causes
• Pain like a thunder clap • Maximum intensity immediately • May be accompanied by loss of consciousness and progression to coma • Severe, progressive • Lasts several hours or days • May develop rapidly	Diffuse or occipital pain	• Seizures • Fever, usually high • Nuchal rigidity • Photophobia • Positive Kernig's sign • Positive Brudzinski's sign • Decreased level of consciousness	• Meningeal irritation from meningitis or encephalitis
• Severe, ripping pain in one side of face • Pain described as searing, burning, or stabbing • Onset abrupt • Pain lasts a few seconds to a few minutes	Along a branch of the trigeminal nerve: around eyes and over forehead; upper lip, nose, and cheek; side of the tongue and lower lip	• Physical examination usually normal • Patient typically identifies a trigger zone (a small area of the face, lips, gums, or forehead affected by such stimulants as brushing teeth, chewing, talking, smiling, and exposure to cold)	• Trigeminal neuralgia
• Dull, achy pain occurring days after a concussion or mild head injury • Lasts for weeks to months	No specific area	• History of concussion or mild head injury • Difficulty concentrating • Malaise • Mood alterations • Fatigue • Dizziness • Loss of balance • Double vision • Physical examination usually normal	• Postconcussion syndrome

- *Medications.* Drugs containing nitrates and others such as cyclosporine are known for causing headaches. With nitrates, headaches become less severe as the patient's tolerance to the medication increases.

Nosebleeds

If your patient complains of nosebleeds, investigate the symptom further by asking her the following questions:

- Would you call the amount of bleeding scant or copious? How long does it take for the nosebleed to stop?
- What color is the blood? Is it bright red, dark red or brown, or is it blood-tinged fluid? Do the droplets have a bloody center with a clear halo?
- Does the bleeding come from one or both nostrils?
- Do you have recurrent nosebleeds, or is this the only one you've had?
- Do you have other symptoms? Do you have congestion or headaches? Do your nasal passages burn? Do you bleed easily in other areas of your body?
- When do you get the symptoms? Does the bleeding seem worse at a particular time of day or year? Does it seem to follow a particular activity, such as nose blowing?
- Was there any recent trauma or insertion of a foreign body in your nose? Have you recently inhaled any chemicals or other strong agents? Do you blow your nose often?
- Do you use nasal oxygen therapy?
- Is the air in your home or at work very dry?
- Which medications do you take, and why do you take them?

Focusing your assessment

When examining a patient who has nosebleeds, focus your assessment as follows:

- Inspect the nasal cavity with a bright light and speculum to confirm the bleeding and locate the site.
- Check the patient's skull, and look for recent head trauma.
- Assess the skin, and look for areas of bruising or bleeding that could indicate a bleeding disorder.
- Check your patient's blood studies for elevated prothrombin time (PT) or decreased platelet count.

Possible causes

- *Injury or lesion.* In the anterior-inferior septum, injury or lesion causes profuse bleeding.
- *Skull injury.* This injury, especially to the basal skull, may cause CSF to leak through the nares.

- *Hypertension.* Increased blood pressure may cause fragile nasal capillaries to break and bleed.
- *Hepatic diseases.* These diseases cause thrombocytopenia (decreased platelets) and an elevated PT, decreasing the blood's ability to clot.
- *Medications.* Such medications as warfarin, heparin, or aspirin decrease the blood's ability to clot.
- *Dry, hot environments or unhumidified oxygen therapy.* Both may dry out mucous membranes and cause capillaries to break and bleed.

Neck pain and stiffness

If your patient complains of neck pain or stiffness, investigate the symptom further by asking her the following questions:
- Did the pain occur gradually or suddenly?
- Is the pain associated with any activity or trauma? If so, describe the activity or trauma in as much detail as you can. If the pain is associated with an activity, does this activity require your head to be in a fixed position for a period of time?
- Is the pain constant or intermittent?
- Have you experienced associated limb pain, numbness, or weakness?
- Is the pain in front or in back of your neck?
- Do you have a fever? What about a rash, headache, or nausea?
- What, if anything, alleviates the pain?

Focusing your assessment

When examining a patient who complains of neck pain or stiffness, focus your assessment as follows:
- Assess neck range of motion. Look specifically for nuchal rigidity and positive Kernig's and Brudzinski's signs, possible signs of meningeal irritation.
- Assess strength of contraction of the trapezius and sternocleidomastoid muscles.
- Inspect for laceration, swelling, or bruising of the neck. Assess for torticollis (contraction of the muscles on one side of the neck).
- Check the muscle strength of both arms for flexion and extension.
- Check the reflexes of the upper extremities for symmetry.
- Palpate the neck muscles for soreness and tenderness.
- Palpate the lymph nodes for enlargement and tenderness.

Possible causes

- *Injury from strain or whiplash.* Pain occurs in the anterior or posterior parts of the neck but usually diminishes over time.
- *Fracture of cervical vertebrae from osteoporosis, injury, or tumor.* Spinal cord injuries result in some loss of sensation, movement, and function below the site of injury.

- *Infection, especially meningitis.* Other symptoms include fever, photophobia, decreased level of consciousness, and headache. (See ▓ *Meningitis.*)
- *Musculoskeletal disorders.* Disorders such as a herniated cervical disk, ankylosing spondylitis, osteoporosis, osteoarthritis, or rheumatoid arthritis may cause neck pain and stiffness. Pain tends to be chronic, waxing and waning in intensity.

Sore throat

If your patient complains of a sore throat, investigate the symptom further by asking her the following questions:
- Do you drink alcohol or use tobacco?
- Do you live in a dry environment? Do you work in an environment that contains chemical irritants?
- Do you use your voice constantly (as a singer, perhaps, or a teacher)?
- Do you have a history of allergies or persistent cough?
- Have you had recent surgery or an emergency that required endotracheal intubation?

Focusing your assessment

When examining a patient who complains of a sore throat, focus your assessment as follows:
- Inspect the throat for redness, inflammation, swollen mucous membranes, and exudate.
- Assess the patient's ability to swallow.
- Check for mild fever, headache, and muscular discomfort.
- Listen to the quality of the patient's voice. Check for hoarseness.

Possible causes

- *Viral or bacterial pharyngitis.* Evidence includes erythema and swelling of the throat and tonsils. Fever, exudate, and severe erythema commonly accompany bacterial infections.
- *Malignancy.* The risk is highest for a smoker or former smoker. Hoarseness commonly accompanies malignancy.
- *Allergy or chemical irritation.* Exposure to offending toxins may result in a sore throat.
- *Injury.* Endotracheal intubation, nasogastric tube insertion, or overuse of the voice from shouting or singing may injure the throat. Hoarseness or loss of voice often accompany injury.

DISORDER CLOSE-UP

MENINGITIS

In meningitis, blood-borne microorganisms, such as bacteria, enter the central nervous system and inflame the meninges, which cover the brain and spinal cord. This acute inflammation can affect all three meningeal membranes: the dura mater, arachnoid membrane, and pia mater. Typically, meningitis is triggered by other infections, such as otitis media, upper respiratory tract infections, or pneumonia. When the microorganisms move from the blood to the cerebrospinal fluid (CSF), albumin and white blood cells follow, causing the CSF to thicken and accumulate in the subarachnoid space. Eventually, the accumulation of CSF raises the intracranial pressure and causes nerve cell compression in the brain and spinal cord. Symptoms of meningitis typically appear 1 to 7 days after the onset of the primary infection, but they can be delayed for up to 3 weeks.

Although meningitis can result from bacteria, fungi, chemical irritation, or tumors, a viral infection is the most common cause. Viral meningitis, also called aseptic meningitis, usually develops in the late summer and early fall, commonly affecting children and adults under age 30. The most common viruses include enteroviruses, the coxsackie virus, mumps virus, herpesvirus, and arboviruses. These viruses enter the body through the oral, oral-fecal, or respiratory pathways. Once in the body, these viruses replicate and spread to the brain through the blood stream.

Bacterial meningitis usually follows a bacterial infection that has occurred elsewhere in the body caused by *Neisseria meningitidis, Streptococcus pneumoniae, Staphylococcus* and *Diplococcus* organisms, and *Haemophilus influenzae*. Bacterial meningitis also may occur after inadvertent introduction of bacteria during neurosurgical procedures, lumbar puncture, spinal anesthesia, or from trauma.

Health history
- Severe headache
- Stiff neck and back
- Malaise
- Photophobia
- Chills
- Altered level of consciousness, such as confusion and delirium
- History of recent bacterial infection, such as respiratory tract, ear, or sinus
- Nausea and vomiting (more common with viral meningitis)

Characteristic findings
Expect your physical findings to vary among patients with meningitis, depending on the extent and severity of the disease. It is often difficult to distinguish between bacterial and viral meningitis on the patient's symptoms alone. Use the following information to help distinguish between expected and unexpected findings.

Inspection
- Altered level of consciousness
- Opisthotonos
- Petechial, purpuric, or ecchymotic rash on lower portion of body with meningococcal meningitis
- Papilledema (on ophthalmoscopic examination)

Palpation
- Nuchal rigidity
- Kernig's sign
- Brudzinski's sign
- Hyperactive, symmetrical deep tendon reflexes

Vital signs
- Sudden onset of temperature elevations as high as 104° F (40° C) with viral meningitis

Complications
- Visual impairment
- Optic neuritis
- Cranial nerve palsies
- Deafness
- Personality changes
- Paresis or paralysis
- Endocarditis
- Coma
- Cerebral infarction
- Unilateral or bilateral sensory hearing loss (in children)
- Epilepsy (in children)
- Mental retardation (in children)
- Hydrocephalus (in children)

EXAMINING
THE EYES AND EARS

Although an eye or ear problem rarely causes acute illness, it can result in considerable discomfort. If it impairs vision or hearing, it can also lead to psychosocial problems, such as difficulty communicating, trouble perceiving visual or auditory stimulation, or the inability to function independently. Additionally, a vision or hearing impairment may make the patient especially anxious.

That's where your assessment skills come in. A nurse's ability to evaluate a patient's eye or ear disorder quickly and accurately can go a long way toward restoring his health, easing his discomfort, and calming his fears.

This chapter provides the information and skills you'll need to examine the eyes and ears effectively and respond appropriately to your patient's needs. In addition to describing the required techniques and tools, it presents normal and abnormal assessment findings. Then it explains how to focus the history and physical examination to investigate specific eye and ear complaints.

Inspection and palpation are the essential techniques you'll use to assess the eyes and ears. With many patients, you'll also conduct vision and hearing tests, and, if you're qualified to do so, you may view internal structures of the eyes and ears, using an ophthalmoscope and an otoscope.

EYE EXAMINATION STEPS AND FINDINGS

To perform an accurate assessment, you must be thoroughly familiar with basic eye anatomy. This is particularly crucial if you don't examine eyes routinely during your daily nursing practice. (See ▌ *Intraocular Structures.*)

Before beginning, review the patient's chief complaint and check his history for disorders that may affect the eyes, such as diabetes mellitus, hypertension, or acquired immunodeficiency syndrome (AIDS). Also be sure to consider his age, overall condition, allergies, and current medication regimen.

To ensure a smooth procedure, gather the following equipment: penlight, ophthalmoscope, Rosenbaum pocket vision screener or Snellen chart, clean opaque card for covering one eye, pupil gauge, cotton-tipped applicator and wisp of cotton, small metric ruler, sterile fluorescein strips, and a cobalt-blue light to aid corneal examination—if available and needed.

As you begin the examination, keep in mind that the eye is an integral part of the brain. This means eye problems may have a neurologic component.

Inspection

Conduct the eye assessment in a quiet, well-lit room with the patient sitting up and facing you. Be sure to note if he's wearing contact lenses.

Start by inspecting the eyes, eyelids, and eyebrows for position, shape, symmetry, and movement. Measure the intercanthal space, which is the distance between the medial canthi (the angles at the medial margin of the eyelids across the bridge of the nose). Inspect for proptosis (also called exophthalmos), which is an abnormal protrusion of the eyeball.

Check the upper and lower lid margins for integrity, color, texture, and position. Ask the patient to close his eyes, and see whether the closed lids completely cover his eyes. Then inspect the orientation of the eyelids and eyelashes, noting if they turn outward or inward. Observe how often the patient blinks, and note any abnormal features of the blinking.

Next, inspect the conjunctiva for clarity, discharge, and inflammation. To assess the palpebral conjunctiva (the portion that lines the inside of the eyelids), gently pull down on the lower lid, and ask the patient to look up as you examine the exposed area. To inspect the bulbar conjunctiva (the portion that covers the sclera), gently pull upward on the upper lid and ask the patient to look down as you assess the exposed area. If he complains of pain or irritation beneath the upper eyelid, evert the eyelid to inspect the conjunctiva. (See ▨ *Performing Eyelid Eversion,* p. 112.)

Now move on to the lacrimal apparatus, checking for adequate tear production and eye lubrication. Then inspect the sclera, noting its color and looking for scleral thinning, indicated by a bluish-gray tinge or bulging (which represents the choroid showing through the sclera).

ANATOMY REVIEW

INTRAOCULAR STRUCTURES

This illustration shows many of the important structures of the eye.

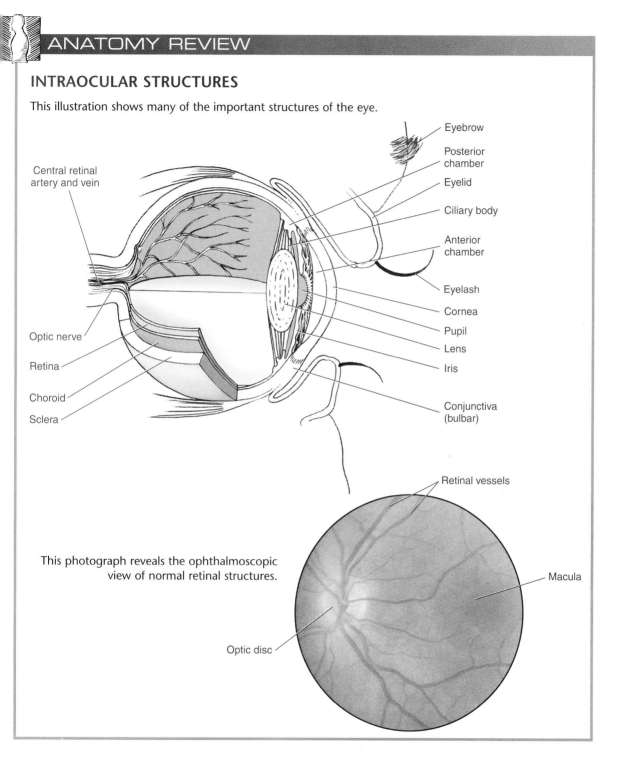

Eyebrow

Posterior chamber

Eyelid

Ciliary body

Anterior chamber

Eyelash

Cornea

Pupil

Lens

Iris

Conjunctiva (bulbar)

Central retinal artery and vein

Optic nerve

Retina

Choroid

Sclera

Retinal vessels

Macula

This photograph reveals the ophthalmoscopic view of normal retinal structures.

Optic disc

EXAMINATION TIP

PERFORMING EYELID EVERSION

You may need to evert the patient's upper eyelid when inspecting the palpebral conjunctiva. Before starting, have the patient remove contact lenses if he wears them.

Gently grasp your patient's eyelashes and instruct him to look down. With your free hand, use a cotton-tipped applicator stick to press gently above the upper eyelid fold while pulling the lid margin up by the lashes. As you maintain pressure on the everted lid, shine the penlight across the conjunctival surface.

When you've finished inspecting the conjunctiva of the everted lid, release the lid margin. The eyelid should return to its normal position when the patient looks up. If it doesn't, gently pull the eyelashes forward.

Inspect the cornea by shining your penlight at an oblique angle onto it from the temporal side of the eye. Look for clouding, opacity, and injury.

If your patient is unconscious or has a problem with cranial nerve (CN) V (the trigeminal nerve), you'll need to check the corneal reflex—a function of CN V. To do this, lightly touch the cornea with a wisp of cotton and check for appropriate blinking. In other patients, this test is rarely performed because it can cause discomfort.

To detect strabismus (deviation of one eye), perform the corneal light reflection test. Shine a penlight on the bridge of the patient's nose, and note where the spots of light fall and whether the light falls on the same location on each eye.

Next, inspect the iris, noting its shape and pigmentation. (See *Essentials of the Eye Examination*.)

PRIORITY CHECKLIST

ESSENTIALS OF THE EYE EXAMINATION

Use this checklist to make sure you cover the most important steps when conducting an eye examination.

❐ Inspect position, shape, and movement of eyes and associated structures.

❐ Check extraocular movements, including the six cardinal positions of gaze.

❐ Inspect eyelids for color, texture, integrity, closure, lesions, inversion, eversion, and drooping.

❐ Inspect eyelash distribution, orientation, and granulation.

❐ Check eyeball surface for lubrication, tearing, redness, and swelling.

❐ Inspect cornea for clarity, surface integrity, reflex (if needed), and light reflection.

❐ Check pupil size, shape, light response, accommodation, and red reflex.

❐ Palpate for firmness, mobility, texture, and smoothness of eyelids and orbital rim.

❐ Palpate punctum for tenderness and discharge.

❐ Test visual acuity.

❐ Perform the confrontation test.

Ophthalmoscopic examination

❐ Check lens clarity.

❐ Inspect vitreous humor for opacities, floaters, precipitates, and blood.

❐ Inspect optic disc color, shape, borders, and physiologic cup.

❐ Check retinal vessels, macula, and fovea.

Pupil examination

With normal room light, measure your patient's pupils using a pupil gauge. Document the result in millimeters and compare the measurements of both eyes. Then assess pupil shape.

Next, check pupil accommodation by having the patient look at an object across the room. As he does this, check for pupil dilation. Then, ask him to stare at your finger as you hold it about 10 cm in front of him. Check for pupil constriction and equal convergence of both eyes on your finger.

LIFESPAN CONSIDERATIONS

A normal variation that begins around age 40, reduced accommodation (presbyopia) results from loss of lens elasticity and weakened ciliary muscles in the iris. As a result, the individual has difficulty seeing nearby objects without corrective lenses.

Assess the pupils' reaction to light. To evaluate direct pupillary response, stimulate one eye by briefly shining your penlight toward the pupil. Observe the reaction of the stimulated pupil as light is applied. To evaluate consensual pupillary response, stimulate the eye a second time, this time watching the response of the other (nonstimulated) pupil. Repeat the test with the other eye.

Extraocular muscle assessment

To evaluate the function of extraocular muscles and the cranial nerves that control them, ask the patient to follow your finger with his eyes as you move it through each of the six cardinal positions of gaze. (See *Six Cardinal Positions of Gaze Test.*)

LIFESPAN CONSIDERATIONS

To check the six cardinal positions of gaze in a young child, use an appealing object, such as a doll or stuffed toy, instead of your finger.

Visual acuity testing

If your patient has a specific eye complaint, especially vision loss, test his visual acuity by using a vision-screening card, such as the Rosenbaum pocket vision screener, and a vision chart, such as the Snellen chart. If he normally wears corrective lenses, make sure he's wearing them during this test.

To test far vision, place the chart on a wall that's 20 feet from the patient. Note the line on the chart at which the patient can accurately read the letters with each eye. Record the numerical fraction that's to the left of that line, for example 20/20. To test near vision, hold a pocket card at a distance of 14 inches from the patient. Record the distance equivalents to the right of the line at which the patient can accurately read.

If he can't read the largest letters on the card, hold up several fingers, and ask him how many he sees. If he can't see your fingers or answers incorrectly, wave your hand in front of his face to determine if he can detect the hand movement. If he can't, shine a penlight into his eyes to see if he can perceive light. Document his best response.

Visual field testing

Evaluate your patient's visual fields and peripheral vision by conducting the confrontation test.

Standing 2 to 3 feet directly in front of the patient, with your eyes level with his eyes, ask him to stare straight ahead and meet your gaze. Then ask your patient to cover his left eye while you cover your right eye. Slowly bring your fingers from beyond the limits of the visual fields in all four quadrants and instruct him to tell you when he can first see them.

SIX CARDINAL POSITIONS OF GAZE TEST

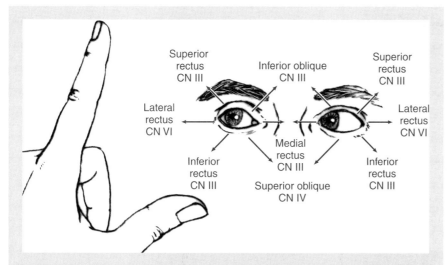

To assess your patient's extraocular muscle function, ask him to watch your finger as you move it through the six cardinal positions of gaze. Begin by holding your index finger about 12 to 18 inches directly in front of him. Then move your finger through each of these maneuvers:
• From the midline to his right side
• Upward, staying to the right of the midline
• Downward, staying to the right of the midline
• Left, across the midline
• Upward, staying to the left of the midline
• Downward, staying to the left of the midline
   Make sure the patient moves only his eyes, not his head, when following the movement of your finger. Observe for conjugate (parallel) eye movement and note any abnormalities, such as deviation of one eye or nystagmus. Ask him to report any diplopia or blurred vision during this test.

Repeat the test with his left eye by asking him to hold his hand over his right eye and gaze into your right eye as you close your left. Again, test his visual fields. If you see your fingers in your peripheral vision before he does, your patient may have restricted visual fields.

   Document your findings by making a circle on a piece of paper. Think of the circle as the edge of a normal visual field. Then, at each of your testing locations, record the perimeter of the patient's vision. Also record the locations of any areas of vision loss inside the visual field.

Normal findings
• Eyes, eyelids, and eyebrows symmetrical in shape and position and
   freely mobile. The eyes should align with the top of the pinnae.

The skin of the eyelids should be loose, thin, and elastic. In an elderly patient, loose, hanging skin may cover a portion of the lid (dermatochalasis).

- Eyelids free from inflammation and scales.
- Edges of the upper and lower eyelids frame the upper and lower margins of the irises when the patient's eyes are open. The opening between the lids is wide enough to allow light through to the pupil.
- Eyelashes curve outward from eyelid margins lying snugly against the eyeball. The lashes on the upper lid turn upward; on the lower lid, they turn downward. The lashes are usually longer and more abundant on the upper lid than the lower lid.
- Eyelashes free of mucus and scales.
- Conjunctiva transparent and free of discharge or hyperemia (reddened, dilated vessels). The eyeball surface appears moist and well lubricated.
- Sclera white and translucent.

LIFESPAN CONSIDERATIONS

In the elderly, sclera may appear bluish because of thinning.

CULTURAL CONSIDERATIONS

In dark-skinned patients, sclera may be yellowish or slightly pigmented with brown spots.

- Corneal reflex brisk, indicating intact function of CN V.
- Corneal surface smooth, transparent, and free of precipitates or irregularities. In an elderly patient, you may note corneal arcus (arcus senilis), a grayish-white ring around the cornea.
- Corneal light reflection at the same place on each cornea in the light reflection test, indicating equal eye positioning.
- Irises flat and circular, with similar pigmentation in both eyes.
- Pupils round, from 3 to 5 mm in size. A slight difference in size (less than 1 mm) between pupils is common.
- Pupils respond equally and briskly to light on direct and consensual tests.
- Pupils dilate appropriately when focusing on close objects and constrict and converge equally.
- Eyes congruent (parallel) in all positions while testing the six cardinal positions of gaze.

- Corrected visual acuity 20/20 or, if that's not possible, 20/30 to 20/40.
- Full visual fields, without restriction or defects. (See 📄 *What to Expect When Examining the Eyes.*)

Abnormal findings
- Proptosis or exophthalmos, possibly associated with Graves' disease. If unilateral, it may indicate an underlying tumor.
- Incomplete eyelid closure (lagophthalmos), from exophthalmos or weakness of CN VII (the facial nerve), as well as periorbital swelling.
- Eyelids everted at the margins. This condition, called *ectropion,* may result from the loss of skin elasticity with age.

NORMAL FINDINGS

WHAT TO EXPECT WHEN EXAMINING THE EYES

Use this brief review to confirm normal findings when examining the eyes.

- Orbits symmetrical in placement, shape, and position; eyeballs freely mobile.
- Eyelids smooth, nontender, and free of discharge (ectropion or entropion may be seen in elderly patients).
- Tear ducts nontender and free of discharge.
- Eyelashes free of granulation, scales.
- Surface lubrication and moisture adequate.
- Conjunctivae clear and moist.
- Sclerae white and opaque.
- Corneas smooth and transparent.

- Irises flat and circular, with even bilateral pigmentation.
- Pupils round and equally reactive to light, with proper accommodation.
- Lenses clear.
- Vitreous transparent.
- Optic disc flat and slightly oval or round; nasal aspect slightly darker pink.
- Optic nerve border distinct; temporal border may have grayish crescent.
- Physiologic cup paler than optic disc.
- Retina of uniform red-orange color; macula darker than retina.

- Eyelids inverted. This condition, called *entropion,* commonly results from aging or from palpebral conjunctival scarring.
- Drooping eyelid (ptosis), associated with Horner's syndrome (a neurologic condition caused by a spinal cord lesion), myasthenia gravis, or weakness of CN III (the oculomotor nerve).
- Involuntary spasm of the orbicularis oculi muscle in the eyelid. Called *blepharospasm,* this condition may result from phenothiazine medications (such as chlorpromazine), a foreign body in the eye, or infection.
- Eyelid swelling, possibly related to a wide range of medical conditions, including inflammation, allergic reaction, infection, heart failure, renal disease, hypothyroidism, and Graves' disease.

- Red eyelid margins, with dried mucus clinging to the lashes, suggesting blepharitis, a chronic bilateral inflammation of the eyelid margins usually accompanied by itching, burning, and irritation. Causes of blepharitis include staphylococcal infection, seborrheic dermatitis, allergy, and psoriasis. Chronic blepharitis may be associated with gout, diabetes mellitus, and ectropion.
- Acute pustular infection involving an eyelash follicle, meibomian cyst, or sebaceous gland of the eyelid. Called a stye or a hordeolum, this infection typically results from a staphylococcal organism.
- Chalazion, an obstruction of the meibomian glands, appearing as a localized, beadlike swelling on the eyelid. Recurrent chalazions may warrant surgery for removal and biopsy to rule out malignancy.
- Soft, yellowish, raised, waxy lesion on or beneath the eyelid. This finding is called *xanthoma* (or xanthelasma) *palpebrarum*, tumors often occurring in groups. Although sometimes benign, they're commonly associated with hyperlipidemia.
- Inflammation and dilation of the conjunctival blood vessels, typically resulting from conjunctivitis, an inflammation of the conjunctiva caused by bacteria, viruses, allergies, certain drugs, or environmental factors.
- Sudden onset of bright red blood in a discrete area outside the conjunctival vessels, from subconjunctival hemorrhage. Typical causes of this condition include heavy sneezing or coughing, trauma, hypertension, and clotting disorders such as hemophilia.
- Inadequate tear production (dry eye syndrome), possibly resulting from a systemic condition, such as Sjögren's syndrome, Stevens-Johnson syndrome, pemphigoid syndromes, or systemic lupus erythematosus.
- Corneal haziness or cloudiness from edema, possibly resulting from an acute increase in intraocular pressure (IOP) or keratitis.
- Red eye, accompanied by increased tearing, a foreign body sensation, moderate-to-severe eye pain, decreased visual acuity, and photophobia. This condition results from corneal abrasion, best identified by fluorescein staining. (See *Checking for Corneal Abrasions.*)
- Irregularly shaped or "keyhole" pupil, possibly resulting from surgical removal of a portion of the iris. Another cause of pupil irregularity is an adhesion resulting from iritis (inflammation of the iris). A square pupil, an unusual finding, may result from use of an iris clip lens, a type of intraocular lens.
- Unequal pupil diameter (anisocoria). Usually, this condition is congenital, although it's sometimes associated with cranial nerve palsy.
- Pinpoint pupils, possibly resulting from topical miotic ophthalmic drugs (such as pilocarpine), systemic drugs (such as opiates), Horner's syndrome, damage to the pons, migraines, or cluster headaches.

CHECKING FOR CORNEAL ABRASIONS

If you routinely care for patients with ophthalmic conditions, you'll probably perform corneal staining to check for possible corneal abrasions. This procedure involves the use of fluorescein, a fluorescent dye available in sterile filter-paper strips.

To use a fluorescein strip, wet it with a drop of sterile water or saline solution, and then touch it to the patient's palpebral conjunctiva. Have the patient blink a few times to distribute the fluorescein solution over the cornea.

Then shine a light over the cornea, preferably a bright penlight with a cobalt-blue filter. Any defects in the corneal epithelium will appear bright green.

- Dilated pupils, possibly resulting from topical mydriatic ophthalmic drugs (such as atropine), some systemic drugs (dexfenfluramine and scopolamine), or CN III palsies.
- Pupil moderately dilated and nonreactive to light, possibly signaling acute angle-closure glaucoma. A medical emergency, it may be accompanied by eye redness and pain, decreased visual acuity, blurred vision, pressure felt over the eye, corneal clouding, seeing halos around lights, and nausea and vomiting.
- Pupil dilated and fixed or slow to respond to light. Called *tonic pupil* (or *Adie's pupil*), this condition is caused by a disturbance of autonomic innervation to one eye, and often impairs accommodation, resulting in blurred vision. It may be accompanied by decreased deep tendon reflexes.
- Lack of parallel eye movement or deviation of one eye, indicating an abnormality of the extraocular muscles.
- Involuntary oscillating eye movements called nystagmus, possibly resulting from a disorder of the labyrinth (inner ear) or the vestibular portion of CN VII. It also may result from a metabolic disorder, drug toxicity, or cerebellar disease.
- Vision of 20/40 or less with corrective lenses, possibly caused by opacities in the cornea, lens, or vitreous humor or dysfunction of the visual pathway (retina or brain). This may be caused by cataracts or systemic disorders, such as hyperglycemia.
- Loss of central vision caused by macular degeneration.
- Blind spots noted during confrontational testing, possibly resulting from vision field loss caused by glaucoma.
- Loss of vision on one side of both visual fields. Called *homonymous hemianopia*, this condition results from occlusion of the cerebral arteries.

Palpation

To palpate the eye, have the patient sit comfortably or lie in a semi-Fowler's position. Using your thumb and index finger (or your index and middle fingers), gently palpate the eyelid and orbital rim, evaluating for firmness, mobility, texture, and smoothness. Then apply gentle pressure on the punctum, the tiny opening in the margin of each eyelid that opens into the lacrimal duct.

Normal findings
- Eyeball firm, smooth, and yielding slightly to pressure (somewhat like a soft rubber ball).
- Eyelid and puncta nontender and free of discharge.

Abnormal findings
- Eyelid edema, cysts, and crepitus, suggesting mucocele, an infection resulting from sinusitis or obstructed sinus drainage.
- Tenderness of the lids, possibly resulting from such disorders as seborrheic dermatitis.
- Purulent discharge expressed from the punctum. This finding indicates dacryocystitis or infection of the nasolacrimal duct.
- A palpable mass in the punctum, possibly indicating adenoma or adenocarcinoma.

Ophthalmoscopic examination

Assessment of the retina and optic disc requires an ophthalmoscope. For most patients, this examination is done only as part of the initial screening, unless the patient has a known or suspected problem involving the retina, macula, or optic disc.

Before attempting to examine a patient, make sure you're comfortable using the ophthalmoscope. Mastering this device and interpreting the findings require practice and skill. (For more information on the ophthalmoscope and its use, see Chapter 1.)

Although the ophthalmoscopic examination is much easier to conduct when the patient's pupils are dilated, with practice you may be able to view the optic nerve and macula through an undilated pupil (especially in a lightly pigmented eye) in a dimly lit room. You or your patient may wear contact lenses during this examination. Your patient shouldn't wear eyeglasses; you should wear them only if you're markedly astigmatic or myopic.

Begin by dimming the room lights. To check for a red reflex, which means the lens is free of clouding and opacities, ask the patient to stare straight ahead at a fixed point at eye level on the wall across the room.

EXAMINATION TIP

If you lose track of the red reflex, the light source has probably moved from the pupil to the iris or sclera. When this happens, redirect the ophthalmoscope and aim it at the pupil.

Caution him to keep his eyes still. Then approach him at an angle, starting about 15 inches away, moving toward him until the ophthalmoscope almost touches his eyelashes. Set the lens dial of the ophthalmoscope at 0, and focus the light on the pupil of one eye. You should be able to see the red reflex as a distinct orange-red glow. Repeat the steps with the other eye.

To view the retina and its structures, adjust the lens dial to the minus range if the patient is myopic and to the plus range if he's hyperopic or aphakic. Turn the dial until the retina comes into clear view, and observe the color of the retina, checking for opacities, floaters, precipitates, and blood. Note any hemorrhages, exudates, or aneurysms in the background. Also inspect retinal veins and arteries for pallor, hemorrhage, distention, tortuousness, narrowing, and obliteration.

To view the optic disc, which is located on the nasal half of the retina, ask the patient to look straight ahead and focus on an object with his unexamined eye. If the disc doesn't come into view at first, follow the retinal arteries and veins to the point where they converge. Inspect the disc for a yellowish-orange to pink color, a slightly oval or round shape, and distinct borders (although these may be blurred on the nasal side). The temporal border may exhibit a grayish crescent, particularly in a myopic eye.

Observe the size of the physiologic cup, the yellow or white depression in the center of the optic disc. Compare the horizontal diameter of the physiologic cup to that of the optic disc. Locate the macula by looking temporal to the optic nerve to an area free of blood vessels. Highly light-sensitive, the macula may appear darker and slightly yellower than the retina. The patient may be unable to tolerate light focused on the macula for more than a few seconds.

Finally, view the fovea, a slight depression in the center of the macula used for sharpest vision. You may see a foveal reflex, a pinpoint white light reflected back to the ophthalmoscope.

Next, assess the lens, vitreous humor, and retinal structures. Begin by setting the lens dial of the ophthalmoscope in the plus range. Then inspect the lens for clarity and opacities. To assess the vitreous humor, observe for opacities, floaters, precipitates, and blood.

Normal findings
- Red reflex bright and regular.
- Crystalline lens clear, translucent, and free of opacities.
- Retina uniform red-orange tinge. It may appear darker and pigmented in dark-eyed and dark-skinned patients.
- Macula free of blood vessels.
- Physiologic cup half the horizontal diameter of the optic disc.
- Vitreous humor clear, transparent, and free of precipitates and opacities.

Abnormal findings

- Red reflex loss, possibly resulting from vitreous opacities, such as a hemorrhage.
- Lens opacity, usually indicating cataracts. Typically, a cataract forms in the center of the lens (nuclear cataract) or at the periphery (cortical cataract).
- Retinal abnormalities, such as granular areas, perivascular exudates, and hemorrhages at the optic fundus. These may result from infection, as with cytomegalovirus (CMV).
- Retinal detachment, pallor, breaks, or folds, possibly resulting from diabetic retinopathy, vascular occlusion, or retinal or macular degeneration.
- Retinal hemorrhages and narrowing, obliteration, dilation, or tortuousness of the retinal vessels, possibly resulting from retinal vascular occlusion or diabetic retinopathy. (See ▥ *Diabetes Mellitus,* pp. 124-125.)
- Retinal exudates, typically resulting from diabetic retinopathy, vascular occlusion, or retinal or macular degeneration.
- Round, white or yellow retinal deposits called drusen, possibly indicating macular degeneration.
- Swollen optic disc with engorged retinal vessels, whitish cotton-wool spots, and a macular "star" caused by exudates, typically resulting from hypertensive retinopathy.
- Bulging optic disc (papilledema), resulting from increased intracranial pressure (ICP) secondary to a brain tumor, meningitis, or pseudotumor.

EXPLORING EYE COMPLAINTS

Common eye complaints include discharge, pain, vision changes, and vision loss. The following section presents pertinent health history questions to ask a patient who reports one of these symptoms, explains how to focus your assessment when examining patients with these complaints, and provides their possible causes.

Eye discharge

If your patient complains of eye discharge, investigate the symptom further by asking him the following questions:

- What color and consistency is the discharge? Is it clear or purulent? Thick or thin?
- Is the discharge coming from one or both eyes?
- Does anything reduce or increase the amount of discharge?
- Is the discharge associated with a particular time of day or activity?

- Does anyone else in your household have eye discharge or other eye symptoms?
- Do your eyes itch or burn?
- Are your eyes sensitive to light?
- Do you wear contact lenses? If so, what method do you use to clean them?
- Do you have a fever, cough, or runny nose?
- Do you have allergies?

Focusing your assessment

When examining a patient who complains of eye discharge, focus your assessment as follows:
- Examine the eye discharge for color, consistency, and amount.
- Inspect the conjunctiva for redness and inflammation.
- Palpate the lacrimal sac for tenderness and try to express additional discharge.
- Test your patient's visual acuity to see if it has been affected by the condition that's causing the discharge.
- If the patient wears contact lenses, examine their condition. If his lens cleaning solution is available, inspect the solution for cloudiness or discoloration.

Possible causes

- *Acute bacterial conjunctivitis.* Sometimes called pinkeye, this infection causes a thick, sticky, purulent or mucopurulent discharge. The conjunctiva appears inflamed, with red, dilated vessels.
- *Viral conjunctivitis.* This infection typically causes a clear or yellow discharge.
- *Allergic conjunctivitis.* This condition typically causes a scant, stringy, white discharge.
- *Corneal injury or infection.* These problems typically cause a watery or purulent discharge. Vessels surrounding the iris may appear inflamed and dilated, and visual acuity may be affected. Corneal injury or infection may result from such conditions as eye trauma, prolonged wearing of contact lenses, or improper contact lens cleaning.
- *Allergy.* Some allergies cause a clear, watery discharge and red, itchy eyes. Symptoms typically arise shortly after exposure to the allergen.

Eye pain

If your patient complains of eye pain, investigate the symptom further by asking him the following questions:
- How would you rate the eye pain on a scale of 0 to 10, with 0 representing no pain and 10 the worst pain you've ever felt?

(Text continues on p. 126.)

DISORDER CLOSE-UP

DIABETES MELLITUS

A chronic disease complex of insulin deficiency or resistance characterized by a disturbance in the metabolism of carbohydrates, proteins, and fats, diabetes mellitus occurs in two forms: type 1, previously termed insulin-dependent diabetes mellitus or juvenile-onset diabetes mellitus, and type 2, previously termed non–insulin-dependent diabetes mellitus or maturity-onset diabetes mellitus. The exact cause of diabetes mellitus is unknown. Genetic factors and a faulty autoimmune response are thought to play a major role in type 1 diabetes mellitus, while genetics and obesity are considered risk factors for type 2 diabetes mellitus.

Pathophysiology

Insulin deficiency or resistance diminishes the use of glucose by the cells, leading to an increased blood glucose level, protein loss from body tissues, and increased mobilization of fats from storage areas. This results in abnormal fat metabolism and lipid deposits in vascular walls, causing atherosclerosis.

As blood glucose level rises, glucose enters the kidney tubules and spills into the urine (usually when the blood glucose level reaches 180 mg/dl). Because glucose can't diffuse through the cell wall without insulin, the osmotic pressure of extracellular fluid rises, causing water to leave the cells and subsequent tissue dehydration. Water is lost in the urine because the osmotic effect of glucose in the kidney tubules prevents tubular reabsorption of fluids. Thus, the patient with diabetes mellitus experiences dehydration associated with hypovolemia.

The body attempts to supply glucose to the cells by shifting from metabolizing carbohydrates to metabolizing fats for energy. This leads to increased ketone production, which results in ketosis. Ketones are excreted in the urine. Sodium is also excreted, causing the blood sodium concentration to decrease. Hydrogen ions then replace sodium, triggering metabolic acidosis.

Type 1 diabetes mellitus

In type 1 diabetes mellitus, a marked decrease or absence of functioning beta cells (the insulin-secreting cells of the pancreas) leads to a lack of insulin and a rise in the blood glucose level. Type 1 diabetes mellitus typically comes on suddenly and causes severe symptoms.

Type 2 diabetes mellitus

In type 2 diabetes mellitus, the pancreas may produce normal, decreased, or even increased amounts of insulin, but the patient has a decreased response to it (insulin resistance). Typically, symptoms are vague and develop gradually.

Health history
Type 1 diabetes mellitus
- Early onset (age 40 or younger)
- Frequent urination (polyuria)
- Extreme thirst (polydipsia)
- Exaggerated hunger (polyphagia)
- Weight loss despite increased food intake
- Extreme fatigue
- Weakness

Type 2 diabetes mellitus
- Late onset (typically older than age 40, although there is an increased prevalence of the disease among children and adolescents between 10 and 19 years old who are obese and have a strong family history)
- Family history of diabetes mellitus
- Obesity
- History of gestational diabetes or delivery of newborn over 9 pounds
- History of other diseases, such as severe viral infection, autoimmune dysfunction, other endocrine disorders, recent stress or trauma, or use of drugs that increase blood glucose levels
- History of frequent infections and slow healing

Normal retina

Retinopathy

- Vaginal itching
- Pruritus
- Polyuria, polydipsia, and possibly polyphagia
- Sexual problems
- Vaginal discomfort
- Vision changes
- Tingling, pain, or numbness in extremities

Characteristic findings

Expect physical findings to vary among patients with diabetes mellitus, depending on the extent and severity of the disease. Use the following information to help distinguish between expected and unexpected findings:

Inspection
- Retinopathy
- Cataract formation
- Skin changes on legs and feet
- Muscle wasting, loss of subcutaneous fat, fruity breath odor (with ketoacidosis) in type 1 diabetes mellitus

Palpation
- Poor skin turgor
- Dry mucous membranes

- Decreased peripheral pulses
- Cool skin
- Decreased reflexes

Vital signs
- Orthostatic hypotension

Complications
- Diabetic ketoacidosis in type 1 diabetes mellitus
- Hyperosmolar nonketotic coma syndrome in type 2 diabetes mellitus
- Cardiovascular disease
- Peripheral vascular disease
- Cerebrovascular disease
- Retinopathy
- Nephropathy
- Diabetic dermopathy
- Peripheral neuropathy (numbness or pain in extremities)
- Autonomic neuropathy (gastroparesis, nocturnal diarrhea, impotence, hypotension)
- Skin, urinary tract, and vaginal infections

- Are your eyes unusually sensitive to light?
- Have you had a severe headache, nausea, or vomiting since the eye pain began?
- Have you experienced any vision changes? For instance, double vision or reduced visual clarity?
- Do you see flashes of light?
- Have your eyes been tearing excessively?
- Have you noticed any discharge coming from your eyes?

Focusing your assessment

When examining a patient who complains of eye pain, focus your assessment as follows:

- Inspect the conjunctiva, check for discharge, and assess the pupils and their reaction to light.
- Using an ophthalmoscope, check for red reflex and examine the optic disc.

Possible causes

- *Acute angle-closure glaucoma.* This disorder causes severe eye pain accompanied by blurred vision or sudden vision loss, severe headache, and nausea and vomiting. The patient may report seeing colored halos around lights. Circumcorneal redness is also common. Expect to find the affected pupil dilated and nonreactive to light. The ophthalmoscopic examination may reveal an enlarged physiologic cup. (See ⏰ *Responding to Acute Angle-Closure Glaucoma.*)
- *Acute keratitis.* This condition typically causes mild-to-severe eye pain accompanied by blurred vision, increased tearing and blinking, and unusual sensitivity to light. The patient also may report a foreign body sensation, such as sand, in his eye.
- *Infectious conjunctivitis.* This condition may cause mild-to-moderate eye pain, typically accompanied by discharge, sticky, encrusted eyelids, and reddened conjunctiva.
- *Uveitis.* This disorder typically causes eye pain and conjunctival inflammation, misshapen pupils, and slightly blurred vision. Ophthalmoscopy may reveal corneal inflammation and opaque deposits.
- *Injury by a foreign body.* This injury typically causes sudden, severe eye pain and a foreign-body sensation. The conjunctiva usually appears inflamed, and the eye tears excessively. Usually, removing the foreign body relieves the pain. An irregularly shaped pupil may indicate a penetrating ocular injury. The pupil may also become miotic.

Vision changes

If your patient reports a change in vision, investigate the symptom further by asking him the following questions:

- Do objects appear blurry?

ACTION STAT

RESPONDING TO ACUTE ANGLE-CLOSURE GLAUCOMA

Sudden onset of severe, throbbing eye pain and unilateral vision loss are classic symptoms of acute angle-closure glaucoma. If your patient complains of these symptoms, you must act fast to avert optic nerve damage and permanent blindness.

What to look for

Typical clinical findings may include:

- Sudden onset of severe, throbbing eye pain (usually unilateral)
- Sudden loss of vision, usually accompanied by nausea and vomiting
- Pain radiating to the face and head along CN V (the trigeminal nerve)
- Dilated conjunctival and episcleral vessels around the corneoscleral limbus
- Steamy or hazy cornea
- Fixed and moderately dilated pupil (4 to 5 mm)
- Shallow anterior chamber
- Extremely high intraocular pressure (IOP) as determined by tonometry (60 mm Hg or higher)
- Premonitory symptoms, such as blurred vision, decreased visual acuity, seeing colored halos around lights, and pain in the head

What to do immediately

If you suspect your patient has acute angle-closure glaucoma, notify the physician immediately. Then take the following steps to help reduce IOP and manage other symptoms:

- Give an osmotic beverage, such as 50% glycerin in water and lime or lemon juice. Usually, the physician prescribes 4 to 6 ounces given over cracked ice, to be sipped slowly through a straw. In many cases, giving an osmotic beverage terminates the attack.
- Be prepared to administer an IV carbonic anhydrase inhibitor (such as acetazolamide) as prescribed.

- If the carbonic anhydrase inhibitor is ineffective, expect to give an IV osmotic (1 to 2 g/kg of mannitol 20% solution in water).
- Administer ophthalmic beta-blockers (such as timolol maleate) as prescribed. These drugs lower IOP by reducing aqueous humor formation and improving aqueous outflow.
- As IOP decreases, administer a miotic (such as pilocarpine) as prescribed to improve aqueous outflow.
- Administer analgesics as prescribed to manage eye pain.
- Give antiemetics as prescribed to control nausea and vomiting.
- Administer an ophthalmic topical steroid (such as prednisolone) as prescribed to reduce inflammation.
- Frequently assess the patient's pain, vision, and associated symptoms, such as nausea.

What to do next

Once your patient has been stabilized, you'll need to:

- Frequently monitor his cardiovascular, pulmonary, gastrointestinal, and mental status.
- Administer pilocarpine as prescribed to maintain a low IOP.
- Give 250 mg of acetazolamide (Diamox) orally 2 or 4 times daily as prescribed to control IOP.
- Keep his head elevated at least 45 degrees to control IOP.
- Assess him for fear and anxiety and allow him to express his fears and anxieties regarding potential vision loss.
- Provide support, information, and comfort measures as needed.
- Keep him informed of planned procedures, and tell him the name and purpose of all prescribed medications.
- Prepare him for surgery (such as laser or surgical iridectomy) as needed.

- Do you see flashes of light, halos around lights, or floating spots in front of your eye?
- Have you been seeing double? If so, are the images side by side or on top of one another? Do double images occur in one eye or both eyes?
- Have you noticed recent drooping of the eyelids?
- Have you been tiring easily or feeling weak?

Focusing your assessment

When examining a patient who complains of vision changes, focus your assessment as follows:
- Inspect the eyelids for symmetry and appearance.
- Perform the six cardinal positions of gaze test to evaluate the extraocular muscles.
- Conduct an ophthalmoscopic examination to check for the red reflex and assess the retina.
- Test visual acuity.

Possible causes

- *Refractive error.* Most vision changes occur gradually and indicate the need for a refractive correction. Patients with a refractive error simply need a prescription for corrective lenses.
- *Detached retina.* Signs and symptoms include seeing flashes of light or floating spots in front of one eye. (The "floaters" occur as the retina pulls away from the choroid and vitreous humor leaks between the two layers, causing blood and tissue particles to "float" in the visual field.) The ophthalmoscopic examination typically reveals absence of a red reflex, an orange or red crescent-shaped retinal tear, and black retinal vessels. As symptoms progress, the patient may describe the sensation of a shade being pulled down over the affected eye. Unless treated, vision in that eye will be lost. Retinal detachment may result from head injury, eye inflammation, severe myopia, diabetic retinopathy, or age-related changes in the vitreous chamber.
- *Cranial nerve impairment.* Horizontal diplopia—seeing side-by-side double images—indicates impairment of CN III or CN VI (the abducens nerve). Vertical diplopia—seeing one image above the other—signals impairment of CN III or CN IV (the trochlear nerve). Diplopia is caused by the inability of the extraocular muscles to control eye movements. The problem may be intermittent or constant, may affect near or far vision, and may occur in one or both eyes.
- *Head injury.* If your patient with double vision has suffered a recent head injury, investigate for early signs of increasing ICP, such as appetite loss, nausea, and vomiting.
- *Neuromuscular disorder.* If his diplopia has had a gradual onset, find out if your patient has other possible signs or symptoms of a neuromuscular disorder, such as myasthenia gravis or multiple

sclerosis (for instance, ptosis, eyelid drooping, or generalized muscle weakness).
- *Lens impairment.* Double vision in only one eye suggests a problem with the lens and generally points to a cataract.
- *Diabetes mellitus.* Signs and symptoms include blurred vision, caused by the effects of fluctuating blood glucose levels on the lens. Also, be alert to reports of diplopia, possibly signaling alterations in the oculomotor nerves caused by hyperglycemia. High blood glucose levels can also cause vascular congestion in the eyes, resulting in the appearance of halos, flashing lights, and dark spots.

Vision loss

If your patient complains of vision loss, investigate the symptom further by asking him the following questions:
- Do you have no vision at all, or can you see lights or shadows?
- When did you first notice the vision loss?
- Did it start suddenly or gradually?
- Is your vision impaired all of the time or mostly at night?
- Have you lost vision only in a part of your visual field? For instance, can you see objects directly in front of you but not those to the left and right without moving your head?
- Do you have a chronic medical condition, such as diabetes mellitus, hypertension, or AIDS, or a chronic eye condition, such as glaucoma or cataracts? If so, what medication do you take?

Focusing your assessment

When examining a patient who complains of vision loss, focus your assessment as follows:
- Inspect the cornea for clarity, opacities, and irregular reflex.
- Evaluate the conjunctiva for redness and excessive tearing.
- Using an ophthalmoscope, inspect the retina for hemorrhages, tears, and exudate, and the optic disc for swelling (a sign of papilledema).
- Perform the confrontation test to check for visual field defects.
- Test your patient's visual acuity. If he can't read the largest letters on the eye chart, ask if he can see your hand movement. If he can't, shine a penlight into his eyes, and ask if he can detect the light.

Possible causes

- *Diabetic retinopathy.* A common complication of diabetes mellitus, diabetic retinopathy causes gradual vision loss from damage to or occlusion of retinal blood vessels. (See 🔖 *Determining Causes of Acute Vision Loss,* p. 130.)
- *Cataracts.* Progressive opacification of the crystalline lens, usually with age, can cause a gradual loss of vision.

DETERMINING CAUSES OF ACUTE VISION LOSS

Acute vision loss may be temporary or permanent and may range from slightly impaired vision to total blindness. Use the following table to help determine the cause of your patient's vision loss.

Characteristics	Possible findings	Probable causes
• Sudden vision loss • Floating spots or flashes of light preceeding vision loss • Sensation of shade being pulled over eye	• No red reflex • Detached retina that bulges inward and appears translucent and rippled	• Retinal detachment
• Sudden vision loss • Sensation of shade being pulled over eye • History of hypertension, diabetes mellitus, or heart disease	• Loss of normal transparency of retina • Diffuse retinal hemorrhages • Dilation of retinal capillaries • Macular edema	• Retinal vein occlusion
• Central vision loss • Progressive blurring of vision	• Cloudy lens • White pupil	• Nuclear cataract
• Central vision loss • Report that vertical lines appear wavy and middle of visual field is fuzzy, smudged, or empty • Possible loss of color vision	• Proliferation of accessory blood vessels on retina • Drusen (hyaline excrescences) • Intraretinal or subretinal hemorrhages	• Macular degeneration
• Peripheral vision loss • Severe eye pain • Nausea and vomiting • Halos seen around lights	• Reddened eye • Mid-dilated, nonreactive pupil • Hazy cornea • Enlargement of physiologic cup	• Acute angle-closure glaucoma
• Spotty vision loss, especially at night • Scotomas (blind spots in visual field)	• Reduction in the visual field	• Lesion in retina or visual pathway
• Poor night vision • Dry skin and hair; ear, sinus, respiratory, urinary, and digestive infections; inability to gain weight; nervous disorders; skin sores	• Corneal dryness and ulceration (xerophthalmia)	• Vitamin A deficiency
• Night blindness followed by slow loss of peripheral vision, leading to tunnel vision • Possible hearing loss	• Shrinkage of optic disc (optic atrophy), narrowing of retinal arterioles, and spotty pigmentation of retina	• Retinitis pigmentosa
• Sudden, transient vision loss • Sensation of shade being pulled over eye	• Small, glistening, yellowish red crystals at the bifurcation of the retinal arteries	• Amaurosis fugax, a disorder associated with carotid stenosis, temporal arteritis, migraines, or papilledema

- *Age-related macular degeneration.* The loss of pigmentation in epithelial photoreceptor cells in the macula causes progressive loss of central vision. Upon examination of the retina, you may note round, yellow or white deposits.
- *Acute angle-closure glaucoma.* This condition typically causes severe eye pain and acute vision loss.
- *Advanced open-angle glaucoma.* This condition causes gradual, painless vision loss in which the patient develops tunnel vision.
- *Retinal vein or artery occlusion.* When a thrombus blocks blood flow in a retinal vein or artery, it causes sudden, painless vision loss.
- *Vitreous hemorrhage.* When blood fills the vitreous cavity, it may cause acute vision loss. This is typically associated with diabetic retinopathy.
- *Retinal tearing or hemorrhaging.* This problem usually causes acute vision loss. The patient may describe a dark curtain being drawn over the vision in one eye. This can be caused by aphakia, myopia, diabetes mellitus, or trauma.
- *Neurologic conditions.* Those that affect the optic nerve can cause acute vision loss including occipital lobe lesions, transient ischemic attacks, and vascular occlusions.
- *Renal disease.* This problem can cause acute vision loss as a result of papilledema or hemorrhages seen with pyelonephritis, glomerulonephritis, and diabetic nephropathy.
- *Cardiovascular problems.* Carotid stenosis and other cardiovascular problems can cause acute vision loss as a result of atherosclerotic changes that interrupt the blood supply to the eyes or hypertensive retinal disease.
- *Vitamin A deficiency.* This condition typically causes poor nighttime vision.

EAR EXAMINATION STEPS AND FINDINGS

Ear disorders range from treatable conditions, such as acute otitis externa (inflammation of the external ear canal), to more severe disorders, such as Ménière's disease (a chronic disease of the inner ear). Besides causing pain, an ear disorder can affect hearing and interfere with the patient's ability to perform daily activities.

To conduct an efficient physical assessment of the ear, you must be familiar with basic ear anatomy, especially if an ear examination isn't a routine part of your practice. (See ▌ *Structures of the Ear,* p. 132.)

For best results, seat the patient comfortably and ensure adequate room lighting. You'll need a penlight for inspection and an otoscope if you plan

ANATOMY REVIEW

STRUCTURES OF THE EAR

This illustration shows the structures of the external, middle, and inner ear.

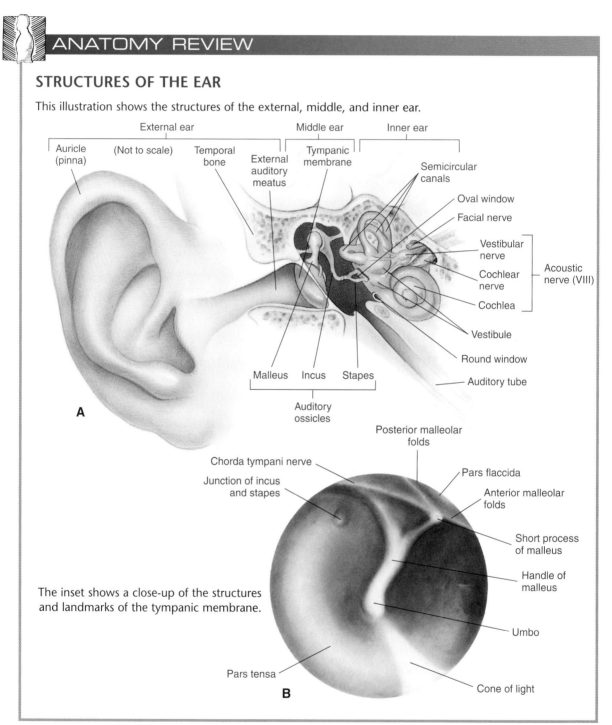

The inset shows a close-up of the structures and landmarks of the tympanic membrane.

A, from Thibodeau, G. & Patton, K. (2003). *Anatomy and Physiology* (5th ed.). St. Louis: Mosby. **B,** from Seidel, H. M., Ball, J. W., Dains, J. E., & Benedict, G. W. (2003). *Mosby's Guide to Physical Examination* (5th ed.). St. Louis: Mosby.

to examine the middle ear. If you're going to test the patient's hearing, choose a quiet area free of distractions.

Inspection and palpation

For optimal speed and efficiency, inspect and palpate the external ear at the same time. With your patient facing you, observe ear size and placement and assess the color and integrity of the skin on the ears. Then examine external ear structures, the auricle (pinna) and its parts (lobule, tragus, antitragus, helix, and antihelix). Observe the position of the ears on the head by imagining a line between the eye's outer canthus and the ear's pinna.

Next, palpate the auricle, checking for freedom of movement, tenderness, and lesions. Palpate behind the external ear for lesions and tenderness, and feel the preauricular and postauricular lymph nodes for tenderness and enlargement.

Using a penlight, inspect the external auditory canal. Check for nodules, cysts, abrasions, discharge, lesions, inflammation, and obstruction. (See 📖 *Essentials of the Ear Examination.*)

Normal findings

- Auricles similar in size and placement. They should move freely and painlessly. Elderly patients may have more prominent auricles.
- Auricles free of scales, redness, and inflammation.
- Skin over the ears dry, clean, and the same color as the skin on rest of the body.

PRIORITY CHECKLIST

ESSENTIALS OF THE EAR EXAMINATION

Use this checklist to make sure you cover the most important steps when examining the ears.

- ❑ Check ear size, placement, skin color, texture, and integrity.
- ❑ Inspect auricles for mobility, color, discharge, cysts, nodules, lesions, and tenderness.
- ❑ Check auditory canal for nodules, cysts, abrasions, discharge, lesions, inflammation, obstruction, cerumen impaction, and tenderness.
- ❑ Inspect preauricular and postauricular lymph nodes for size, consistency, and tenderness.
- ❑ Check auditory canal for patency, integrity, cerumen impaction, swelling, bony overgrowths, redness, drainage, and pain.
- ❑ Inspect tympanic membrane for color, integrity, cone of light, bony landmarks, bulging, erythema, perforation, drainage, fluid, air, and lesions.

- Earlobes (lobules) soft and flexible. In an elderly patient, they may be pendulous.
- Pinna aligned with outer canthus of the eye, deviating no more than 10 degrees vertically.
- Preauricular and postauricular lymph nodes either nonpalpable or small, soft, and nontender.
- External auditory canal free of nodules, cysts, and drainage.
- Buildup in cerumen not impacted in the canal, although it may be present. Cerumen may be flaky, and its color may vary from creamy pink to black or brown. In an elderly patient, cerumen may appear dry from a lack of active sebaceous glands. (See 🗐 *What to Expect When Examining the Ears.*)

Abnormal findings
- Dry, scaly skin on the external ear or in the auditory canal, indicating psoriasis or seborrhea.
- Skin breakdown, abrasions, or erosions, possibly resulting from pressure caused by a person lying on his side for prolonged periods.
- Eroded areas behind the external ears, sometimes developing from the pressure of oxygen tubing in patients who need chronic nasal oxygen therapy.
- Painful crusted lesions on the helix, possibly representing squamous cell carcinomas caused by frequent sun exposure. If the lesions metastasize, nearby lymph nodes may be enlarged.
- Hard nodules, or calculi, on the auricle rim or outside the opening of the external auditory canal, possibly representing gouty tophi. When you apply pressure to them, they may express uric acid, a white, crystalline substance.

NORMAL FINDINGS

WHAT TO EXPECT WHEN EXAMINING THE EARS

Use this brief review to confirm normal findings when examining the ears.

- Auricles equal in size and placement, symmetrically positioned, and freely mobile.
- Skin over ears clean, dry, and same color as other skin; free of scales, redness, and inflammation.
- Preauricular and postauricular lymph nodes nonpalpable or small, soft, and nontender.
- External auditory canal patent and free of nodules, cysts, drainage, inflammation or obstruction; cerumen present but not excessive or impacted.
- Tympanic membrane intact, shiny, translucent, and pearly gray; cone of light present; bony landmarks visible.

- Low-set ears, usually seen with Down syndrome or congenital renal disorders.
- Tenderness of the external ear on palpation and movement, possibly resulting from otitis externa and accompanied by enlargement and tenderness of the postauricular lymph nodes.
- Foreign body obstructing the auditory canal. A pea, a bead, even an insect may completely or partially obstruct the canal. More common in children than adults, foreign bodies may become trapped in the canal and remain lodged there until removed. Sometimes, a foreign body leads to tympanic perforation.

Otoscopic examination

To view the internal ear structures, you'll need an otoscope. Before performing this examination, make sure you feel comfortable using this device. With practice, you'll be able to view the incus, umbo, and the handle and short process of the malleus through the otoscope. (For details on using the otoscope, see Chapter 1.) When examining a child, enlist the help of a parent or guardian. (See 🔖 *Performing an Otoscopic Examination in a Child,* p. 136.)

Before you begin, inspect the auditory canal for signs of inflammation and obstruction. If you note either condition, don't insert the otoscope because doing so could cause further irritation or force a foreign object farther into the canal.

If you've determined that you can safely insert the otoscope, pull the outer portion of the auricle up, back, and slightly outward (when examining an adult).

EXAMINATION TIP

Holding the otoscope with the handle up can provide greater stability during the exam. When you insert the speculum into the ear canal in this manner, you can brace your hand against the patient's head to prevent injury.

Then examine the external canal, which normally contains hair and cerumen. If necessary, remove excess cerumen to improve your view of the tympanic membrane.

Next, gently insert the speculum of the otoscope into the inner portion of the canal. As you inspect the tympanic membrane, look for a cone of light—a triangular reflection visible in the left lower quadrant of the left ear and the right lower quadrant of the right ear. Then locate bony landmarks, such as the incus, umbo, and the handle and short process of the malleus.

PERFORMING AN OTOSCOPIC EXAMINATION IN A CHILD

Examining children's ears can challenge your assessment skills. If the child presents with symptoms of ear pain, he'll likely already be uncomfortable and frightened. Therefore, as you proceed with the examination, speak in soothing tones and prepare to enlist the help of a parent or guardian. Use the following guidelines to help keep the assessment on track:

• Save the otoscopic examination for last. Perform less invasive parts of a physical examination first to help establish rapport with the child and avoid upsetting him early on.

• If the child is small enough, have him sit facing inward on his parent's or guardian's lap. Then, ask the parent or guardian to restrain the child by wrapping his or her arm around the child's body, with the other arm holding his head.

• If the patient is too big for a lap, have him lie either supine or prone on an examination table. Ask the parent or guardian (and possibly a third person) to help restrain the child's head and legs, if needed. Under these conditions, expect to lie across the child's torso to immobilize it, as you insert the otoscope.

• If the child is younger than 3 years of age, straighten the ear canal by grasping the lower part of the pinna and pulling down and back. That's because the ear canal is shorter and straighter at this age. As the child ages, the ear canal becomes more "S" shaped. So for a child older than 3, expect to pull the upper part of the pinna up and back, as you would for an adult.

• As you insert the speculum of the otoscope in the ear canal, try to brace the lateral aspect of your hand (the one holding the pinna) against the child's head to prevent injury if the child suddenly moves.

• If the child is crying or screaming, the increased blood flow to the tympanic membrane may give it a red appearance. If you're skilled with the use of a pneumatic otoscope, use it to detect a lack of tympanic membrane movement—a sign of otitis media.

• When you've completed the otoscopic examination, comfort the child, or return the child to his parent or guardian for reassurance.

If you have trouble seeing the tympanic membrane or its structures, gently reposition the speculum to get a better view. (Inner ear structures—such as the vestibule, semicircular canal, and cochlea—aren't visible for examination.)

Normal findings
• Tympanic membrane intact and pearly gray.
• Visible bony landmarks, such as the incus, umbo, and handle and short process of the malleus, visible. In an elderly patient, these landmarks may be more pronounced because of sclerosis or atrophy.

Abnormal findings
• Lesions in the canal, possibly representing boils or herpes vesicles.
• Cerumen impaction, possibly blocking your view of the tympanic membrane. The impacted cerumen may vary in color and appear either shiny and wet or dry and hard.

CULTURAL CONSIDERATIONS

Caucasians and African Americans tend to have cerumen that's wet and dark, while Asians and Native Americans often have cerumen that's gray, dry, and flaky.

- Reddened tympanic membrane with purulent, foul-smelling ear drainage, suggesting acute otitis externa.
- Bulging, reddened, or perforated tympanic membrane, possibly resulting from acute otitis media. This condition may be accompanied by dilated tympanic blood vessels and loss of bony landmarks. Another sign of otitis media is absence of the cone of light because of bulging or retraction of the tympanic membrane.
- Perforated eardrum, appearing as a hole in the center of the tympanic membrane or extending to its margins. Drainage may seep through the perforation. If the perforation stems from an infection, such as otitis media, you may see a reddened ring around it.
- Serous, amber fluid and air in the tympanic membrane, resulting from serous effusion. This condition is caused by viral infection or barotrauma experienced during diving or air flight.
- Vesicles on the tympanic membrane, typically reflecting bullous myringitis, a viral infection that often accompanies acute otitis media and may cause bloody ear discharge.

EXPLORING EAR COMPLAINTS

Common ear complaints include ear pain, ear discharge, hearing loss, and vertigo. The following section presents pertinent health history questions to ask a patient who reports one of these symptoms, explains how to focus your physical examination appropriately, and lists possible causes for each complaint.

Ear pain
If your patient complains of ear pain, investigate the symptom further by asking him the following questions:
- When did you first notice the pain?
- Is the pain constant or intermittent?
- How would you rate it on a scale of 0 to 10, with 0 representing no pain and 10 representing the worst pain you've ever felt?
- Does anything seem to make the pain better or worse?
- Have you recently been exposed to very loud noise, suffered an ear or a head injury, or had a foreign object inserted in your ear?

- Have you experienced fever, chills, or upper respiratory symptoms lately?
- Have you noticed any hearing loss, ringing in the ears, or dizziness?
- Do you have a sensation of fullness in your ears?
- Have you noticed any ear discharge? If so, what color was it? Was it clear or cloudy? Did it appear bloody?

Focusing your assessment

When examining a patient who complains of ear pain, focus your assessment as follows:

- Take the patient's temperature to check for fever (possibly indicating an ear infection).
- Palpate the external ear and mastoid process for tenderness.
- Assess the preauricular and postauricular lymph nodes for enlargement and tenderness.
- Using an otoscope, check the auditory canal for redness, drainage, trauma, and lesions (such as vesicles or papules).
- Gently insert the speculum and examine the canal from the meatus to the tympanic membrane. Assess the tympanic membrane for redness, bulging, perforation, and loss of bony landmarks. Also check for vesicles, fluid, or air bubbles.

Possible causes

- *Acute otitis externa.* This condition can cause severe ear pain that typically worsens on palpation and is accompanied by a mild hearing loss; tinnitus; dizziness; purulent, foul-smelling ear discharge; and enlarged, possibly tender, postauricular lymph nodes. Otoscopic findings include inflammation of the auditory canal, possibly with abrasions or lesions, and a reddened tympanic membrane.
- *Bullous myringitis.* This disorder may cause sudden, severe ear pain with bloody ear discharge. Vesicles may appear on the tympanic membrane.
- *Acute otitis media.* This condition causes ear pain, fever, and chills. If the tympanic membrane ruptures, the patient may describe a popping sensation in his ear, followed by some relief from the pain. Otoscopic examination may reveal bulging, redness, and possibly perforation of the tympanic membrane, with loss of bony landmarks and dilation of tympanic vessels. After membrane rupture, the ear canal appears normal and is nontender on palpation.
- *Serous effusion.* This condition causes ear pain, accompanied by serous amber fluid and air behind the tympanic membrane, mild hearing loss, a popping sensation, and a feeling of fullness in the ear.

Ear discharge

If your patient complains of ear discharge, investigate the symptom further by asking him the following questions:

- What color and consistency is the discharge? Is it clear, purulent, or bloody? Is it thick or thin?
- Is the discharge coming from one ear or both ears?
- When did you first notice the discharge?
- Does anything seem to make it better or worse?
- Does the discharge tend to appear during a specific time of day or during or following a particular activity, such as swimming?
- Do you have any ear pain?
- Have you recently had a head injury, been exposed to loud noise, or inserted a foreign object into your ear?

Focusing your assessment

When examining a patient who complains of ear discharge, focus your assessment as follows:

- Take your patient's temperature. Ear discharge accompanied by fever may indicate an ear infection.
- Observe any ear discharge for color, clarity, consistency, and odor.
- If your patient has experienced a recent head injury, keep in mind that fluid draining from the ear could be cerebrospinal fluid (CSF). Use a test strip to check the drainage for high glucose levels.
- Examine the external ear and middle ear for tympanic perforation, inflammation, and lesions.

Possible causes

- *Otitis externa.* This condition causes a purulent, foul-smelling ear discharge.
- *Bullous myringitis.* This condition may cause bloody ear discharge.
- *Head injury.* A head injury may allow CSF to leak from the ear. The discharge will be clear, thin, watery, and odorless. It will contain high glucose concentrations.

Hearing loss

If your patient complains of hearing loss, investigate the symptom further by asking the following questions (Note: If the hearing loss is severe, you may have to ask your questions in writing or by using another form of nonverbal communication.):

- Can you hear some sounds? Or is your hearing completely lost?
- Have you lost hearing in both ears?
- Did the hearing loss occur suddenly or gradually?
- Does anything seem to make the condition better or worse?
- Do you have ear pain or discharge?
- Do you have a sensation of pressure or fullness in your ears?

- Do you get frequent ear infections?
- Have you recently been exposed to loud noises or inserted a foreign object in your ear?
- Are you taking any medications?

Focusing your assessment

When examining a patient who complains of hearing loss, focus your assessment as follows:
- Inspect the external auditory canal for discharge and cerumen impaction.
- Using an otoscope, examine the tympanic membrane for perforation, redness, bulging, scarring, or an air-fluid level (which indicates air bubbles).
- Use the whisper test or ticking-watch test to assess the extent of the patient's hearing loss.
- Perform Weber's test and the Rinne test to check for sensorineural and conductive loss.

Possible causes

- *Injury.* Many injuries can cause hearing loss, including exposure to loud noise, tympanic perforation, repeated infections of the middle ear, cerumen impaction, or serous effusion (indicated by air bubbles behind the tympanic membrane).
- *Age-related changes.*

LIFESPAN CONSIDERATIONS

In older adults, hearing loss commonly is sensorineural and results in difficulty hearing high-pitched sounds or the sound combinations "oso" and "ofo." Whatever its cause, hearing loss requires further evaluation.

(See *Determining Causes of Hearing Loss,* p. 141)

Vertigo

If your patient complains of vertigo, an abnormal sensation of movement or spinning, investigate the symptom further by asking him the following questions:
- How many episodes of vertigo have you had?
- When did the first episode occur?
- How often do the episodes happen? How long do they last?
- Can you describe the sensation in detail? For instance, do you feel as if you're spinning around the room or as if the room is spinning around you?
- Does anything decrease the sensation or make it stop, such as sitting or lying down? Does anything make it worse, such as a particular movement?

INTERPRETING ABNORMAL FINDINGS

DETERMINING CAUSES OF HEARING LOSS

Hearing loss may have a sudden or gradual onset and may involve one or both ears. Use the following table to help pinpoint the cause of your patient's hearing loss.

Characteristics	Possible findings	Probable causes
• Progressive hearing loss (usually unilateral) • Sudden, recurrent attacks of vertigo accompanied by nausea and vomiting • Tinnitus (may be constant or intermittent) • Pressure or fullness in affected ear	• Loss or impairment of thermally induced nystagmus (as shown by caloric testing) • Decreased air and bone conduction (as shown by audiometry) • Nystagmus • Unilateral or bilateral sensorineural hearing loss	• Ménière's disease
• Hearing loss of gradual onset • Possible nausea and vomiting	• Bilateral hearing loss affecting both auditory and vestibular portions of inner ear	• Ototoxicity from such drugs as salicylates, aminoglyco-sides, diuretics, or antineoplastic agents
• Hearing loss most pronounced when source of sound is near auditory canal • Tinnitus • Dizziness • Possible facial numbness and asymmetry	• Sensorineural hearing loss • Tumor within ear (as shown by magnetic resonance imaging or computed tomography)	• Acoustic neuroma (tumor of CN VIII)
• Unilateral hearing loss • Pain, tinnitus, and fullness or pressure in affected ear	• Cerumen buildup in auditory canal • Inability to visualize tympanic membrane	• Excessive or impacted cerumen
• Unilateral hearing loss • Acute onset of severe vertigo • Nystagmus • Tinnitus • Nausea and vomiting	• Sensorineural hearing loss • Serous or purulent ear drainage	• Labyrinthitis

- Have you ever lost consciousness or fallen during an episode of vertigo?
- Have you noticed a recent hearing loss, ringing in your ears, or involuntary eye movements?
- Have you experienced recent nausea or vomiting?

Focusing your assessment

When examining a patient who complains of vertigo, focus your assessment as follows:

- Rule out other disorders that cause light-headedness or fainting, such as cardiac arrhythmias.

- Check blood pressure with the patient lying down, sitting, and standing. A drop of 20 mm Hg or more in systolic pressure when the patient rises from a lying or sitting position suggests orthostatic hypotension, a cause of dizziness often related to hydration status and use of such medications as antihypertensives.
- Auscultate heart sounds to help rule out cardiac arrhythmias and other heart problems. Check for rhythm irregularities and extra heart sounds (S_3 or S_4) or murmurs.
- If possible, obtain an electrocardiogram.
- Evaluate the patient's respiratory rate and pattern. Hyperventilation, resulting in hypocapnia (carbon dioxide deficiency in the blood), or hypoxia (reduced oxygen supply to tissues), can cause light-headedness or dizziness.
- Check for nystagmus, which may reflect a vestibular (inner ear) disturbance. To do this, have the patient tilt his head backward and forward or move it from side to side while sitting. Watch for involuntary, rhythmic eye movements, which may be horizontal, vertical, or rotating. Then have him lie flat and turn onto one side and then the other. Ask whether these movements produce vertigo or nausea. Be prepared in case they cause vomiting.

Possible causes
- *Acute labyrinthitis.* An inflammation of the labyrinth of the inner ear, this condition begins suddenly and lasts hours or days. It can cause nystagmus, which you may observe as the patient moves his head forward and backward or left to right. Occasionally, acute labyrinthitis causes nausea and vomiting.
- *Ménière's disease.* This disorder produces chronic, recurrent episodes of vertigo accompanied by tinnitus, pressure or fullness in the ears, and nausea or vomiting. Although it may wax and wane in severity, it ultimately progresses, leading to unilateral or bilateral sensorineural hearing loss.
- *Benign positional vertigo.* A patient with this condition experiences sudden, transient vertigo when he rolls over to the side or lifts his head. Symptoms come on suddenly and last only seconds to minutes. Nausea and vomiting occasionally may occur, but hearing isn't affected. Sometimes, benign positional vertigo indicates vertebrobasilar insufficiency or cervical spine dysfunction.
- *Acoustic neuroma.* A benign tumor, acoustic neuroma causes repeated episodes of vertigo, imbalance, unsteady gait, tinnitus, and sensorineural hearing loss. The tumor develops from CN VIII (the acoustic nerve) and grows in the auditory canal. Symptoms may progress to include paresthesias and gait disturbances.

EXAMINING
THE CHEST AND BACK

Perhaps nowhere else in the body will your assessment skills receive as rigorous a workout as they will here, at the thorax. To accurately assess your patient's chest and back, you'll need sound knowledge of almost all the major body systems, including the cardiac, respiratory, and musculoskeletal systems, as well as the digestive, neurologic, and renal systems. (See *Structures of the Thorax,* pp. 144 to 148.)

In addition, you'll need to be able to differentiate quickly between signs and symptoms that warn of serious, potentially life-threatening disorders, such as angina pectoris, myocardial infarction, lung cancer, and obstructive lung disease, as well as those resulting from less acute disorders, such as a chronic musculoskeletal problem or a transient renal condition. But regardless of what's causing the patient's problem, you'll need to ensure that he gets the proper care.

Because the chest and back involve so many body systems, you'll also need to incorporate your examination findings with corresponding findings in other regions of the patient's body. For example, if you auscultate an abnormal heart sound that's consistent with heart failure, you'll want to look for peripheral edema—another sign of heart failure—when you assess the lower extremities later.

ANATOMY REVIEW

STRUCTURES OF THE THORAX

The following illustrations present an overview of anterior and posterior thoracic landmarks and structures, the lungs, and the heart. Be sure you're familiar with all the structures of the thorax before undertaking a thorough assessment of your patient.

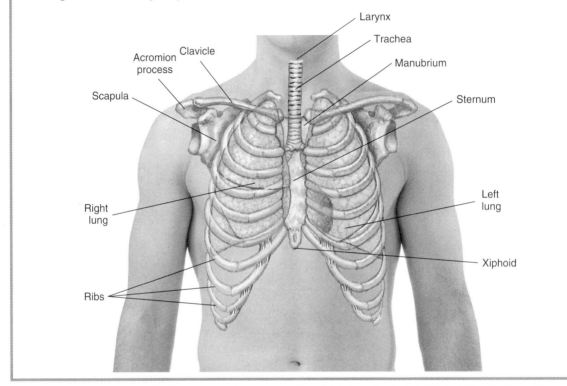

From Thompson, J. M., McFarland, G. K., Hirsch, J. E., & Tucker, S. M. (2002). *Mosby's Clinical Nursing* (5th ed.). St. Louis: Mosby.

Throughout your assessment, be sure to keep pertinent points of your patient's health history in mind and focus on specific complaints your patient has identified while giving his history. This chapter presents focused assessment instructions for a range of chief complaints, including chest pain, back pain, cough, hemoptysis, dyspnea, orthopnea, wheezing, and breast lumps.

Assessing your patient's thorax will require you to use the complete range of assessment techniques: inspection, palpation, percussion, and auscultation. This chapter outlines important procedures for each one, along with normal and abnormal findings for the thorax. You may want to combine some assessment steps for efficiency and accuracy; for example,

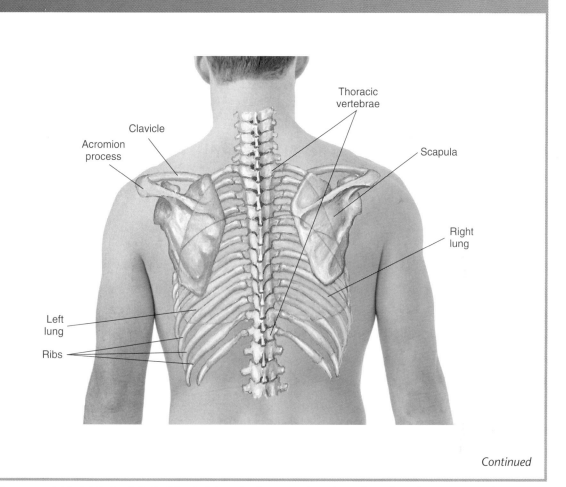

Thoracic
vertebrae

Clavicle

Acromion
process

Scapula

Right
lung

Left
lung

Ribs

Continued

From Thompson, J. M., McFarland, G. K., Hirsch, J. E., & Tucker, S. M. (2002). *Mosby's Clinical Nursing* (5th ed.). St. Louis: Mosby.

performing inspection and palpation simultaneously before you move on to percussion and auscultation. By using your skills and your knowledge wisely, you can give your patient the expert physical examination he needs.

EXAMINATION STEPS AND FINDINGS

Before starting your examination of a patient's chest and back, assemble the equipment you'll need. Make sure you have examination gloves, a stethoscope, a centimeter ruler, and a washable marking pen.

(Text continues on page 148.)

ANATOMY REVIEW

STRUCTURES OF THE THORAX—cont'd

Anterior landmarks

Posterior landmarks

Right anterior axillary line

Left anterior axillary line

Clavicle

Sternum

Xiphoid process

Costal angle

Right midclavicular line

Midsternal line

Left midclavicular line

Left midscapular line

Vertebral line

T 1

Right midscapular line

Scapula

Anatomy of the heart

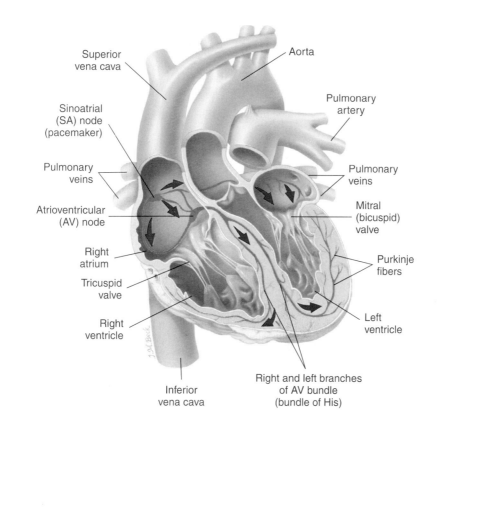

From Thibodeau, G. & Patton, K. (2003). *Anatomy and Physiology* (5th ed.). St. Louis: Mosby.

Continued

ANATOMY REVIEW

STRUCTURES OF THE THORAX—cont'd

Anatomy of the lungs

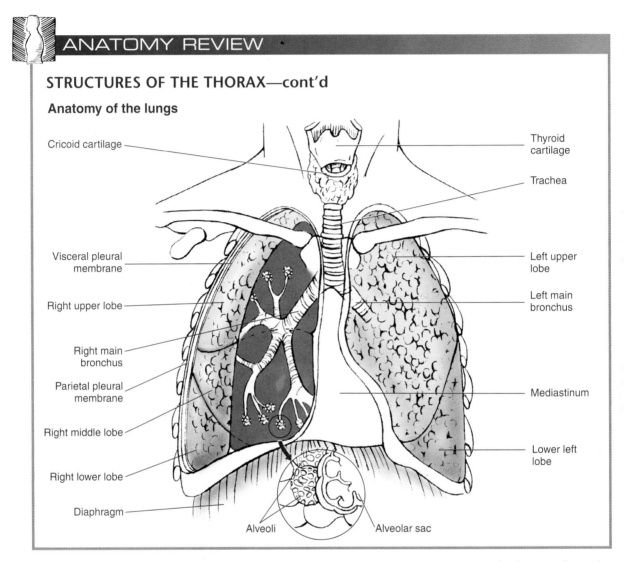

Cricoid cartilage

Visceral pleural membrane

Right upper lobe

Right main bronchus

Parietal pleural membrane

Right middle lobe

Right lower lobe

Diaphragm

Alveoli

Thyroid cartilage

Trachea

Left upper lobe

Left main bronchus

Mediastinum

Lower left lobe

Alveolar sac

Next, make sure you have an appropriate room in which to perform the examination. It should be quiet and private, warm enough to keep the patient comfortable, and well lit. Bright, tangential lighting is important to highlight chest movement. Many nurses find that a revolving stool on casters offers a comfortable, mobile seat during the procedure.

Inspection

Begin your examination with the patient sitting upright, unsupported if possible, and undressed to the waist. If your patient is too ill to sit upright, assistance may be necessary to support him. You'll want to work from the upper chest downward, comparing one side to the other. (See 📷 *Key Examination Steps for the Chest and Back*.)

Chest

Inspect your patient's chest from the front, from the side, from behind, and standing over his shoulder, looking down over the anterior chest. Inspect the skin of the chest wall for cyanosis or pallor, scars, wounds, bruises, lesions, nodules, or superficial venous patterns. Observe for red or reddish-blue coloration, excoriation, or exudate.

Note the shape and symmetry of the thorax from the front and back. Estimate the anterior-posterior (AP) diameter compared to the transverse diameter.

LIFESPAN CONSIDERATIONS

Older adults can develop convexity of the thoracic spine—called kyphosis. This posterior curvature of the spine increases the thoracic anterior-posterior diameter and shortens the thorax.

PRIORITY CHECKLIST

KEY EXAMINATION STEPS FOR THE CHEST AND BACK

Use this checklist to make sure you cover the most important steps when examining the chest and back.

- ❐ Inspect skin integrity and color.
- ❐ Inspect shape and symmetry of the chest.
- ❐ Inspect the spine and scapula. Look for spinal deformities and unequal scapular height.
- ❐ Watch accessory muscle use.
- ❐ Inspect the precordium for pulsations.
- ❐ Assess anterior-posterior and lateral dimensions of the thorax.
- ❐ Palpate chest and back for masses or deformity.
- ❐ Assess range of motion of the back and spinal column.
- ❐ Perform a full breast examination.
- ❐ Assess the location of the apical impulse.
- ❐ Palpate the anterior chest for thrills, masses, and deformities.
- ❐ Check for tactile fremitus.
- ❐ Palpate or use blunt percussion at the costovertebral angle.
- ❐ Measure and evaluate respiratory excursion.
- ❐ Percuss the lateral back and chest to assess underlying structures of the thorax.
- ❐ Auscultate the anterior chest for heart sounds.
- ❐ Auscultate to assess lung sounds.
- ❐ Measure diaphragmatic excursion.
- ❐ Auscultate the chest and back for presence and quality of breath sounds.
- ❐ Evaluate voice resonance.

Look at the angle of the costal margins at the xiphoid. Observe your patient's muscular development and nutritional status by noting the presence of underlying fat and the prominence of his ribs.

Assess your patient's respiratory rate, depth, and rhythm or pattern of breathing. (See *Assessing Your Patient's Respirations*.)

Do this without your patient's knowledge, so you'll be sure he's breathing in his usual manner. Compare the length of the inspiratory and expiratory phases. Note any symptoms of distress. As the patient breathes, watch for symmetry of chest wall movement, costal versus abdominal breathing, the use of accessory muscles, bulging or retraction of the intercostal spaces (ICSs), and pulsations or heaving. Observe for the

ASSESSING YOUR PATIENT'S RESPIRATIONS

Use the illustrated patterns below to assess and identify your patient's respirations.

Eupnea		Normal
Tachypnea		Rapid rate
Bradypnea		Reduced rate
Apnea		Absence of breathing
Hyperventilation		Deep respirations, near normal rate
Kussmaul's respiration		Fast and deep, with no pauses
Cheyne-Stokes respiration		Cyclic pattern of apnea and varied breathing
Biot's respiration		Fast and deep, with periods of apnea
Apneustic respiration		Long, gasping inspirations, with ineffective expirations

cardiac impulse in the apical area, medial to the midclavicular line in the fourth and fifth ICSs.

Inspect the breasts of both male and female patients with their arms hanging loosely at their sides. Then compare the patient's breasts, noting their size, color, symmetry, contour, texture, striae, venous patterns, dimpling, and the presence of edema or areas of redness.

LIFESPAN CONSIDERATIONS

Females usually have fully developed breasts by age 14, but by age 40, breast tissue begins to atrophy as glandular tissue shrinks. At this age, supporting ligaments begin to relax, and the breasts appear to "drop" or hang more loosely.

Examine the areolae for shape, color, and texture. Observe the nipples for color, size, inversion or eversion, retraction, deviation, or evidence of bleeding, cracking, or discharge. Ask your female patient to raise her arms over her head, press her hands against her hips, and then lean forward from the waist. Assess her breasts again, briefly, in each position. Finally, lift her breasts to assess their lower and lateral aspects.

CULTURAL CONSIDERATIONS

The age of breast development and the appearance of the breasts vary among ethnic groups. For example, African-American girls tend to develop breasts at an earlier age than other ethnic groups and also have a higher prevalence of supernumerary nipples. Asian females tend to have smaller breasts than other ethnic groups. The color of the nipples and areolae may also vary among ethnic groups—they're usually darker in dark-skinned individuals—but in general the nipples are the same color as the areolae.

During your breast examination, observe the patient's axillary and supraclavicular regions for bulging, retraction, discoloration, or edema. Also inspect the axillae for signs of rash or infection.

Back

Start by having your patient expose his entire back. Ask him to fold his arms across his chest, and then move behind him. Inspect the skin of his back for texture, lesions, scars, or sinus tract openings (tubelike, inflammatory structures that suggest infection). Observe the skin over the iliac crests and sacrum for redness and other signs of breakdown. Note any redness or nodules near the coccyx. In bedridden patients, look for edema in the sacral region.

Note the shape of the thorax and any deformities. Observe the bony framework, including the scapulae, and the angle at which the ribs slope from the vertebrae.

Now ask your patient to extend his arms in front of him and lower them slowly to his sides. Watch to see whether his scapulae protrude outward from his back more than normal. This condition is called *winged scapulae*. While the patient breathes, inspect the movement of his posterior chest wall for symmetry, bulging, or retraction of the ICSs.

Now ask your patient to stand. Look at his overall body posture. Assess his spinal column for alignment. Make sure the thoracic and lumbar areas curve appropriately. Observe for any abnormal curvature, such as lateral displacement. Compare the contour of the patient's shoulders and symmetry of heights of his shoulders and iliac crests.

Normal findings
- Skin smooth and generally uniform in color, depending on exposure to the sun. No cyanosis.
- No lesions, nodules, or superficial venous patterns.
- Thorax basically symmetrical, with an AP diameter less than the transverse diameter. Shape varies somewhat with the patient's body build.
- Costal angle 90 degrees, widening on inspiration.
- Respiratory rate 12 to 20 breaths per minute.
- Respirations regular and quiet, neither too shallow nor too deep.
- Inspiratory phase half as long as the expiratory phase.
- Chest expansion symmetrical in onset and depth during respiration, without the use of accessory muscles. Males tend to breathe abdominally, using the diaphragm, whereas females tend to use the costal cage.
- ICSs neither retracted nor bulging.
- Cardiac impulse visible in about half of adults. It may be displaced upward in pregnancy or to the right in dextrocardia (a rare anomaly in which the heart is located in the right side of the chest).
- Breast shape convex in females and even with the chest wall in males. Right and left breasts may differ in size. Skin texture is smooth and contour uninterrupted. Striae may be visible from previous changes in breast size but should be bilaterally similar.
- Breasts free from dimpling, edema, or red areas.
- Areolae round or oval and comparable in size. Color can range from pink to brown, depending on skin tone and pregnancy history. Texture should be smooth, although a peppering of Montgomery's tubercles is normal.
- Nipples the same color as the areolae. They're either everted or have a long-standing history of inversion. They are bilaterally equal, with no deviation. They display no retraction, bleeding, cracking, or discharge.

- Axillary and supraclavicular regions free of rash, bulging, edema, or infection.

Abnormal findings
- Jaundice, indicating liver dysfunction or biliary obstruction.
- Cyanosis or pallor, possibly indicating compromised tissue oxygenation.
- Scars, possibly resulting from past injury or surgical intervention.
- Bruises, possibly suggesting trauma or a bleeding disorder. If the patient has a wound, note its location, shape, size in length and depth, and the condition of any dressing.
- Lesion or nodule that has changed shape, color, size, or texture, has become ulcerated, or has started bleeding or itching. Although it may be benign, as in pigmented nevi or fatty deposits, these signs typically suggest malignancy.
- Spinal deformities causing asymmetry of the thorax, suggesting scoliosis (lateral curvature of the spine), kyphosis (convex curvature of the spine), or another spinal disorder.
- Barrel-shaped thorax, possibly resulting from underlying respiratory disease.
- Structural deformities, such as pigeon chest (prominent sternal protrusion) or funnel chest (indentation of the lower sternum).
- Protruding ribs, possibly indicating malnutrition.
- Tachypnea (increased respiratory rate), possibly indicating decreased blood oxygen levels, metabolic disease, anxiety, broken ribs, pleurisy, liver enlargement, or central nervous system disease.
- Bradypnea (decreased respiratory rate), possibly indicating neurologic and electrolyte disturbances, infection, or oversedation.
- Abnormal respiratory pattern, possibly indicating serious underlying disease. Examples include Cheyne-Stokes (crescendo-decrescendo), Kussmaul's (rapid, deep), and Biot's (irregular, with periods of apnea).
- Prolonged expiratory phase, possibly indicating asthma.
- Use of accessory muscles, tachypnea, orthopnea, nasal flaring, pursed lips, and cyanosis, indicating respiratory distress. (See *Detecting Respiratory Warning Signs,* p. 154.)
- Localized intercostal retraction during inspiration, possibly resulting from an obstruction in the large bronchi.
- Generalized intercostal retraction during inspiration, indicating emphysema, asthma, or chronic bronchitis.
- Intercostal bulging during expiration, suggesting emphysema, asthma, or massive pulmonary effusion.
- Asymmetry, resulting from a collapsed lung or a mass.
- Pulsations or heaving of the precordium, possibly indicating ventricular enlargement, valve disease, or aneurysm.

DETECTING RESPIRATORY WARNING SIGNS

If your patient is in respiratory distress, you'll be able to observe several characteristic signs.

A person who's having trouble breathing, and who's using accessory muscles to do so, will look anxious. His nostrils will flare. He'll look cyanotic around the mouth. You'll see the sternocleidomastoid muscles visibly contracting.

You should also see retractions of the suprasternal notch, the intercostal areas, and the substernal area. Finally, you'll notice that the patient's chest is expanded more fully than normal.

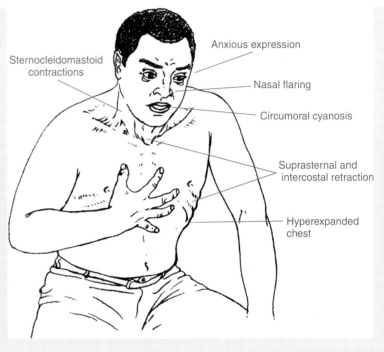

Sternocleidomastoid contractions

Anxious expression

Nasal flaring

Circumoral cyanosis

Suprasternal and intercostal retraction

Hyperexpanded chest

- Areas of redness or tenderness on the female breast, possibly indicating mastitis.
- Edema of the female breast, resulting from lymphatic blockade (from infection or carcinoma) or from radiation treatment.
- Dimpling (peau d'orange) or unilateral discoloration or venous patterns on the female breast, possibly indicating malignancy.
- Gynecomastia (enlargement of the male breast).
- Mastitis, cysts, or nodules involving the female or male breast.
- Visible lymph nodes or edema in the axillary or supraclavicular regions, possibly indicating metastatic disease or infection.
- Axillary rash, possibly stemming from a deodorant allergy or yeast infection.

Palpation

Palpation of the chest and back takes place with your patient in the same upright position as inspection. In fact, you might consider combining inspection and palpation to decrease the time required to complete your assessment.

Chest

Begin palpation by examining your patient's breasts. Make sure your hands are warm. Palpation of the male breasts can be brief but should not be omitted. Ask your female patient if she regularly performs a self-examination. Give her instructions or reinforce her technique as you examine her breasts. Emphasize the importance of breast self-examinations in detecting cancer early in its development. (See *Performing a Breast Examination,* p. 156.)

Continue by palpating the lymph nodes of the axillae in both male and female patients. To examine the right axillary lymph nodes, support your patient's right forearm with your right arm and put the palm of your left hand into the axilla. Use the palmar surface of your fingers to roll the soft tissue downward against the chest wall and muscles of the axilla. Explore all sections of the axilla, and put your patient's arm through the full range of motion during your examination. Then repeat the process for the other axilla.

Now palpate the supraclavicular lymph nodes. First, bend your patient's head forward to relax the sternocleidomastoid muscle. Then hook your fingers over the clavicle and palpate the entire supraclavicular area. Using both hands, palpate symmetrical areas of the thoracic muscles and skeleton. Feel the rib cage for symmetry, elasticity, and tenderness. Palpate the sternum and xiphoid process.

While palpating, pay attention to the patient's skin. Note its temperature, moistness, and turgor. Be alert for edematous areas. Note any pulsations, bulging, masses, depressions, or unusual movement.

Now palpate for conditions that relate to your patient's respiratory status. Assess for crepitus—a crackly, crinkly sensation—in the subcutaneous tissue, either localized or over the anterior thorax. Feel for vibrations during inspiration. Evaluate chest wall vibrations as the patient repeats certain sounds. (See *Palpating for Tactile Fremitus,* p. 157.)

Assess respiratory excursion with your patient in the supine position. Place your thumbs along the patient's costal margins and your fingers along the lateral rib cage. Slide your thumbs medially, and raise a loose skinfold. As your patient inhales deeply, note how far your thumbs are separated by the chest expansion. Check the symmetry of respiratory movement.

If you suspect a problem with your patient's lung expansion, assess respiratory excursion at two places on his anterior thorax and one on the posterior thorax. Even if you don't suspect a problem, be sure to assess respiratory excursion on the posterior thorax.

Now palpate for conditions that relate to your patient's cardiac status. With your patient in the supine position, stand at his right side and palpate the precordium using the palmar surface of your right hand. Begin at the apex, the fifth left ICS. Move to the left sternal border and then to the base (second left ICS). Feel for thrills (fine, rushing vibrations) or pulsations.

PERFORMING A BREAST EXAMINATION

To perform a breast examination, palpate each breast systematically with the pads of your fingers. Be sure to examine the entire breast, including the tail of Spence. If you feel lumps or lesions, be sure to describe fully their size, location, texture, mobility, and whether they are painful to the patient.

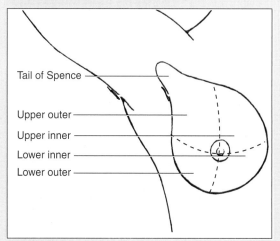

1. Before you begin, divide the breast into imaginary segments. If you find a lump or lesion, use these terms to describe its location.

2. Palpate gently but firmly in a counterclockwise pattern, starting at the outside of the breast and working slowly inward.

3. Now palpate the tail of Spence. Repeat the circular pattern, pushing deeper and more heavily. Don't lift your fingers off the breast as you move from point to point.

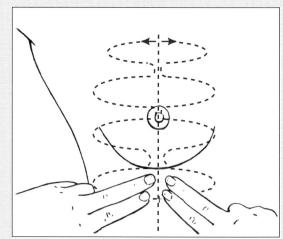

4. As an alternative, you can use a parallel, washboard pattern. Finally, gently compress the nipple between your fingers to check for discharge.

PALPATING FOR TACTILE FREMITUS

To palpate for tactile fremitus, place the palmar surfaces of both hands on the right and left sides of your patient's anterior thorax, at the second intercostal space (ICS).

Ask your patient to say "99" and keep repeating it as you gradually move your hands over the patient's chest, systematically comparing the lung fields. Start at the center. Move toward the periphery, then back toward the center. Gently displace a female patient's breasts, as necessary.

Repeat this procedure on the patient's back, starting from the top of the suprascapular area to the interscapular, infrascapular, and hypochondriac areas at the level of the 5th ICS and 10th ICS, right and left of the midline.

You should feel vibrations of equal intensity on either side of the midline. Tactile fremitus is palpated most commonly in the upper chest near the bronchi. It's typically strongest around the second ICS, although the vibrations may vary in intensity with the patient's chest wall structure and voice intensity and pitch.

If you feel increased tactile fremitus in one or both lungs, your patient may have inflammation, infection, congestion, or consolidation of a lung or part of a lung. If tactile fremitus is diminished or absent in one or both lungs, this may indicate the presence of pleural effusion or pneumothorax.

Note the location of the cardiac impulse, the point of maximum impulse. Positioning your patient on his left side may help you locate the cardiac impulse.

LIFESPAN CONSIDERATIONS

The point of maximum impulse may be more difficult to palpate in an older adult with increased thoracic anterior-posterior diameter.

Palpate the epigastric area for pulsation.

Now, with the patient in the supine position, complete your examination of the female breast. Have the patient raise her arm over her head. Place a small pillow under that shoulder and palpate the breast as described earlier. Repeat for the opposite side.

Back

Continue your examination with your patient in an upright position, standing or sitting. Face his back. Palpate the posterior thorax, noting any bulging, depressions, sinus tracts, nodules, masses, areas of tenderness, vibration on inspiration, or unusual movement. Palpate the scapulae, ribs, and thoracic spine for flexibility and tenderness.

Evaluate tactile fremitus in the posterior chest, comparing symmetrical areas of the lungs. Note any localized areas of increased or decreased fremitus. Move downward while noting where fremitus ends.

Assess respiratory excursion by placing your thumbs at the level of the 10th rib on either side of the vertebrae. The palms of your hands should lightly contact the posterior-lateral surface of the rib cage. Slide your thumbs medially to raise a loose skinfold between your thumbs and the spine. Watch your thumbs diverge during quiet, normal breathing, and then ask your patient to inhale deeply. Feel for the range and symmetry of respiratory movement.

Palpate the costovertebral angle by placing the palm of your hand over the right costovertebral angle and striking your hand with the ulnar surface of the fist of your other hand (also known as blunt percussion). Repeat over the left costovertebral angle. Normally, the patient should perceive this procedure as a dull thud. Make note if the patient feels any tenderness or pain. (See *Checking for Costovertebral Angle Tenderness.*)

With your patient standing, check his range of spinal motion. Watch from behind while your patient bends forward (flexion). You can also place two to three fingers of the same hand adjacent to the spinal processes as he bends forward. Note their separation. Also inspect the spine again for normal and abnormal curvature.

Now ask your patient to bend back at the waist as far as possible (hyperflexion). Then have him bend to each side as far as possible and

---

CHECKING FOR COSTOVERTEBRAL ANGLE TENDERNESS

Check for tenderness at the costovertebral angle by percussing it during your assessment of your patient's posterior thorax.

Percussion at this site should not be painful to your patient. However, if the area does feel tender, you may need to consider other diagnostic tools to determine the source of discomfort, which may be kidney infection.

rotate his upper trunk in a circular motion. Finally, ask him to lean forward and rest his weight on the examination table, with his arms straight and with hands palms-down. Palpate the paravertebral muscles and along the spinal processes. Note any tenderness, herniated disks, or muscle spasms.

Normal findings

- In females, breast tissue dense, firm, and elastic. Generalized nodularity and tenderness is common during the menstrual cycle.
- Axillary and supraclavicular lymph nodes not palpable.
- Rib cage bilaterally symmetrical; ribs slightly elastic but sternum, xiphoid process, and thoracic spine inflexible.
- Scapulae equal in height, with no "winging" upon movement.
- Ribs extended at about a 45-degree angle to the vertebrae.
- Skin smooth, without lesions, scars, or sinus tract openings; skin over bony prominences intact; no redness or edema.
- Skin warm and dry or slightly moist if the patient is anxious or has a fever; normal turgor with no edema.
- No crepitus or vibration palpated on inspiration.
- Fremitus prominent and symmetrical over large bronchi, except for a slight increase over the right upper lobe. Fremitus varies with the intensity and pitch of the patient's voice and chest wall structure and thickness.
- Thorax expanded at least 5 cm and symmetrical in adults.
- Costovertebral angle with no tenderness or pain.
- Cardiac impulse gentle and brief, aligned with the midclavicular line in the fifth left ICS. It may be displaced upward in pregnancy or located on the right side in dextrocardia.
- Abdominal aortic pulsation palpable in the epigastric region of a thin patient.
- Diaphragm slightly higher on the right side because of the liver.
- Spinal curve convex (outward) at the thorax area and concave (inward) at the lumbar area.
- Spinal column with no lateral curvature.
- Shoulders and iliac crests equal in height.
- Back symmetrically flat, with a lumbar concavity convex on flexion. Expect forward flexion of 75 to 90 degrees. Spinous processes should separate. Hyperflexion is normally 30 degrees. Lateral bending is normally 35 degrees. The trunk should rotate 30 degrees in each direction.
- Spinous processes with no tenderness or muscle spasms.

Abnormal findings

- Nodules in the female or male breast, possibly indicating malignant tumor, benign cyst, or fibroadenoma. (See *Breast Cancer,* p. 160.)

DISORDER CLOSE-UP

BREAST CANCER

Breast cancer is the leading cause of cancer deaths among females in the United States and Europe. Its exact cause is unknown. However, it has been linked to a number of risk factors, including a family history of breast cancer, early menarche, delayed pregnancy, and such environmental factors as exposure to radiation and use of hormone therapy.

Malignant cells usually originate in the epithelial tissue of the breast. The majority develop in the ductal system; the minority develop in the lobar system. The upper outer quadrant is the most common site of cancer. About half of all breast cancers are found here and in the tail of Spence.

The uncontrolled growth of cancer cells within the breast tissue begins with a single cell that divides, or doubles, in 30 to 210 days. After 16 such doublings, the mass reaches a size of 1 cm or more. At this stage, it can be clinically detected. As it continues to grow, the tumor may attach to the chest wall. It also may spread to the regional lymph nodes, primarily the axillary nodes. The cells metastasize easily, breaking away from the main tumor and traveling through the lymphatic system and blood stream to other sites, such as the lungs, liver, and bones.

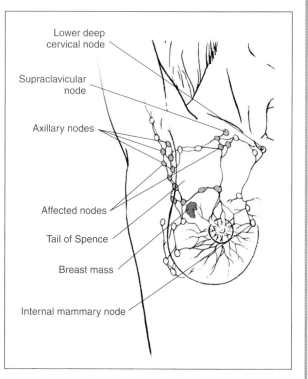

Health history
- Painless lump or mass in the breast
- Thickening of breast tissue
- Family history of breast cancer, especially among first-degree relatives, such as sisters, mother, and daughters.
- Premenopausal female over age 45
- History of long menstrual cycle, early menarche, or late menopause
- First pregnancy after age 35
- History of radiation exposure or estrogen hormone therapy
- History of preexisting fibrocystic breast disease

Characteristic findings
Expect your physical examination findings to vary among patients with breast cancer, depending on the extent and severity of the disease and its progression. Use the information that follows to help distinguish between expected and unexpected findings.

Inspection
- Nipple discharge (clear, milky, or bloody)
- Nipple retraction
- Scaling around nipple area
- Dimpling of breast tissue and peau d'orange appearance
- Increased vascularity
- Pain or tenderness
- Arm edema (may indicate advanced disease)

Palpation
- Hard lump, mass, or thickening of tissue
- Expression of fluid from nipple
- Enlarged supraclavicular and axillary lymph nodes, with possible palpable lumps

Complications
- Infection
- Bone metastasis, with decreased mobility and possible fractures
- Central nervous system metastasis
- Respiratory system metastasis

- Lymph node enlargement, possibly indicating infection or malignancy. Biopsy may be needed.
- Chest asymmetry, possibly resulting from thoracic deformities or pneumothorax.
- Tenderness in pectoral muscles, costal cartilages, or ribs, possibly indicating musculoskeletal inflammation, local trauma, tumor, or underlying pleural inflammation (as with pneumonia or pulmonary infarction).
- Crepitus, indicating air in the subcutaneous tissue from a rupture somewhere in the respiratory system. It may occur with emphysema or pneumothorax.
- Intermittent bubbling sound only on inspiration and clearing with a cough, suggesting coarse crackles.
- Scraping or grating sound on inspiration and possibly expiration, suggesting a pleural friction rub, caused by inflammation of the pleural surfaces.
- Absent or decreased fremitus, suggesting bronchial obstruction, pneumothorax, pleural effusion, pulmonary edema, emphysema, or chest wall edema or increased thickness.
- Increased fremitus, revealing areas of consolidation (as in pneumonia), heavy bronchial secretions, a tumor, or compressed lung tissue.
- Respiratory excursion that reveals loss of symmetry or impairment of thoracic movement, suggesting underlying disease of the lung and pleura on one or both sides.
- Forceful or widely distributed cardiac impulse, signaling increased cardiac output (as in anemia, hyperthyroidism, or fever) or left ventricular enlargement.
- Thrills, possibly resulting from valve disease.
- Pulsations in locations other than the cardiac impulse region, possibly indicating right ventricular enlargement, pulmonary artery dilation, or abdominal aortic aneurysm.
- Skin breakdown, especially in bedridden patients and over bony prominences, possibly resulting in pressure ulcers.
- Dependent edema in the sacral area of a bedridden patient.
- Barrel-shaped thorax, associated with respiratory disease or possibly aging.
- Chest structure abnormalities, possibly resulting from thoracic kyphoscoliosis.
- Winged scapulae, indicating injury to the nerve of the anterior serratus muscle.
- Horizontal slope to the ribs, possibly indicating emphysema.
- Asymmetrical thoracic expansion during respiration, possibly resulting from a collapsed lung or a mass.
- Intercostal bulging or retraction, possibly indicating pulmonary disease or bronchial obstruction.

- Poor posture, with causes ranging from osteoporosis to poor personal habits.
- Abnormal spinal curvature, possibly suggesting scoliosis, kyphosis, or lordosis. Scoliosis (lateral curvature) can be structural or functional and is becoming more common. Kyphosis (accentuated convex thoracic curvature) may be observed in aging adults, especially females. Lordosis (accentuated concave lumbar curvature) occurs in pregnancy and obesity.
- Abnormalities in shoulder contour and height, suggesting spinal column misalignment or shoulder dislocation.
- Unequal heights of the iliac crests, possibly suggesting legs of different lengths or a deformity in the hips.
- Persistence of lumbar concavity and failure of the spinous processes to separate on flexion, suggesting arthritis of the spine (spondylitis).
- Decreased spinal mobility, possibly resulting from degenerative joint disease or ankylosing spondylitis.
- Spinal tenderness, possibly suggesting rheumatoid arthritis, osteoporosis, infection, or malignancy involving the spine.
- Herniated intervertebral disks, producing tenderness of the spinous processes, intervertebral joints, sacroiliac notch, and sciatic nerve, as well as paravertebral muscle spasm and tenderness.
- Costovertebral tenderness, possibly indicating kidney infection.

Percussion

Percussion of the chest and back is used to identify the left ventricular border of the heart, the depth of diaphragmatic excursion in the upper abdomen during breathing, the border between the right lung and the liver, and the border between the left lung and the stomach. Percussion can be used to help identify disorders that impair lung ventilation, such as stomach distention, hemothorax from postthoracotomy bleeding, lobar consolidation, and pneumothorax.

Chest

Begin by having your patient lie on his back in a comfortable position. You'll be percussing from the supraclavicular area to the midabdominal area and out to the sides. If your female patient has large breasts, have her lift them while you percuss the area. If she can't do so, you'll need to displace each breast with your nondominant hand as you percuss with your dominant hand. Avoid percussing over the clavicles, breast tissue, and heart. Beginning with the supraclavicular areas, alternating from one side to the other. (See ⬛ *Percussing the Chest and Back.*)

Work your way down the anterior chest, percussing over each ICS. Remember to percuss over the same area on each side for comparison.

At the point on the right side where the sound changes from resonant to dull, you are percussing over the border between the lungs and the liver.

EXAMINATION TIP

PERCUSSING THE CHEST AND BACK

When percussing your patient's chest and back, work your way back and forth across the thorax in a systematic fashion, comparing one side of the body to the other as you go. Keep in mind that you'll follow the same pattern when auscultating breath sounds. The following illustrations show typical percussion patterns for assessing the chest and back.

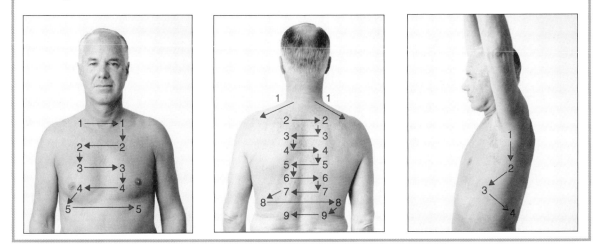

As the diaphragm contracts with each inspiration, the lungs descend, and the border between the lungs and the liver moves down a few inches. This is called diaphragmatic excursion. (See *Measuring Diaphragmatic Excursion,* p. 164.)

As you percuss down the left side of the chest, the sound changes from resonant to tympanic over the gastric air bubble of the stomach. Although X-rays are more accurate, percussion can be used to identify the border of the left side of the heart. You can use percussion to determine whether your patient's heart is enlarged or displaced.

With your patient lying on his back, place his left arm over his head and rest it on a pillow. Locate the fourth left ICS along the axillary line. It should be just below the axilla. Starting at the axillary line, percuss medially toward the sternum, in the ICS. When the sound changes from resonant to dull, you have identified the cardiac border. Use a pen to mark this point.

Now repeat the procedure, starting at the fifth left ICS. Then use the sixth left ICS. Each time, mark the location where the sound changes. For a more detailed assessment, you can start at the second or third ICS. Because the right cardiac border is hidden by the sternum, it can't be percussed in most cases.

MEASURING DIAPHRAGMATIC EXCURSION

To assess diaphragmatic excursion, you'll need a centimeter ruler and a washable marking pen. With your patient seated upright with his back exposed, ask him to take a deep breath and hold it. Then begin percussing at the base of his right scapula and move downward toward his diaphragm.

When you detect a change from resonance to dullness, you'll have found your first anatomical landmark. Tell your patient to breathe and place a mark at this site before continuing to the next step.

Now, ask your patient to exhale as much as possible and hold it. This time, begin percussing at your first landmark, and move upward on the posterior thorax toward the scapula. When you notice a change from dullness to resonance, you'll have found the second landmark. Place a mark at this site, and repeat this technique on the other side of the patient's posterior thorax, so you can compare measurements on the right and left sides.

Once you obtain your two landmarks, measure the distance from one line to the other to determine diaphragmatic excursion. Normal excursion distance is 3 to 5 cm. Keep in mind that the diaphragm is usually higher on the right than on the left because of the position of the liver.

Back

Ask your patient to sit with both arms crossed in front or resting on a bedside table. Move to the other side of the bed to percuss your patient's back. If possible, have your patient lean forward into his lap, with arms crossed and neck flexed. By separating the scapulae and ICSs, this position exposes more lung. Remember not to percuss over the scapulae or the spine.

As you percuss the back, you'll again move from side to side to compare and contrast your findings. Percuss between the ICSs on each side. When you reach the lower back area, stand somewhat to the side rather than directly behind your patient. This hand position will feel more natural, and you'll produce a clearer sound. Remember that, because your patient is breathing and the diaphragm is moving, you may not percuss a distinct diaphragmatic border.

With the same procedure you used for the anterior chest, measure for diaphragmatic excursion. Finally, ask your patient to rest his arm on his head, and percuss along the midaxillary line at 2-inch intervals.

Normal findings

- Band of resonance about 2 inches wide (also known as Krönig's isthmus) between the neck and shoulder on each side as you percuss the apices.

- Resonant sounds over the lungs until you reach the diaphragm. This will be at about T10 on your patient's back. It may be one ICS higher on the right side because of displacement by the liver.
- Area of dullness to the left of the sternum between the third ICS and fifth ICS that is produced by the heart.
- Dullness over the diaphragm.
- Diaphragmatic excursion about 1¼ to 2¼ inches and almost equal in length on both sides.

Abnormal findings

- Dullness over the lungs during percussion, possibly indicating a mass or consolidation. The dullness of right middle-lobe pneumonia typically occurs behind the right breast. (See 🔲 *Pneumonia,* p. 166.)
- Hyperresonance over the lungs, indicating hyperinflated or emphysematous lungs. Hyperresonance heard on only one side may indicate a pneumothorax.
- High diaphragmatic excursion on one side, suggesting a pleural effusion or high diaphragm, possibly resulting from diaphragmatic (phrenic nerve) paralysis, stomach distention (left side), hepatomegaly (right side), or significant atelectasis.
- Bilaterally low diaphragm level at rest, indicating a depressed diaphragm, usually from a severely hyperinflated chest associated with emphysema or asthma.
- Unilaterally low diaphragm level at rest, resulting from tension pneumothorax.

Auscultation

Ask your patient to sit up straight. If he can't sit up, have him lie down and roll to one side and then the other side. Raise the head of the bed 30 to 45 degrees. In either position, ask him to remain still and breathe normally while you auscultate heart and breath sounds. Before listening, prepare the patient and his environment for optimal results. (See 🔲 *Auscultating Heart and Breath Sounds: Tips for Success,* p. 167.)

Heart sounds

The heart makes characteristic sounds that reflect its activity. By auscultating these sounds carefully and identifying abnormal sounds accurately, you can detect a number of serious cardiac disorders. (See *Sounds of the Cardiac Cycle,* p. 168.)

Before beginning auscultation, warm the diaphragm and bell of your stethoscope by rubbing them between your hands. You'll use the diaphragm to hear higher-pitched heart sounds, such as S_1, S_2, murmurs of aortic and mitral regurgitation, pericardial friction rubs, and lung sounds.

PNEUMONIA

Pneumonia is an acute lung inflammation caused by an infection with one or more organisms, such as bacteria, viruses, and fungi. Pneumonia also may result from aspiration of food, fluids, or vomitus or inhalation of toxic or caustic chemicals, smoke, dust, or gases. The disorder may occur as a complication of immobility and chronic illnesses, and it often follows influenza. Pneumonia can involve lung tissue in part or all of a lobe, or it can occur diffusely.

Pneumonia is most likely to occur when normal defense mechanisms are weakened or overcome. This is especially likely in a patient who has a decreased level of consciousness, is immunocompromised, or has a portal for microorganisms, such as an endotracheal tube.

In bacterial pneumonia, bacteria initiate a massive inflammatory reaction in the alveoli. When chemical mediators cause pulmonary capillaries and other vessels to dilate, they become more permeable to fluid, fibrin, and red and white blood cells, creating exudate. The exudate-filled airways and alveoli cause the normally air-filled lung tissue to consolidate, stiffen, and impair gas exchange. If pneumonia affects large areas of lung tissue, hypoxemia and respiratory failure can ensue.

In viral pneumonia, interstitial inflammation and desquamation occur in the bronchiolar epithelial and goblet cells and bronchial mucous glands, impairing mucociliary clearance. Eventually, the alveoli fill with exudate, which can diminish gas exchange. While viral pneumonia is usually mild and self-limiting, the patient can develop a secondary bacterial pneumonia.

Health history
- History of influenza
- History of exposure to noxious gases
- Immobilization
- Decreased level of consciousness
- Nasogastric tube feedings
- Endotracheal intubation and mechanical ventilation
- Complaints of fever, chills, sweats
- Headache, fatigue
- Chest pain
- Cough

Characteristic findings
Expect your physical examination findings to vary among patients with pneumonia depending on the extent and severity of the disease. Use the following information to help distinguish between expected and unexpected findings.

Inspection
- Productive cough with sputum (color varies with type of infection)
- Dyspnea

Palpation
- Increased tactile fremitus
- Unequal chest expansion

Percussion
- Dullness over affected area
- Decreased respiratory excursion on affected side

Auscultation
- Crackles (coarse)
- Wheezes (sonorous)
- Egophony
- Bronchophony
- Whispered pectoriloquy

Vital signs
- Tachycardia
- Tachypnea
- Fever

Complications
- Septic shock
- Hypoxemia
- Respiratory failure
- Empyema, lung abscess
- Bacteremia
- Endocarditis, pericarditis
- Meningitis

EXAMINATION TIP

AUSCULTATING HEART AND BREATH SOUNDS: TIPS FOR SUCCESS

Auscultating heart and breath sounds can provide valuable information about your patient's health. However, because these sounds are not always easy to locate or to isolate from each other, a certain degree of skill and knowledge is required to perform this important component of the physical examination. Use these tips to auscultate heart and breath sounds quickly and thoroughly.

General tips

- Make sure the patient is warm and relaxed to minimize shivering and movement, which can increase abnormal sounds.
- Avoid listening over clothing; place the stethoscope directly on the skin.
- If the patient has a hairy chest or back, moisten the hair to avoid extraneous sounds that you could mistake for abnormal heart or breath sounds.
- Try to minimize ambient sounds by closing the door to the hallway and turning off unnecessary machines. If the patient is mechanically ventilated, consider asking a colleague to manually ventilate the patient while you auscultate.
- Find anatomical landmarks, such as intercostal spaces, to determine where you're listening at each point. Remember that many sounds, such as bronchial breath sounds, are normal only in certain locations.

Heart sounds

- With the patient in a supine position, instruct him to hold his breath momentarily as you listen for heart sounds. Signal him when to resume breathing.
- Listen to the entire precordium by inching from one spot to another to make sure that you've covered the major auscultatory areas.
- Take time to evaluate each area carefully before moving on. Once you've auscultated each area using the diaphragm, repeat the procedure using the bell of the stethoscope.
- When using the bell, remember to apply it to the chest wall lightly because excessive pressure will turn the bell into a diaphragm.

Breath sounds

- Have the patient sit upright—if possible—to listen to the anterior, lateral and posterior thorax. Position his arms overhead to listen to the lateral sites and folded across his chest for the posterior sites.
- Use a zigzag motion when moving your stethoscope to each position to compare sounds on each side.
- Pay careful attention to areas where palpation and percussion revealed abnormal findings. If the patient has dyspnea, auscultate these abnormal areas first—for example the lung bases—in case he fatigues during the examination.

LIFESPAN CONSIDERATIONS

Heart sounds may be more faint in an older adult with increased thoracic anterior-posterior diameter.

You'll use the bell to hear low-pitched sounds, such as S_3, S_4, and diastolic murmurs. As you auscultate, you'll need to be familiar with chest landmarks to aid in positioning the stethoscope and documenting your findings. (See *How and Where to Listen for Heart Sounds*, p. 169.)

SOUNDS OF THE CARDIAC CYCLE

The sounds you hear while auscultating your patient's heart reflect the physical events happening inside your patient's chest. In a normal heart, those events produce two characteristic heart sounds: S_1 and S_2.

Just before S_1, the mitral and tricuspid valves are open, and most of the blood in the atria is filling the relaxed ventricles. The atria then contract slightly, pushing about 30% more atrial blood into the ventricles. This atrial contraction is called the atrial kick.

Now the ventricles contract, beginning the period called systole. Pressure in the ventricles increases rapidly, forcing the mitral and tricuspid valves to close. The *lubb* sound produced by the closing of the valves, S_1, is the first sound you hear in the cardiac cycle in a patient with a normal, healthy heart. Although the mitral valve closes about 0.02 to 0.03 seconds before the tricuspid valve, the time difference is so small that you hear only one sound.

As ventricular pressure continues to increase, it causes the aortic and pulmonic valves to open, and blood is pumped out of the heart into the lungs and aorta. Once the ventricle ejects most of its blood, pressure begins to fall, and the aortic and pulmonic valves snap shut. The *dubb* sound produced by the closing of the valves, S_2, marks the beginning of diastole. The *dubb* of S_2 is slightly more highly pitched than the *lubb* of S_1.

S_1 and S_2 split

If enough time elapses between the closing of valves that normally close simultaneously, you may hear what's called a split S_1 or S_2. The first part of the split sound is closure of the left-sided heart valves (aortic or mitral); the second part is closure of the right-sided heart valves (pulmonic or tricuspid). S_1 splitting may be normal or may indicate a conduction disorder, such as right bundle-branch block. S_2 splitting that increases with inspiration and almost disappears with expiration is called physiologic splitting and is normal.

Begin auscultation with your patient's heart rate. To determine the heart rate (apical pulse) and rhythm, place the diaphragm of your stethoscope over your patient's point of maximum impulse (PMI), which is located at about the fifth ICS, left midclavicular line. You may need to palpate along this area to find the strongest pulse. Listen for 30 to 60 seconds, noting the rate, rhythm, quality of sound, and any extra or unusual sounds.

If your patient has a pacemaker, you'll need to know its normal settings and whether it's a demand or fixed device. This is one way of determining whether or not the pacemaker is malfunctioning. For example, if you auscultate your patient's heart rate at 50 beats per minute (bpm), and you know his pacemaker is set to activate when the ventricular rate is less than 60 bpm, you can suspect that his pacemaker is malfunctioning.

Describe the patient's rhythm as "regular," "regularly irregular," or "irregularly irregular." In ventricular trigeminy, where every third beat is a premature ventricular contraction (PVC), you might hear *lubb-dubb, lubb-dubb-lubb* in a pattern that repeats itself. This would be considered a regularly irregular rhythm. Atrial fibrillation, in which there is no pattern to the ventricular beats, is an example of an irregularly irregular rhythm.

HOW AND WHERE TO LISTEN FOR HEART SOUNDS

The table below provides tips on how to position your patient, what part of your stethoscope to use, and where to listen for specific heart sounds.

Heart sound	Patient position	Stethoscope part	Where to listen
S_1 (1st heart sound)	Any position	Diaphragm	• Entire precordium • Heard best at apex
S_2 (2nd heart sound)	Sitting or supine	Diaphragm	• Aortic area at 2nd right intercostal space (ICS) to the right of the sternum • Pulmonic area at 2nd left ICS to the left of the sternum
S_3 (3rd heart sound)	Supine or left lateral recumbent	Bell	• Apex
S_4 (4th heart sound)	Supine or left semilateral	Bell	• Apex
Murmur	High Fowler's and leaning slightly forward	Diaphragm and bell to differentiate between high-pitched and low-pitched sounds	• Entire precordium • Heard best over affected valve's auscultation site
Rub	Any position	Diaphragm	• Entire precordium • Heard best at 3rd ICS, left sternal border

If your patient has an irregular rhythm, you'll hear the heart rate speed up and slow down as you listen. To get an accurate rate, you'll need to listen for a full minute and carefully count the beats.

Keep in mind that some patients, such as those with a history of atrial fibrillation, normally have an irregular rhythm. To assess it accurately, you'll need to know your patient's baseline rhythm and heart rate range. If you have trouble hearing the heart rate, find your patient's carotid pulse, and palpate it as you listen with the stethoscope. You'll hear the first heart sound, S_1, at the same time you feel the pulse.

Next, listen for heart sounds over the aortic, pulmonic, mitral, and tricuspid areas. (See *Identifying Key Cardiac Auscultatory Areas,* p. 170.)

Continue using the diaphragm of your stethoscope. Have your patient breathe normally. Spend 10 or 15 seconds over each area. Take longer if you hear something unusual.

Work your way down the left sternal border as you listen over each ICS between the second and fifth ribs. Remember that heart sounds may not be detected in exactly the same location with every patient. Additionally, the angle of the heart can shift slightly in the chest if the patient has left or right ventricular hypertrophy, which will displace the best location to listen to the tricuspid and mitral valves.

IDENTIFYING KEY CARDIAC AUSCULTATORY AREAS

When listening for normal and abnormal heart sounds, it helps to locate the aortic, pulmonic, tricuspid, and mitral valve auscultatory areas, as well as areas to where sounds can be transmitted, such as Erb's point. To identify these key areas, palpate and count the intercostal spaces (ICSs). Remember that you can easily locate the second ICS by sliding your fingers laterally from the manubriosternal junction—where the sternum meets the second rib. As you move toward the heart's apex, you may need to displace breast tissue with your nondominant hand to accurately count the ICSs.

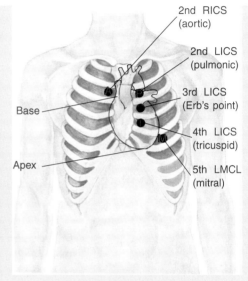

2nd RICS (aortic)

2nd LICS (pulmonic)

3rd LICS (Erb's point)

4th LICS (tricuspid)

5th LMCL (mitral)

Base

Apex

From Wilson, S. F. & Giddens. J. F. (2001). *Health Assessment for Nursing Practice* (2nd ed.). St. Louis: Mosby.

Initially, focus on the S_1 sound. It will be loudest over the mitral and tricuspid areas. Listen to its intensity and for the presence of splitting. This is best heard at the left sternal border.

Next, focus on S_2, which is loudest over the aortic and pulmonic areas. To try to hear a split S_2, have your patient hold his breath for a few seconds while you listen. Then have him exhale, and listen again. You should hear the split during inspiration, and it should disappear during expiration. If the split occurs during inspiration *and* expiration, it's called fixed splitting.

Now check for S_3 and S_4, the extra heart sounds. S_3 is called a ventricular gallop. This faint, low-pitched sound is heard directly after S_2 and results from early, rapid filling of the ventricle with blood at the very beginning of diastole. It's heard best over the mitral valve area and sounds like *lubb-dup-ah*.

S_4 is called an atrial gallop. It's a low-frequency sound that occurs in conditions of increased ventricular stiffness. It's heard late in diastole, or just before S_1, and sounds like *ta-lup-dubb*. It may be hard to distinguish split heart sounds from S_3 and S_4. An occasional patient has both an S_3 and an S_4, producing a quadruple rhythm. If the heart is beating fast, you'll hear one loud extra sound called a summation gallop.

To listen for an S_3 or S_4, have your patient roll partly onto his left side. This position helps accentuate a left-sided S_3 or S_4. Using the bell of your stethoscope, listen over the PMI. To help you determine whether you're hearing a split sound or an S_3 or S_4, have your patient sit up, lean forward, and inhale. Listen for the split S_2. Then listen while the patient exhales. If the split doesn't change, it may be either an S_3 or a fixed physiologic split.

S_4 is much harder to distinguish from a split S_1, but it's heard immediately before the S_1. Usually, a split heart sound is faster, and each part of the split has the same pitch. S_3 or S_4 may have a slightly lower pitch. Note the location you best hear the sounds and the timing, pitch, intensity, and effect of respirations. If the extra sounds differ from the "S" sounds in quality, pitch, and duration, you may be hearing a murmur. Also be aware that you may hear other sounds, including clicks, snaps, and rubs.

Murmurs. Murmurs are turbulent sounds made as blood flows across a sclerotic (stiff) or incompetent valve or through an abnormal heart wall opening. The turbulence is caused by disturbed blood flow through a small or rigid orifice. The smaller the orifice, the more resistance it creates and, often, the louder the murmur.

Most murmurs are associated with valve diseases, such as stenosis or insufficiency. Stenotic valves prevent forward blood flow. With valve insufficiency, or prolapse, the leaflets close improperly, resulting in backward blood flow.

Murmurs also can be caused by nonvalvular conditions, including ventricular septal defects (VSDs), sclerotic or aneurysmal arteries, hyperkinetic states, anemia, pregnancy, patent ductus arteriosus, narrowing of the aorta, and hypertrophic obstructive cardiomyopathy (HOCM), also known as idiopathic hypertrophic subaortic stenosis (IHSS).

Characterize a murmur by its timing, location, radiation, quality, pitch, shape, and duration. Start by identifying the murmur as systolic or diastolic. To do so, palpate your patient's carotid pulse as you listen. Systolic murmurs occur with S_1, or immediately after you feel the pulse, before S_2. Usually, they are harsh, high-pitched sounds in a *lubb-shh-dubb* pattern. If the patient has valve disease, the sound is produced either from forward flow through stenotic valves open during systole (the aortic and pulmonic) or from backward flow through closed but insufficient valves (the mitral and tricuspid). These are classified as ejection or regurgitant murmurs. Keep in mind that certain conditions or age-related changes can produce innocent systolic murmurs. (See *Understanding Causes of Innocent Murmurs,* p. 172.)

A diastolic murmur is heard after S_2. It's a much softer, lower-pitched sound in a *lubb-dubb-shh* pattern. Diastolic murmurs are produced either from forward blood flow through a stenotic mitral or tricuspid valve or from backward blood flow through an insufficient aortic or pulmonic valve.

LIFESPAN CONSIDERATIONS

UNDERSTANDING CAUSES OF INNOCENT MURMURS

Some murmurs have no apparent pathological cause and are therefore known as innocent murmurs. These innocent murmurs occur during systole and result from normal, physiologic changes related to age or pregnancy. Use this chart to help identify an innocent murmur and its cause.

Patient characteristics	Description of murmur	Possible cause
Children and adolescents	Early to midsystole, grade I or II, medium pitch, blowing, short, and nonradiating; best heard in 2nd intercostal space (ICS), left sternal border (LSB)	Forceful myocardial contractions coupled with increased blood flow
Children, ages 3 to 7 years	Musical or vibrating, nonradiating murmur that becomes softer when the child is inactive and quiet, and louder with activity; best heard in 3rd or 4th ICS, LSB (also known as Still's murmur)	Increased velocity of blood flow across aortic valve. Possible bands crossing the left ventricular outflow tract
Pregnant women	Systolic ejection murmur grade II to grade IV; may grow more intense with either inspiration or expiration. Best heard in 2nd ICS, right sternal border (RSB).	Increased blood volume related to pregnancy
Older adults	Early systole, grade I or II; best heard in second ICS, RSB	Increased length, tortuosity, and stiffening of aorta

The aortic and mitral valves are affected most often because of the high pressures on the left side of the heart.

Focus on the location, radiation, quality, pitch, shape, and duration of the murmur. Identify the place on the chest where you can hear the murmur best. Note whether the sound radiates to other chest areas. As you listen, remember the direction of blood flow, and try to follow the sound with your stethoscope. Include this direction in your documentation.

Note the quality of the murmur. Describe it as swooshing, heaving, whistling, musical, rumbling, roaring, or blowing. Use the most descriptive terms to document what you hear. You may need to be creative. Describe the pitch as high, medium, or low.

Next, describe the shape of the sound, a measure of the murmur's intensity over a period of time. It's described in four ways: crescendo (soft to loud), decrescendo (loud to soft), crescendo-decrescendo (gets loud, then gets softer), plateau (same loudness throughout).

Most murmurs can be heard with the diaphragm of your stethoscope. However, if your patient has a low-pitched, soft, blowing murmur, you'll hear it best if you use the bell of your stethoscope.

Keep in mind that the intensity of a murmur does not always correlate with your patient's condition. Consider a small VSD, for example. It may produce a loud murmur because the blood must travel through a small opening at high pressure. If the defect enlarges, the murmur will become softer because blood flow will meet less resistance. However, the larger defect may place your patient in greater hemodynamic compromise.

Finally, describe the murmur's duration and the place you hear it in the cycle. If you hear it only with ejection, document it as a systolic ejection murmur. You also can describe a murmur as "early," "early to mid," "mid," "mid to late," or "early to late," followed by the word systolic. If you hear the murmur throughout the cycle, document it as pansystolic or holosystolic.

Clicks. A click is an extra systolic sound usually associated with mitral valve prolapse. The best way to hear it is to ask your patient to sit up, lean forward, and exhale while you listen over the apex of his heart or the left sternal border. Use the diaphragm of your stethoscope. Having your patient squat or lie in the left lateral recumbent position will also help to bring out this sound. Clicks are usually mid or late systolic. Occasionally, they're early. Ask your patient to bear down (Valsalva's maneuver), and listen to see if the click intensifies.

If through your stethoscope you hear a click that sounds like cracking bone, usually at the end of inspiration and sometimes with expiration, you're probably hearing a sternal click. This is especially likely if your patient has recently had heart surgery with a thoracotomy. In fact, if the sternum hasn't fused yet, you may be able to palpate the sternal click.

Do not confuse this sternal click with a heart sound. If you suspect sternal instability could be causing your patient's click, palpate for it first. Then, as you auscultate, you'll be aware of it. You can feel it by having your patient take a deep breath and cough as you place the palm of your hand over the incision area.

If your patient has a mechanical heart valve, you'll hear a valve click that can sound somewhat like a ticking clock. It will have a different quality than the click of mitral valve prolapse.

Snaps. An opening snap is a very early diastolic sound caused by the opening of a thickened mitral valve. When diseased valve leaflets close, they may have a tendency to stick together. As the valve opens, the separation produces a snapping sound, something like a boat sail being suddenly filled with a gust of wind. This sound radiates toward the apex of the heart. It's softer with inspiration and louder with expiration. Its high-pitched snapping quality will help you distinguish it from an S_3 or a split S_2. It's usually accompanied by a diastolic murmur.

To hear this sound, have your patient lean onto his left side. Ask him to exhale. Starting at the left sternal border, move the diaphragm of your stethoscope toward the apex of the heart as you listen.

Rubs. A pericardial friction rub is a scratchy, scraping sound that gets louder when your patient exhales and leans forward. To hear it, listen with the diaphragm of your stethoscope over the third ICS at the left sternal border.

Commonly, the sound you hear will have two components, although occasionally it will have three. That's because the heart moves three times in the cardiac cycle: during atrial systole, ventricular systole, and ventricular diastole.

Atrial systole occurs immediately before ventricular systole, so they often combine to produce a single component of the sound. Ventricular diastole then produces another component.

Normal findings
- S_1 and S_2 sounds producing the *lubb-dubb* associated with normal valve closing.
- Ventricular rate between 60 and 100 bpm in a resting adult.
- Ventricular rate less than 60 bpm (bradycardia) in some young adults, athletes, or patients taking heart-slowing medications, such as beta-blockers.
- Rhythm consistent and regular, without extra beats.
- Systolic murmur in a young child.
- Valve click in a patient who has had a valve replacement.

Abnormal findings
- Heart rate less than 60 bpm, possibly indicating increased intracranial pressure (late sign), cardiac arrhythmias (such as heart block), parasympathetic or vagal stimulation, baroreceptor (carotid artery) stimulation, digitalis toxicity, or pacemaker malfunction.
- Heart rate more than 100 bpm (tachycardia), possibly indicating dehydration, sepsis, anxiety or sympathetic stimulation, cardiac arrhythmias (such as atrial fibrillation or ventricular tachycardia), hemorrhaging, effects of epinephrine and similar drugs, chemical stimulation (caffeine or nicotine), thyrotoxicosis, hypoxia, anemia, or heart failure.
- Irregular heart rhythm, possibly resulting from atrial fibrillation, premature or delayed ventricular contractions, premature atrial contractions, or heart block. (See ▩ *Correlating Pulse and Heart Sounds.*)
- Absent or muffled heart sounds, possibly resulting from blood or fluid collected in the pericardial sac. Even a small amount of fluid can cause a life-threatening emergency.
- Fixed split S_2, possibly associated with right ventricular failure.

EXAMINATION TIP

CORRELATING PULSE AND HEART SOUNDS

When assessing a patient with extra heart sounds, you may get a better understanding of those sounds when you correlate them with the patient's pulse.

To perform the procedure, you'll need your stethoscope and a quiet room. As you auscultate for heart sounds over the patient's apex, use your other hand to gently palpate the carotid artery at the same time. The carotid artery is best because it's closest to the heart.

As you auscultate, remember that S_1 is the sound you hear at virtually the same time you feel the patient's pulse.

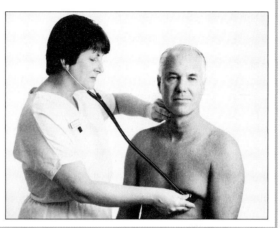

- Audible S_3, possibly an early sign of heart failure in patients over age 30. It's common in people under age 20 and is best heard in those with slow heart rates. It may be caused by the rapid filling of ventricles or slow filling of a ventricle that's already overfilled, as seen with heart failure.
- Audible S_4, possibly resulting from myocardial infarction and ischemia and hypertension. It may be caused by the vibration of the forceful atrial contraction required to move blood into a stiff ventricle.
- Murmur, typically indicating valve disease, such as stenosis, insufficiency, incompetence, or regurgitation. Nonvalvular conditions that cause murmurs include VSDs, sclerotic or aneurysmal arteries, hyperkinetic states, anemia, pregnancy, HOCM, patent ductus arteriosus, and coarctation (narrowing) of the aorta. (See 📖 *Determining the Cause of Murmurs,* p. 176.)
- Click, or a sharp, high-pitched sound with a "clicking" quality, usually suggesting mitral valve prolapse.
- Opening snap, usually resulting from rheumatic heart disease.

Breath sounds

After listening for heart sounds, move on to breath sounds. The air flowing in and out of the structures of the lungs produces different types of sounds. They're described by location, duration, pitch, and quality.

INTERPRETING ABNORMAL FINDINGS

DETERMINING THE CAUSE OF MURMURS

When you auscultate a murmur during your assessment of heart sounds, keep in mind that a murmur can have several causes that are usually related to an alteration in a valve or other cardiac structure. To help pinpoint the probable cause, be sure to describe the murmur's pitch, quality, shape, and whether it occurs during systole or diastole. Also, look for any accompanying signs and symptoms or disorders. Use this chart to guide you.

Characteristics	Locations	Possible findings	Probable causes
High-pitched, blowing, holosystolic murmur, plateau-shaped	Heard best at apex of the heart with patient lying on left side; may radiate to axilla and back	Tachycardia, S_3 or S_4 heart sounds, split S_2; myocardial infarction (MI), papillary muscle rupture, endocarditis, heart failure	Mitral regurgitation
Medium-pitched, blowing, holosystolic murmur, increased intensity with inspiration, plateau-shaped	Heard best at 4th intercostal space (ICS), left sternal border (LSB), or area of xiphoid process	Fatigue, jaundice, anorexia; MI, endocarditis, heart failure	Tricuspid regurgitation
High-pitched, blowing, decrescendo diastolic murmur	Heard best at LSB, 2nd right ICS or 3rd left ICS while patient leans forward, holding his breath	Tachycardia, S_3; fatigue, cough, dyspnea on exertion, orthopnea, paroxysmal nocturnal dyspnea, pulmonary edema; endocarditis	Aortic regurgitation
High-pitched, blowing, decrescendo diastolic murmur	Heard best at LSB, 2nd right ICS or 3rd left ICS while patient leans forward, holding his breath	Dyspnea, pulmonary hypertension, jugular venous pulsation with increased v waves; endocarditis, cardiac trauma	Pulmonic regurgitation
High-pitched, loud, harsh holosystolic murmur	Heard best at 3rd to 5th ICSs along LSB	Dyspnea, chest pain, syncope, acute heart failure, shock; palpable precordial thrill, hypotension	Ventricular septal defect

When you begin, expect to follow an organized, systematic pattern, as you did for percussion.

As you listen through the precordial area, you'll hear bronchial and bronchovesicular breath sounds. (See *Identifying Characteristic Breath Sounds in the Chest and Back,* p. 178.)

These sounds give you information about the upper and middle airways of the patient's lungs. Although many common pulmonary problems occur in the lobes of the lungs, the patency of the upper airways is vital. If your patient is intubated, has recently been extubated, is asthmatic, has a tracheostomy, has had upper airway trauma or surgery, has had a

Characteristics	Locations	Possible findings	Probable causes
Medium-pitched, harsh, midsystolic murmur, crescendo-decrescendo or diamond-shaped	Heard best at 2nd left ICS; may radiate to left shoulder and upward	Delayed capillary refill, cyanosis, possible palpable thrill, 2nd ICS, LSB; congenital heart disease	Pulmonic stenosis
Medium-pitched, harsh, midsystolic murmur, musical when heard at apex; crescendo-decrescendo or diamond-shaped	Heard best at 2nd right ICS; radiates to neck and down LSB or apex	Syncope, angina, exertional dyspnea, possible palpable thrill, 2nd ICS, right sternal border (RSB); left ventricular hypertrophy, rheumatic heart disease, atherosclerosis, congenital heart disease	Aortic stenosis
Low-pitched sound with rumbling quality, mid- and late-diastolic murmur; decrescendo-crescendo-shaped; intensifies with expiration	Heard best over 5th ICS along midclavicular line; radiates very little; best heard with bell of stethoscope	Fatigue, exertional dyspnea, atrial fibrillation, right parasternal lift, decreased pulse amplitude; may also have mitral regurgitation; rheumatic heart disease	Mitral stenosis
Low-pitched sound with rumbling quality, mid- and late-diastolic murmur; decrescendo-crescendo-shaped; intensifies with inspiration	Heard best over 4th ICS along LSB; radiates very little; best heard with bell of stethoscope	Fatigue, hepatomegaly, decreased pulse amplitude, increased jugular venous pulsation; rheumatic heart disease, right atrial myxoma	Tricuspid stenosis

pneumonectomy or a collapsed lung, or has had any condition involving tracheal or bronchial irritation, you may need to pay special attention to breath sounds in this area.

Begin your auscultation of breath sounds with the anterior chest. Raise your patient to the semi-Fowler's position, with the head of the bed at a 45- to 90-degree angle. Adjust the angle of the bed to the position most comfortable for him. If your patient has emphysema or chronic obstructive pulmonary disease (COPD), he may be more comfortable leaning over the bedside table, with his lips pursed and his arms resting on a pillow. As an alternative, you could ask him to sit on the edge of the bed and

IDENTIFYING CHARACTERISTIC BREATH SOUNDS IN THE CHEST AND BACK

As air enters the lungs through the upper airways, it produces different sounds at different locations based on the diameter of the airway, airway pressure, and vibrations. Depending on where you place your stethoscope on the thorax, normal breath sounds have varied pitch, intensity, and duration. To find the expected location of bronchial, bronchovesicular, and vesicular breath sounds, refer to these illustrations.

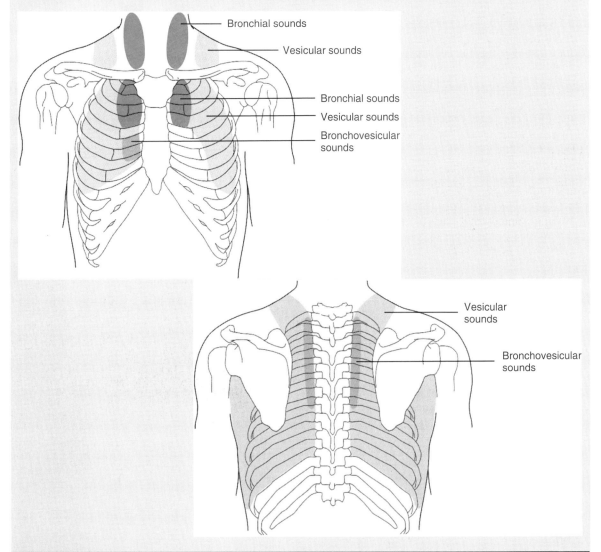

From Barkauskas, V. H., Baumann, L. C., & Darling-Fisher, C. S. (2002) *Health and Physical Assessment* (3rd ed.). St. Louis: Mosby.

dangle his feet. If your patient is short of breath, encourage him to take slow, deep breaths. Show him how to perform pursed-lipped breathing, if necessary.

If possible, encourage your patient to sit upright, look straight ahead with his chin up, and take deep breaths through his mouth. This will ensure maximum lung inflation with each breath. Ask your patient to take a breath each time you place your stethoscope on his chest. Listen for at least one full breath in each location. Be aware of your patient's comfort level. If he becomes light-headed, let him rest before you continue.

Start by listening over the trachea. Move the stethoscope from side to side, in the same position on each side, working your way down the chest. Repeat the pattern on the back. This method is used to compare and contrast what you're hearing from one side to the other.

Bronchial (sometimes called tracheal) breath sounds are loud, high-pitched, harsh, and hollow. To hear them, listen with the diaphragm of your stethoscope just medial to the cricoid cartilage and above the supraclavicular notch as your patient takes a deep breath. Typically, the inspiratory phase is about half the duration of the expiratory phase.

As you listen over your patient's bronchial area, you should also hear bronchial breath sounds. Listen over the right bronchus and then the left. Place the diaphragm of the stethoscope just above the clavicles on each side of the sternum, between the scapulae and over the manubrium. Because the right bronchus is more parallel to the sternum than the left, bronchial sounds may be more prominent on the right side. You'll hear high-pitched, blowing, muffled sounds. If you're listening to an intubated patient, expect to hear breath sounds over each bronchus. If you don't, the endotracheal tube may have slipped into one of the bronchi and only one lung is being aerated. Notify the physician immediately if this occurs.

You can auscultate bronchovesicular sounds at the apex of the right lung anteriorly, and posteriorly to both sides of the spine, between the scapulae. They're similar in quality to bronchial sounds but begin to take on a vesicular quality as you listen along the sides of the chest. Inspiration and expiration length will be equal.

Vesicular sounds are heard over most of the peripheral lung fields, in the areas away from the larger airways. They're soft, relatively low-pitched sounds that last throughout inspiration and fade quickly as expiration begins. Inspiration is three times the length of expiration, and the quality is breezy or swishing. As you move down the rib cage, listen to the right side, then to the left. Use similar locations on each side. As you reach the sides of the chest and bottom of the rib cage, you should hear vesicular breath sounds.

Also be sure to listen for adventitious (added) breath sounds. (The terminology has been changing over the years and is still evolving.) Breath sounds are divided into two categories: crackles (noncontinuous sounds) and wheezes (continuous sounds). Wheezes are divided into two categories: sibilant wheezes (formerly called wheezes) and sonorous wheezes (formerly called rhonchi). Listen for both normal and adventitious sounds, and document the type, duration, and location in the respiratory cycle.

Crackles and wheezes. Crackles are distinct, noncontinuous sounds of two types: fine and coarse. Fine crackles are thought to be caused by two mechanisms. One type of crackling sound occurs when alveoli in the lung bases "pop" open during inspiration, as with atelectasis or pulmonary fibrosis. The other type of crackle occurs in patients with pulmonary edema, probably from air bubbling through fluid. When you listen, you'll hear crinkling, popping, or even sounds like a slurping straw, usually at the beginning or end of inspiration. Rales and crepitus are older terms for fine crackles.

Typically, crackles that result from fluid are dependent. Fluid settles at the lowest portion of the lungs and the level ascends as the condition worsens. If your patient has been sitting upright, expect to hear them in the lung bases. Alternatively, if your patient has been lying on one side for several hours, the fine crackles will be more prominent in the lung on that side. In the final stages of heart failure, auscultation typically reveals continuous crackles, along with sibilant and sonorous wheezes (the so-called washing-machine chest).

If your patient has diffuse interstitial fibrosis, you may hear dry crackles that resemble the sound of crumpling cellophane or Velcro.

Coarse crackles and sonorous wheezes are current terms for what used to be called rhonchi. Although both can be caused by secretions in the tracheobronchial passages, they are dissimilar.

Coarse crackles are not continuous sounds, and they do not have a musical tone. Sonorous wheezes are low-pitched, continuous noises. They can also be heard in the presence of constriction, obstruction, or spasm of the large airways.

When you listen for coarse crackles, you'll hear loud bubbling or gurgling sounds during both inspiration and expiration but more commonly on expiration. These sounds are heard primarily in the trachea and bronchi, but they are also heard in the lower lobes of the lungs.

Expect to hear these sounds if your patient has pneumonia or bronchitis. If your patient cannot easily cough up secretions or has a loose, productive cough, you'll hear coarse crackles with or without a stethoscope. Often they can be remedied by suctioning, having your patient cough, respiratory treatments, or bronchodilators.

If you aren't sure whether you're hearing fine or coarse crackles, listen to your patient's lungs, have him cough a few times, and then listen again. Usually, coarse crackles will clear or diminish after coughing. Fine crackles caused by fluid or secretions will remain unchanged.

Sibilant wheezes are prolonged, high-pitched, musical or whistle sounds resulting from rapid airflow through narrowed airways and intraluminal smooth muscle contractions. They may be polyphonic (consisting of several pitches) or monophonic (a single pitch).

Sibilant wheezes are heard most often during or at the very end of expiration. Sometimes, however, they can be heard throughout the respiratory cycle. If you hear them bilaterally, they may indicate bronchospasm. They may or may not be associated with crackles and are not affected by coughing.

Other breath sounds. Stridor, a loud musical sound produced by upper airway obstruction, is heard commonly during childhood croup and doesn't require a stethoscope. It's typically inspiratory, but it becomes inspiratory and expiratory as the airway becomes more obstructed. To differentiate stridor from wheezes, listen over the trachea below the cricoid cartilage on one side of the neck. Stridor sounds loudest in this location, whereas wheezing is loudest in the chest.

Less commonly, you may encounter such sounds as friction rubs, referred breath sounds, and a mediastinal crunch. A pleural friction rub occurs during or at the end of inspiration and has a high-pitched, scratchy sound. Different from a pericardial rub, a pleural rub is heard with inspiration and disappears after expiration.

To determine whether a rub is pleural or pericardial, listen over the patient's heart while he holds his breath. If you hear a rub with each heartbeat, the rub is pericardial, not pleural.

Also keep in mind that pleural rubs have two components, not three. Occasionally, however, you may encounter a combination of both kinds of rubs, called pleuropericardial rub.

Referred breath sounds are noises heard over an area where you wouldn't normally expect to hear anything, such as on the side where your patient had a pneumonectomy or a lobectomy, or above a tracheostomy. Because sound travels through fluid and tissue, you may hear a faint inspiratory or vesicular sound over that area.

A mediastinal crunch (Hamman's sign) is a precordial crackling or crunching sound heard with each heartbeat, not with respirations. Nevertheless, it's still considered an abnormal breath sound. It has also been described as a high-pitched clicking or whooping. It's best heard with your patient in the left lateral position and usually disappears if your patient moves from the left to the right side.

Voice resonance. Another way to use auscultation to evaluate your patient's lungs is through vocalization, or voice resonance. This technique involves having your patient speak or whisper sounds while you listen to areas of the lungs through his chest and back. Vocal sounds generate vibrations that travel through the lungs and out to the chest wall. As these sounds travel through anatomical structures, their clarity is lost. If they travel through solids or fluids, on the other hand, their clarity remains or increases.

To assess voice resonance, place the diaphragm of the stethoscope over the same areas where you listened for lung sounds. Listen from top to bottom and side to side to compare and contrast sounds. First, ask your patient to say "99." See if the sound stays clear or softens. Next, have your patient say the letter "e." Note if "e" sounds like "e," or more like "a." Finally, have your patient whisper the numerals "1-2-3" while you listen. Note whether you can hear the sounds clearly or whether they become muffled.

Normal findings
- Bronchial breath sounds heard over the trachea and bronchi.
- Bronchovesicular breath sounds heard at the lung's right apex anteriorly and between the scapulae to about the middle of the back. Inspiration is equal to expiration.
- Vesicular breath sounds heard over the peripheral lung fields on the lower third of the back, out to the sides, and above the scapulae. Inspiration is three times the length of expiration.
- Loud and muffled "99" heard over the upper lung fields, becoming softer as you move down the back over the patient's lower lobes.
- Muffled "e" heard as auscultation progresses down the chest.
- Muffled noises heard as your patient whispers "1-2-3." (See ▥ *What to Expect When Examining the Chest and Back.*)

Abnormal findings
- Pericardial friction rub, developing when irritated or inflamed pericardial and epicardial surfaces rub against each other, as from swelling of the pericardium from infection (pericarditis), trauma, cardiac tamponade, uremia, myocardial infarction, and rubbing of mediastinal chest tubes (used for drainage after thoracic surgery).
- Soft, faint, wheezy, or absent breath sounds over the trachea.
- Coarse crackles, wheezing, or absent breath sounds over the precordial area.
- Coarse crackles or sonorous wheezes over the bronchial area, possibly indicating bronchitis when combined with a loose cough.
- Fine crackles, possibly associated with heart failure, pneumonia, or pulmonary fibrosis. If the crackles are caused by heart failure, you'll be able to hear them in the dependent portions of the patient's lungs. (See ▥ *Heart Failure,* p. 184.)
- Sibilant wheezes, usually resulting from edema, secretions, asthma, inhaled or mechanical irritants, or an allergic reaction.
- Bronchial or vesicular breath sounds in atypical areas.
- Absent breath sounds, possibly indicating a collapsed lobe or consolidation.
- Stridor, suggesting upper airway obstruction—as in childhood croup. It also suggests foreign body airway obstruction, laryngeal tumor, or tracheal stenosis.

NORMAL FINDINGS

WHAT TO EXPECT WHEN EXAMINING THE CHEST AND BACK

Use this review to confirm normal findings when examining the chest and back.

Inspection
- Anterior-posterior thorax dimension less than the transverse dimension by nearly half.
- Breasts with no nipple retractions, dimpling, discharge, erythema, or swelling.
- Respirations even, without involving accessory muscles.
- Spinal column straight.
- Bony prominences, with no evidence of skin breakdown.

Palpation
- Warm, dry skin free of lesions, masses, or areas of tenderness.
- Breasts free of lumps.
- Axillary and subclavian nodes nonpalpable.
- Voice vibration (fremitus) equal on either side of the sternum and spine. Fremitus may feel more intense over the second intercostal space (ICS) and the upper airways and less intense or absent over the precordium and lung bases.
- Equal respiratory excursion.

- Point of maximum cardiac impulse at the fifth ICS, and midclavicular line. It occupies a radius of no more than 1 cm.
- No tenderness at costovertebral angle.

Percussion
- Resonance over the lung fields.
- Dullness over the heart.
- Diaphragmatic excursion 3 to 5 cm.

Auscultation
- Bronchial sounds over the trachea.
- Bronchovesicular sounds over the mainstem bronchus and posteriorly between scapulae.
- Vesicular breath sounds throughout the remaining lung fields.
- Voice resonance audible but muffled and best heard medially toward the spine.
- S_1 loudest at the apex of the heart; S_2 loudest at the base. The splitting of S_2 on inspiration is a normal finding.
- Heart rate between 60 and 100 beats per minute while your patient is at rest.
- Heart rhythm regular.

- Mediastinal crunch, resulting from air trapped in the mediastinal space, usually from surgery, trauma, or a punctured lung.
- A clear and audible "99" (bronchophony), suggesting that the sound is traveling through fluid or a mass.
- Audible "a" as your patient repeats "e" (egophony), indicating a pleural effusion or lung consolidation.
- A clear and audible "1-2-3" as your patient whispers it (whispered pectoriloquy), possibly indicating a consolidation.

EXPLORING CHIEF COMPLAINTS

Chief complaints involving the chest and back may represent serious cardiac or respiratory disorders, including pneumonia, myocardial infarction, bronchitis, or heart failure. You should focus your assessment and

DISORDER CLOSE-UP

HEART FAILURE

Heart failure occurs when the heart can't pump enough blood to meet the body's metabolic requirements. Normally, the right and left ventricle work in synchrony to contract and eject blood in a forward fashion. In order to maintain a normal stroke volume—or the amount of blood that the ventricle ejects with each beat—the ventricles must fill and maintain sufficient preload (tension against the ventricular walls). Then, cardiac cells, called myocytes, must contract with enough force to overcome afterload (the pressure or resistance the heart pumps against).

In systolic heart failure, myocardial function is depressed when one or both ventricles can't contract and eject blood sufficiently, despite elevated filling pressures. In diastolic heart failure, stiffened ventricular walls increase tension and end-diastolic pressure, and the ventricles can't relax and expand to accept enough blood to maintain adequate stroke volume.

Heart failure can be acute or chronic and stem from many causes. Most commonly, the cause is ischemic heart disease, including myocardial infarction. Other causes include viral cardiomyopathy, valvular heart disease, and arrhythmias. Usually, heart failure stems from dysfunction of the left ventricle—the heart's main pumping chamber—but it can also result from right ventricular or biventricular failure. Whatever the cause, heart failure is often further complicated by the activation of compensatory mechanisms, including the sympathetic nervous system and the renin-angiotensin-aldosterone system.

When assessing a patient with heart failure, keep in mind that the patient's signs and symptoms are related to either increased blood volume and organ congestion, low organ perfusion, or both. Signs and symptoms of organ congestion include weight gain (often sudden), hepatomegaly, increased jugular vein distention (JVD), peripheral edema, orthopnea and paroxysmal nocturnal dyspnea (PND), and pulmonary crackles. Manifestations of low organ perfusion caused by diminished cardiac output are fatigue, confusion, renal dysfunction, and cool, pale extremities.

Health history
- Shortness of breath
- Chest pain
- Palpitations
- Dyspnea on exertion and at rest
- Activity intolerance
- PND
- Orthopnea
- Cough, usually dry, often at night
- Fatigue and weakness
- Insomnia
- Nocturia
- Confusion or inability to concentrate
- Anxiety

evaluate your patient completely. As always, keep your patient's health history in mind as you assess his chief complaint.

Chest pain

If your patient complains of chest pain, investigate the symptom further by asking him the following questions:
- When did the pain start?
- What were you doing when it started?
- How would you rate the pain on a scale of 1 to 10, with 10 being the worst pain you've ever felt? Is it worse or better now?
- Where in your chest is the pain located?
- Does the pain radiate anywhere?

- Unexplained weight gain
- Complaints of shoes or rings being tight
- Ankle swelling
- Anorexia and nausea

Characteristic findings

Expect your physical examination findings to vary among patients with heart failure depending on the extent and severity of the disease. Use the following information to help distinguish between expected and unexpected findings.

Inspection
- Mental confusion
- Diaphoresis
- Breathlessness
- Orthopnea
- Cough
- Anxiety
- Cyanosis of nail beds and lips
- Neck vein pulsations
- JVD
- Peripheral dependent edema

Palpation
- Enlarged or displaced apical impulse
- Cool, clammy skin
- Hepatomegaly
- Hepatojugular reflex
- Abdominal pain or tenderness

- Splenomegaly
- Abdominal distention

Percussion
- Dullness over lung bases (pleural effusions)
- Increased liver size
- Shifting dullness

Auscultation
- Crackles
- Gallop heart sounds, S_3, S_4
- Sonorous wheezing
- Expiratory wheezing
- Diminished sounds (especially at bases)

Vital signs
- Narrowed pulse pressure
- Tachypnea
- Pulsus alternans
- Tachycardia

Complications
- Pulmonary edema
- Decreased perfusion to major body organs and ischemia
- Myocardial infarction
- Arrhythmias
- Sudden death

- What type of pain is it? Sharp, heavy, radiating, crushing?
- Are you short of breath, sweaty, or nauseated? Do you cough? Do you have a fever?
- Does anything make the pain feel better, such as resting or taking nitroglycerin?
- Does anything make it worse, such as taking deep breaths or coughing?
- Would you describe this pain as being like anything you've ever experienced before?
- Is this a chronic problem? Does the pain occur more frequently or less frequently with exertion? Have you had to cut back on your activities because of it?

Focusing your assessment
When a patient complains of chest pain, focus your assessment as follows:
- Observe your patient's general appearance. Is he short of breath or diaphoretic? A diaphoretic patient with cool extremities may be in cardiogenic shock.
- Check his vital signs. Hypotension and tachycardia may be signs of cardiogenic shock.
- Auscultate heart sounds. Listen for irregularity, gallop, or murmur. A patient with recent infarcts may have a new murmur, indicating a life-threatening ruptured papillary muscle or VSD.
- Examine the neck veins for jugular venous distention, which could indicate heart failure.

DISORDER CLOSE-UP

MYOCARDIAL INFARCTION

A myocardial infarction (MI) occurs when a coronary artery becomes critically occluded, blocking blood flow to part of the cardiac muscle. The occlusion usually stems from a thrombus at the site of a ruptured atherosclerotic plaque or from prolonged vasospasm. If cells are deprived of oxygen and nutrients long enough, irreversible hypoxemic damage causes cell death and tissue necrosis.

Infarcted tissue has a central necrotic area surrounded by an injured zone. The injured zone is surrounded by an ischemic zone. Necrotic cells no longer function metabolically, and they don't produce or conduct electrical energy or participate in mechanical contraction. Tissue in the ischemic and injured areas, however, remains viable. Quick return of blood flow can minimize the amount of tissue lost. You can use the patient's electrocardiogram (ECG) to help determine the size and location of the three zones.

Health history
- History of atherosclerosis, coronary artery disease, or hyperlipoproteinemia
- Family history of heart disease
- Smoking
- History of hypertension

- Sedentary lifestyle, obesity
- Complaints of crushing, substernal chest pain radiating to left arm, jaw, neck, or shoulder blades
- Complaints of indigestion or heartburn
- Increasing frequency of angina
- Feeling of impending doom
- Fatigue
- Nausea and vomiting
- Shortness of breath

Characteristic findings
Expect your physical examination findings to vary among patients with MI, depending on the extent and severity of the disease. Use the information that follows to help distinguish between expected and unexpected findings.

Inspection
- Anxiety and restlessness
- Dyspnea
- Diaphoresis
- Jugular venous distention

Palpation
- Cool, mottled skin
- Diminished peripheral pulses

- Auscultate breath sounds. Coarse or fine crackles may indicate heart failure.
- Palpate the chest wall. Point tenderness over the rib cartilage may indicate costochondritis.

Possible causes

- *Myocardial infarction.* The classic symptom of myocardial infarction is persistent crushing chest pain that may radiate to the left arm, jaw, neck, or shoulder blades. Pain associated with exertion or a heavy meal may also indicate ischemia. Rest or nitroglycerin may relieve the pain. An elderly or diabetic patient may have no pain at all. (See *Myocardial Infarction.*)

Auscultation
- S_4 or S_3 heart sounds
- Paradoxical splitting of S_2
- Systolic murmur
- Pericardial friction rub (transmural MI)

Vital signs
- Tachycardia and hypertension (anterior MI)
- Bradycardia and hypotension (inferior MI)

Complications
- Arrhythmias
- Cardiogenic shock
- Heart failure
- Rupture of atrial or ventricular septum
- Ventricular aneurysms
- Cerebral or pulmonary embolism
- Reinfarction
- Post-MI pericarditis

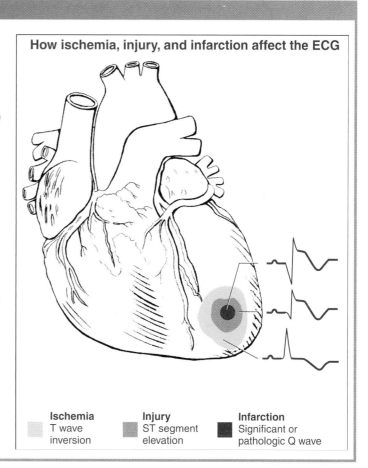

How ischemia, injury, and infarction affect the ECG

Ischemia	**Injury**	**Infarction**
T wave inversion	ST segment elevation	Significant or pathologic Q wave

- *Costochondritis (Tietze's syndrome).* One of the most common causes of chest pain, costochondritis may be associated with trauma or exercise and commonly follows viral illness. With costochondritis, pain usually occurs over the second, third, and fourth costochondral cartilages. Palpation directly over the cartilage generally produces point tenderness. (See ▨ *Determining Causes of Chest Pain.*)
- *Angina pectoris.* Characterized by pressing, squeezing chest pain or tightness, angina pectoris results from inadequate blood flow to the heart muscle. Typically, it's provoked by exertion, stress, or eating. It usually lasts from 1 to 3 minutes, but it can last longer. Nitroglycerin or rest will relieve the pain. (See ▨ *Angina Pectoris,* p. 191)
- *Pericarditis.* Usually a stabbing pain worsened by inspiration, movement, or lying down, pericarditis results from an inflammation of the pericardial sac.
- *Thoracic aortic aneurysm.* Pain associated with an aortic aneurysm extends to the neck, shoulders, lower back, or abdomen but rarely radiates to the jaw or arms.
- *Pulmonary embolism.* Chest pain associated with a pulmonary embolism is usually accompanied by dyspnea. The pain may mimic angina, or it may be pleuritic (worsening with a deep breath). Other signs include tachycardia, hemoptosis, and a low-grade fever. Less commonly, the patient may develop a pleural friction rub, cyanosis, or leg edema.
- *Pneumonia.* The most common signs of pneumonia are pleuritic chest pain, cough, sputum production, chills, and fever. Lung auscultation can vary from fine or coarse crackles to diminished or absent breath sounds.
- *Pneumothorax.* Sudden, sharp pleuritic pain is the classic sign of pneumothorax. The pain is usually accompanied by dyspnea and exacerbated by any movement of the chest wall, such as breathing or coughing. Chest wall movement may be asymmetrical. Breath sounds are often absent over the affected lung.
- *Cholecystitis.* The abdominal pain of gallbladder disease may radiate to the chest, back, or shoulder blades. Pain usually follows a high-fat meal or occurs at night, awakening the patient. Diaphoresis, belching, flatulence, nausea, vomiting, chills, and low-grade fever may also be present.
- *Peptic ulcer.* The pain of a peptic ulcer, usually described as gnawing or burning and worsening with an empty stomach, can radiate to the patient's chest and back, mimicking the pain a person experiences with myocardial ischemia.
- *Hiatal hernia.* Sharp, severe pain precipitated by lying down may be a sign of hiatal hernia. Antacids may relieve it.
- *Acute anxiety.* Chest pain that accompanies stress, in the absence of other physical explanations, may be a result of anxiety.

(Text continues on p. 192.)

INTERPRETING ABNORMAL FINDINGS

DETERMINING CAUSES OF CHEST PAIN

Although commonly associated with heart disease, chest pain can also result from pulmonary, gastrointestinal, musculoskeletal, and psychological disorders. If your patient complains of chest pain, you'll need to quickly focus your examination and intervene appropriately. Use this table to help determine its cause.

Characteristics	Locations	Possible findings	Probable causes
• Squeezing or aching sensation • Feeling of heaviness or burning • Provoked by exertion, emotional stress, eating • Usually lasts 1 to 3 minutes • Relieved by rest or nitroglycerin	• Substernal or retrosternal areas • May radiate to shoulders, arms, neck, lower jaw, or upper abdomen	• Increased heart rate • Increased blood pressure • Distant heart sounds • Atrial and ventricular gallops (S_3, S_4)	• Angina pectoris
• Pressing, squeezing or stabbing sensation • Feeling of tightness, heaviness, or burning • Sudden onset • May last from 30 minutes to several hours • Not relieved by rest, position change, or nitroglycerin • May be associated with nausea and vomiting	• Substernal or retrosternal areas or across the chest • May radiate to shoulders, arms, neck, lower jaw, or upper abdomen	• Anxiety, restlessness • Diaphoresis • Rapid, weak pulse • Fever • Variable blood pressure; initially elevated, unless cardiogenic shock is developing • Irregular heart rhythm • Distant heart sounds • Atrial and ventricular gallops (S_3, S_4) • Systolic murmur	• Myocardial infarction
• Stabbing pain worsened by deep inspiration, movement, or lying down • Sudden onset • May be relieved by sitting up or leaning forward	• Precordial or retrosternal areas • May radiate to shoulders, neck, arms, elbows, back	• Dyspnea • Fever, accompanied by diaphoresis, chills • Irregular heart rhythm • Pericardial friction rub	• Pericarditis
• Stabbing pleuritic pain • Sudden onset • May be relieved by high Fowler's position, other position changes, or chest splinting	• Over affected lung	• Sudden onset of dyspnea • Cough with hemoptysis • Cyanosis • Diaphoresis • Anxiety, restlessness • Low-grade fever • Hypotension • Tachypnea, tachycardia • Wheezing • Accentuated pulmonic heart sound • Pleural friction ruby	• Pulmonary embolus

Continued

INTERPRETING ABNORMAL FINDINGS

DETERMINING CAUSES OF CHEST PAIN—cont'd

Characteristics	Locations	Possible findings	Probable causes
• Severe, tearing pain • Sudden onset • May be associated with nausea and vomiting	• Anterior chest • May radiate to the neck, back, or abdomen	• Hypotension • Diaphoresis • Decreased, unequal, or absent peripheral pulses or weakness • Aortic regurgitation murmur	• Dissecting aortic aneurysm
• Stabbing pleuritic pain • Sudden onset • May be aggravated by movement, breathing, or coughing	• Lateral thorax • May radiate across the chest, over the abdomen, or to the shoulder on the affected side	• Sudden onset of dyspnea • Asymmetrical chest wall movement • Tachypnea • Cyanosis • Tracheal deviation • Tympany on percussion • Hyperresonance on affected side • Diminished-to-absent breath sounds over affected area	• Pneumothorax
• Gripping, sharp colicky pain • Usually precipitated by eating fatty foods or lying down • May lessen in 2 to 3 days and usually resolves within 1 week • May be associated with nausea and vomiting	• Right epigastric area or over abdomen • May radiate to right shoulder	• Splinting during deep inspiration • Low-grade fever • Involuntary guarding of right-sided abdominal muscles • Palpable gallbladder	• Cholecystitis
• Gnawing, burning pain that worsens with empty stomach • Occurs intermittently over a few weeks, subsides, then recurs • Temporarily relieved with food or antacids • May be associated with nausea and vomiting	• Epigastric area • May radiate to the back	• Belching • Abdominal bloating • Weight loss	• Peptic ulcer
• Sharp, severe pain precipitated by heavy meal, bending, or lying down • May be relieved by antacids, walking, or semi-Fowler's position	• Lower chest or upper abdominal areas	• No significant findings	• Hiatal hernia

DISORDER CLOSE-UP

ANGINA PECTORIS

There are three types of angina pectoris. *Stable angina* usually occurs when atherosclerosis narrows one or more coronary arteries and prevents them from dilating to provide increased blood flow to meet increased myocardial oxygen demand—as with exertion or stress. Stable angina is usually transient, lasting less than 5 minutes, and subsides with rest or nitroglycerin. *Unstable angina* occurs when an atherosclerotic plaque ruptures and a thrombus forms that partially occludes the coronary arterial lumen, disrupting blood flow to the myocardium and causing ischemia. The thrombus dissolves within 20 minutes, preventing myocardial necrosis and infarction. Unstable angina occurs with greater frequency, duration (20 minutes or more), and severity and occurs at rest or isn't relieved by rest or nitroglycerin. *Variant (Prinzmetal's) angina,* an atypical form of angina, occurs without an identified precipitating cause, usually at the same time each day, and is associated with coronary artery spasm.

In all three types, reduced coronary blood flow causes reversible myocardial ischemia and characteristic chest pain. Chest pain develops because reduced coronary blood flow and decreased oxygen supply cause cells to switch from aerobic metabolism to anaerobic metabolism.

In anaerobic metabolism, lactic acid builds up in the cells, altering cell membrane permeability and releasing such substances as histamine, kinins, and enzymes. These stimulate terminal nerve fibers in the cardiac muscle, which send pain impulses to the central nervous system. Typically, the pain begins in the chest and radiates down the arms or up the neck.

Health history
- History of coronary artery disease (CAD) or other risk factors for CAD, including hyperlipidemia, hypertension, hyperhomocysteinemia, cigarette smoking, diabetes mellitus, obesity, and a sedentary lifestyle
- Family history of heart disease
- Recent exposure to stress or activity
- Complaints of chest pain, described as tight, squeezing, heavy pressure or constricting sensation beginning beneath the sternum and possibly radiating to the jaw, neck or arm (lasting 1 to 5 minutes and relieved with rest or

Areas of pain from angina

nitroglycerin [stable angina], or lasting longer than 20 minutes and unrelieved with rest or nitroglycerin [unstable angina])

Characteristic findings
- Expect your physical examination findings to vary among patients with angina, depending on the extent and severity of the disease. Use the following information to help distinguish between expected and unexpected findings.

Inspection
- Dyspnea
- Pallor
- Anxiety and fear
- Diaphoresis

Auscultation
- Irregular heart rhythm
- Atrial or ventricular gallop (S_3 or S_4)
- Distant heart sounds

Vital signs
- Tachycardia
- Tachypnea

Complications
- Arrhythmias
- Myocardial infarction
- Sudden cardiac death

Back pain

If your patient complains of back pain, investigate the symptom further by asking him the following questions:
* Where is the pain located?
* When did the pain start?
* Is it getting better or worse?
* Does anything make the pain better or worse, such as changing positions?
* Does the pain radiate into either leg?
* Do you have any numbness?
* Have you had any urinary or fecal incontinence?
* Have you had any recent trauma or injury?
* Have you had a fever recently?
* What treatments have you tried to ease the pain? Heat? Massage?

Focusing your assessment

When a patient complains of back pain, focus your assessment as follows:
* Observe your patient's posture while he's standing. Then ask him to bend over and touch his toes. An asymmetrical body form may indicate scoliosis.
* Auscultate the abdomen for bruits, and look for pulsating masses, which may indicate an abdominal aortic aneurysm.
* Assess the extremities and trunk for any signs of loss of sensation or motor function that may indicate such neurologic compromise as spinal cord compression.
* Have your patient perform full range of motion with his back. Limited range or pain with range-of-motion activities may indicate a problem with a vertebra or disk.
* With your patient lying flat, lift his leg straight up under the ankle (straight leg test). Pain with this motion may indicate a herniated lumbar disk.
* Examine your patient for muscle weakness, decreased muscle tone, and exaggerated or diminished reflexes, which may indicate a spinal tumor.

Possible causes

* *Abdominal aortic aneurysm.* A rapid onset of severe lower back pain, possibly radiating to the chest, suggests a rupture or dissection of an abdominal aortic aneurysm. Your patient may have a pulsating mass in the midepigastrium. Pain may radiate to the posterior thighs. With a dissecting aneurysm, the pain is not relieved by repositioning. If the pain is described as tearing or ripping, and it's located in the anterior thorax and the back between the scapulae, it may indicate a dissecting thoracic aneurysm. Other signs include cold, pulseless lower extremities, and blood pressure differences between arms of greater than 10 mm Hg. (See *Determining Causes of Back Pain.*)

- *Herniated or ruptured lumbar disk.* The pain associated with a herniated lumbar disk is severe and usually radiates unilaterally to the buttock, leg, and foot. Pain is intensified by Valsalva's maneuver, coughing, sneezing, or bending and is often accompanied by muscle spasm.

INTERPRETING ABNORMAL FINDINGS

DETERMINING CAUSES OF BACK PAIN

A common complaint, back pain usually stems from muscle strain or arthritis. However, it can also result from serious conditions, such as vertebral fractures and spinal cord tumors. For that reason, assess your patient's back pain carefully and thoroughly, using the following table to help determine its cause.

Characteristics	Locations	Possible findings	Probable causes
• Pain confined to lower back • No evidence of nerve root involvement (numbness, weakness) • Usually relieved by rest	• Lumbar (L) and sacral (S) areas • May radiate to shoulders	• Unusual posture related to spasm • Paravertebral muscle tenderness • Restricted low-back motion	• Sprain or strain injury related to poor body mechanics • Trauma
• Sudden, severe low-back pain • Muscle spasm • Limited motion	• Lumbar or sacral areas • Thoracic spine	• Radiologic evidence of vertebral bone fractures • Paralytic ileus • Urinary retention	• Vertebral compression fractures • Osteoporosis • Heavy lifting or trauma • Metastatic tumor or myeloma • Metabolic bone disease
• Low-back pain with limited motion • Pain improves with rest	• Lumbar and sacral areas	• Abnormal posture • Pain when straight legs raised • Local muscle weakness, atrophy • Nerve root involvement: radicular pain, paresthesias, twitching, muscle spasms, decreased tendon reflex • L4, L5: pain to posterior thigh, calf, and foot; walking on heels may be difficult • L5, S1: pain in midgluteal region, back of thigh, back of calf down to heel and bottom surface of foot and 4th and 5th toes; walking on toes may be difficult	• Prolapsed or protruded disk • Silent degeneration over several years • Flexion injury • Spinal cord tumor

Continued

INTERPRETING ABNORMAL FINDINGS

DETERMINING CAUSES OF BACK PAIN—cont'd

Characteristics	Locations	Possible findings	Probable causes
• Common in lumbar or cervical spine • Pain centered in spine and increased by activity • Pain relieved by rest	• Lumbar or sacral areas • Cervical and upper shoulder	• Limited motion • Degree of radiologic changes may not correlate with symptoms	• Degenerative joint disease • Osteoarthritis
• Progressive limitation of movement • Morning stiffness	• Area affected varies with type of disorder	• Decreased spinal mobility	• Rheumatoid arthritis: usually older females with pain, stiffness mainly in cervical area • Ankylosing spondylitis: usually young males with pain and fusion in sacroiliac region
• Dull, constant pain • Pain is unrelieved by rest and may be worse at night	• All areas of the spine and back	• Local bone tenderness	• Bone metastases from prostate, breast, lung, thyroid, or kidney cancer • Multiple myeloma
• Severe, stabbing pain	• Low back • Abdomen	• Dysuria, nocturia, urinary frequency, chills and fever in males • Fever, lower abdominal pain, and vaginal pain in females • Nausea and vomiting, fever, and chills	• Gastrointestinal disease, such as peptic ulcer, pancreatitis • Genitourinary disease, such as pyelonephritis, nephrolithiasis, endometriosis, or prostatitis • Abdominal aortic aneurysm

- *Spinal tumors.* Pain that radiates around the trunk or down the limb and can't be relieved by bed rest may indicate a spinal tumor. The patient also may have muscle weakness or wasting, with exaggerated or diminished tendon reflexes. Urinary retention or constipation may also be present.
- *Fractured vertebra.* Pain with a fractured vertebra usually worsens with movement and may radiate to the legs. Mild paresthesia may accompany the pain.

- *Osteoarthritis.* Patients typically describe arthritic pain as deep, aching pain; it's usually relieved by rest. Your patient may complain of morning stiffness and aching during weather changes.
- *Genitourinary problems.* In a female patient, severe back and abdominal pain associated with the menstrual period and dysmenorrhea may indicate endometriosis. In a male patient, low-back pain associated with dysuria, nocturia, urinary frequency, chills, and fever may indicate prostatitis. A pelvic infection should be suspected in any female patient with a fever, lower abdominal pain, and vaginal discharge associated with low-back pain.
- *Lumbosacral strain.* Stiffness, soreness, and generalized tenderness may indicate a lumbosacral strain.
- *Kidney stone.* Severe back pain accompanied by nausea and vomiting, fever, and chills may indicate a stone obstructing a kidney or ureter.

Hemoptysis

If your patient complains of coughing up blood, investigate the symptom further by asking him the following questions:
- When did the hemoptysis begin?
- What color is the sputum? Does it look like fresh blood, old brown blood, or pus-filled sputum with bloody streaks?
- How often do you cough up blood?
- Does it seem to be getting better or worse?
- Have you had any associated symptoms, such as shortness of breath or chest pain?
- Have you had any recent fever or chills?
- Have you had any weight loss or night sweats?
- Have you had any recent chest surgery or trauma?

Focusing your assessment

When a patient complains of hemoptysis, focus your assessment as follows:
- Assess your patient for chest pain. Complaints of new-onset hemoptysis and chest pain may indicate a pulmonary embolus.
- Assess the patient's oral mucosa and nares for signs of bleeding or trauma. Hemoptysis may arise from areas other than the respiratory tract.
- Assess the skin for petechiae or bruising, which may indicate a coagulation disorder.
- Evaluate your patient's current situation. Sudden hemoptysis in a patient undergoing pulmonary artery catheter insertion could indicate pulmonary artery rupture. This is a medical emergency. In an intubated patient, it could indicate tracheal erosion.
- Assess the volume of blood. Hemoptysis of greater than 100 ml in a 24-hour period may be life-threatening.

Possible causes
- *Bacterial infection.* Acute and chronic infections are the most common causes of hemoptysis, especially infections caused by *Staphylococcus, Klebsiella,* and *Pseudomonas* bacteria.
- *Tuberculosis.* Hemoptysis associated with fever or night sweats may indicate tuberculosis.
- *Coagulopathy.* The presence of petechiae or bruising of the skin along with hemoptysis may signify a coagulopathy, leukemia, or thrombocytopenia.
- *Lung cancer.* Hemoptysis in a patient with a history of smoking or occupational exposure to carcinogens may be a sign of lung cancer. Hemoptysis caused by erosion occurs in half of the patients with lung cancer at some point during the disease.
- *Fungal infection.* Most pulmonary fungal infections can cause hemoptysis. Patients who are immunocompromised or have a history of tuberculosis or exposure to it are at a higher risk for fungal infections.

Cough
If your patient complains of a cough, investigate the symptom further by asking him the following questions:
- Is the cough productive or nonproductive?
- If the cough is productive, what color is the sputum?
- When did the cough start?
- Is it getting better or worse?
- Does the cough occur more frequently at a certain time of the day?
- Do you have a fever or chills?
- Are you short of breath?
- Are you taking anything for the cough?
- Do you have any other symptoms (sore throat, runny nose, hoarseness)?
- Have you noticed a recent weight loss or night sweats?
- What type of work do you do? Describe your work environment. Are you or have you been exposed to toxic chemicals, fibers, or fumes (for example, asbestos)?

Focusing your assessment
When a patient complains of a cough, focus your assessment as follows:
- Auscultate the breath sounds. Coarse crackles, bronchial breath sounds, or an area of consolidation may indicate pneumonia. Fine crackles may indicate heart failure. Abnormal breath sounds that clear after coughing indicate secretions rather than heart failure.
- Examine any sputum produced by the cough. Green sputum may indicate a *Pseudomonas* infection. Rust-colored sputum may indicate a *Klebsiella* infection. Scant sputum production may indicate a viral infection.

- Assess the results of pulmonary function testing, including the patient's 1-second forced expiratory volume (FEV_1), peak flow, and vital capacity to detect obstructive pulmonary disease.

Possible causes

- *Asthma.* Although wheezing is the characteristic symptom associated with asthma, your patient may also have an unusually tight-sounding, dry cough, with tenacious mucoid sputum. This cough may be triggered by exposure to cold or exercise.
- *Cigarette smoking.* The most common cause of a chronic cough, cigarette smoking is associated with a cough that is more severe early in the morning. Usually it produces a yellowish-brown mucus. It may disappear as quickly as a month after the patient stops smoking.
- *Air pollution or exposure to irritants.* Sulfur dioxide, nitrogen dioxide, and ozone are common air pollutants that cause a cough. Asbestosis is also a cause. Industrial and agricultural exposure can result in an acute or chronic cough as well. Many coughs related to air pollution begin after work or at night.
- *Bronchogenic carcinoma.* Cough is a major symptom of bronchogenic carcinoma, and often is the first sign of this disease. Suspect lung carcinoma in a heavy smoker with a chronic cough.
- *Bronchitis.* Recent onset of cough and fever could indicate an acute episode of bronchitis. (See 📖 *Bronchitis,* p. 198.)
- *Angiotensin-converting enzyme (ACE) inhibitor use.* A dry cough is a possible side effect of ACE inhibitors, which often are prescribed for heart failure and hypertension.
- *Tuberculosis.* A cough associated with fatigue, weakness, anorexia, weight loss, or night sweats may indicate tuberculosis, especially recurrent disease.

Dyspnea

If your patient complains of dyspnea, or shortness of breath, investigate the symptom further by asking him the following questions:
- Does the shortness of breath occur with rest or with activity?
- If shortness of breath occurs with activity, how much exertion brings it on? Walking 50 feet? 100 feet? More?
- Are you short of breath now?
- What helps the shortness of breath get better?
- Do you have any associated symptoms, such as dizziness or chest pain?
- Is this a new problem or a chronic problem?
- If it's a chronic problem, does it seem to be getting worse?
- Have you seen anyone for this problem? If so, what treatment are you receiving?

DISORDER CLOSE-UP

BRONCHITIS

Bronchitis is an acute or chronic inflammation of the mucous membranes of the bronchi. Acute bronchitis results when the larger bronchi react to an infectious agent by becoming diffusely inflamed and producing excessive amounts of mucus. The airways are otherwise normal. Acute bronchitis is common and usually causes little permanent disability.

Chronic bronchitis, by contrast, is a type of chronic obstructive pulmonary disease (COPD). Obstruction results from inflammation of major and minor airways. The submucosal glands become edematous and overgrown, secreting excess mucus into the bronchial tree.

Usually, chronic bronchitis results from prolonged exposure to bronchial irritants, such as cigarette smoke, air pollution, toxic fumes, and dust. A ventilation-perfusion imbalance develops from resistance in the small airways and because areas of inflammation and retained secretions don't occur uniformly throughout the lungs. Repeated infections with persistent obstruction can lead to scarring, necrosis, and destruction of the small bronchioles.

Health history
- Long-term smoking
- History of frequent upper respiratory infections
- History of exposure to environmental pollutants
- Cough (increasing in frequency and severity), especially at night
- Complaints of exertional dyspnea with increased time needed to recover
- Family history of COPD
- Weight gain

Characteristic findings
Expect your physical examination findings to vary among patients with chronic bronchitis, depending on the extent and severity of the disease. Use the information that follows to help you distinguish between expected and unexpected findings.

Inspection
- Dyspnea
- Productive cough with copious sputum (gray, white, or yellow)
- Use of accessory breathing muscles
- Cyanosis
- Finger clubbing
- Barrel chest (possible)

Palpation
- Pedal edema
- Neck vein distention

Auscultation
- Wheezing
- Prolonged expiratory time
- Decreased breath sounds
- Changes in breath sounds (variable)

Vital signs
- Tachypnea
- Elevated temperature (possible)

Complications
- Cor pulmonale
- Pulmonary hypertension
- Right ventricular hypertrophy
- Acute respiratory failure

Focusing your assessment
When a patient complains of shortness of breath, focus your assessment as follows:
- Check your patient's vital signs and appearance. New-onset shortness of breath can indicate a serious underlying problem. (See *Determining Causes of Dyspnea*.)

INTERPRETING ABNORMAL FINDINGS

DETERMINING CAUSES OF DYSPNEA

A patient with dyspnea has a distressing sensation of air hunger. Because dyspnea can result from a wide variety of cardiac and pulmonary conditions, its etiology can be difficult to identify quickly. Always take a detailed history when assessing a patient with dyspnea. Then use this table to help determine its cause.

Characteristics	Possible findings	Probable causes
• Gradual-onset dyspnea, beginning as exertional • Minimal cough, usually nonproductive	• Varying degrees of respiratory distress • Tachypnea • Prolonged expiration • Expiration often begins with a grunting noise • Posture leaning forward with extended arms • Use of accessory muscles • Hyperresonance to percussion • Decreased breath sounds with faint, high-pitched wheezes at end of expiration • Weight loss • History of smoking • Carbon dioxide retention	• Emphysema
• Gradual-onset dyspnea • Long history of cough and sputum production • Paroxysmal nocturnal dyspnea related to increased sputum production	• History of smoking, obesity, and frequent respiratory infections • Carbon dioxide retention • Coarse crackles and wheezes that change in location and intensity after cough • Late features: cyanosis, clubbing, peripheral edema, neck vein distention, right ventricular failure, cor pulmonale	• Chronic bronchitis
• Episodes of acute dyspnea • Sensation of having a lump in the throat • Hoarseness	• Stridor and retraction of supraclavicular muscles with inspiration • Respiratory distress and failure	• Aspiration of food or foreign object • Allergic reaction, resulting in angioedema • Upper airway obstruction
• Dyspnea with exertion (early), developing into dyspnea at rest • Suffocating or drowning sensation • Cough and wheezing • Paroxysmal nocturnal dyspnea and orthopnea	• Moist inspiratory crackles • Tachypnea • Gallop rhythms and cardiac murmurs • Jugular vein distention • Diaphoresis • Peripheral edema • Pleural effusions	• Heart failure • Myocardial infarction or ischemia • Valvular disease • Cardiomyopathies
• Dyspnea at rest • Hyperventilation	• Sharp, fleeting chest pain, variably located • Frequent sighing • Irregular breathing pattern • Normal breathing during sleep	• Anxiety • Emotional stress
• Acute-onset dyspnea • Wheezing • Cough • Commonly affects children	• Tachypnea with wheezing • Attacks can last minutes to hours • Episodic disease	• Asthma

Continued

INTERPRETING ABNORMAL FINDINGS

DETERMINING CAUSES OF DYSPNEA—cont'd

Characteristics	Possible findings	Probable causes
• Dyspnea at rest • Unexplained sudden breathlessness	• Sharp or stabbing pleuritic pain • Hemoptysis • Tachycardia and tachypnea • Accentuated pulmonic heart sound • Hypotension • ST changes on electrocardiogram • Pleural friction rub • Atelectasis after 24 hours	• Pulmonary embolus
• Dyspnea at rest • Productive cough (mucoid, purulent, or bloody)	• Tachycardia and tachypnea • Decreased respiratory excursion on affected side • Dullness to percussion over area of infection • High-pitched, end-inspiratory crackles • Increased bronchial breath sounds • Fever • Chest pain • Increased tactile fremitus over consolidation area • Confusion or disorientation in elderly patients	• Pneumonia
• Exertional, gradual-onset dyspnea • Nonproductive cough	• Dry basilar crackles best heard at the end of deep inspiration • Fatigue • Malaise • Late: evidence of pulmonary hypertension, clubbing	• Interstitial fibrotic lung disease • Rheumatoid and collagen-vascular disease • Sarcoidosis
• Gradual-onset dyspnea • Productive cough	• Wheezing • Stridor • Fever • Hemoptysis • History of smoking	• Pulmonary neoplasms (primary or metastatic)

- Notify the physician immediately and consider giving oxygen if your patient is tachypneic, diaphoretic, or cyanotic.
- Check your patient's extremities to see if they are cyanotic or cold, which indicates circulatory compromise. Cold, cyanotic extremities with hypotension may indicate hypoperfusion associated with shock.
- Auscultate breath sounds. Crackles and wheezes can indicate heart failure or pulmonary edema.
- Assess your patient for chest pain, which could indicate cardiac ischemia.
- Inspect the chest for tracheal deviation, a sign of pneumothorax or pleural effusion.

- Inspect for barrel chest, a sign of emphysema.
- Check for jugular vein distention and dependent edema, signs of pulmonary edema.
- Assess your patient's mental status. Confusion or a change in mental status may indicate hypoxia.
- Examine your patient's calves for any signs of deep vein thrombosis. A positive Homans' sign (pain when the foot is dorsiflexed) may indicate venous occlusion, which could result in a pulmonary embolus.
- Examine the color of the nail beds, gums, and conjunctivae. Pale membranes and nail beds associated with fatigue may indicate anemia, which could result in shortness of breath.

Possible causes

- *Anemia.* Progressive weakness coupled with shortness of breath and pallor may be signs of aplastic or hypoplastic anemia.
- *Pulmonary hypertension.* Weakness, increasing shortness of breath on exertion, and fatigue may be signs of pulmonary hypertension. Signs of right-sided heart failure such as peripheral edema, ascites, neck vein distention, and hepatomegaly also may be present.
- *Central nervous system lesion.* Lesions in the central nervous system may press on the hypothalamus, causing an increased respiratory rate and a feeling of shortness of breath.
- *Pleural effusion.* With a large pleural effusion, your patient will complain of dyspnea and may have a visible tracheal shift. You'll auscultate diminished or absent breath sounds over the effusion, and you may hear a pleural friction rub.
- *Pulmonary embolism.* Sudden dyspnea that occurs in the setting of a deep vein thrombosis could signal a pulmonary embolism. Left untreated, pulmonary infarction, severe hypoxemia, and death could ensue. Homans' sign may or may not be present.
- *Pneumonia.* Shortness of breath with a fever and cough may warn of pneumonia.
- *Pulmonary edema.* Tachypnea, tachycardia, elevated blood pressure, and shortness of breath are signs of pulmonary edema. Crackles are usually auscultated from the chest. Your patient also may have jugular venous distention and dependent edema.
- *Lung cancer.* Occurring as squamous cell carcinoma, small cell carcinoma, or adenocarcinoma, lung cancer most commonly occurs on the wall or epithelium of the bronchial tree. Prognosis is usually poor but improves with early detection. Lung cancer should be suspected in any patient who smokes and has shortness of breath.
- *Pneumothorax.* Trauma to the chest or a spontaneous leak in the lung membranes that allows air to enter the pleural can cause the lung to collapse, resulting in a pneumothorax. Signs include absent breath sounds on one side of the chest and asymmetrical chest movements. (See *Telltale Signs of Tension Pneumothorax,* p. 202.)

TELLTALE SIGNS OF TENSION PNEUMOTHORAX

An emergency in which the lung collapses from the force of high pressure in the pleural space, tension pneumothorax may result from penetrating chest injury, mechanical ventilation that uses positive end-expiratory pressure, or even chest-tube occlusion.

Signs and symptoms that point to tension pneumothorax include the following:
- Sudden shortness of breath with tachypnea and tachycardia
- Anxiety
- Asymmetrical chest wall movement with mediastinal shift away from the affected side
- Absent or diminished breath sounds on the affected side
- Hyperresonance on the affected side
- Distended neck veins

You must act fast to relieve the pressure causing the tension pneumothorax so the lung will reinflate. Prepare to assist with chest-tube insertion as soon as possible.

- *Emphysema.* A leading cause of death in the United States, emphysema follows recurrent inflammation of the lung walls. Shortness of breath with a barrel chest and clubbing of the fingers are signs of emphysema. (See 📖 *Emphysema.*)

Orthopnea or paroxysmal nocturnal dyspnea

If your patient complains that he needs to sleep propped up on several pillows (orthopnea) or that he awakens at night feeling short of breath (paroxysmal nocturnal dyspnea), investigate the symptom further by asking him the following questions:
- When did you first notice these symptoms?
- How many pillows do you sleep on at night? Have you increased the number recently?
- Do you sleep on extra pillows to help your breathing or for another reason?
- If you awaken at night with shortness of breath, how often do you have the episodes?
- Are the episodes increasing in frequency?
- Do you have any associated symptoms, such as chest pain, leg swelling, or cough?
- Have you gained any weight recently?

Focusing your assessment

When a patient complains of orthopnea or nocturnal dyspnea, focus your assessment as follows:
- Auscultate the lungs for crackles, which may indicate pulmonary edema.

DISORDER CLOSE-UP

EMPHYSEMA

One of two major types of chronic obstructive pulmonary disease (COPD) (which also includes chronic bronchitis), emphysema is a degenerative condition characterized by destruction of alveolar walls, entrapment of air in the spaces beyond the terminal bronchioles, narrowing of small airways, and loss of alveolar elasticity.

Emphysema mainly affects expiration. Because muscles used during inspiration can pull air past most obstructions, air can enter the lungs. But it can't leave as easily and becomes trapped in the alveoli, severely limiting oxygen intake and ultimately leading to hypoxia.

The body uses abdominal and accessory thoracic muscles to force air past the obstruction, slowing expiration. As a result, the patient retains carbon dioxide, which leads to hypercapnia.

Besides overworking respiratory muscles, emphysema strains the heart's right side, which provides pulmonary circulation. The heart compensates for hypoxemia by pumping faster to deliver more blood to the lungs and harder to push blood through constricted capillaries. As a result, the heart's right side hypertrophies (cor pulmonale).

Health history

- Long-term smoking
- Alpha$_1$-antitrypsin deficiency
- Family history of COPD
- Dyspnea during daily activities
- Anorexia
- Feeling of general malaise
- Chronic nonproductive cough

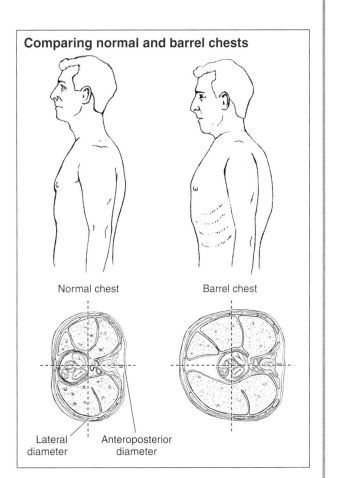

Comparing normal and barrel chests

Normal chest   Barrel chest

Lateral diameter   Anteroposterior diameter

Characteristic findings

Expect your physical examination findings to vary among emphysema patients, depending on the extent and severity of the disease. Use the information that follows to help distinguish between expected and unexpected findings.

Continued

DISORDER CLOSE-UP

EMPHYSEMA—cont'd

Inspection
- Increased anterior-posterior and lateral chest diameters, forming the typical barrel chest
- Forward-leaning posture
- Pursed-lip breathing
- Dyspnea
- Minimal cough (may develop productive cough in late stages secondary to chronic bronchitis)
- Audible expiratory wheeze
- Cyanosis of nail beds and mucous membranes
- Finger clubbing
- Use of accessory muscles during breathing
- Emaciation
- Restlessness and anxiety

Palpation
- Decreased tactile fremitus
- Downward displacement of liver's edge
- Nonpalpable apical pulse

Percussion
- Hyperresonance
- Decreased diaphragmatic excursion

Auscultation
- Wheezing
- Decreased breath and heart sounds
- Decreased voice sounds
- Prolonged expiration

Vital signs
- Elevated temperature
- Increased pulse rate
- Decreased blood pressure
- Pulsus paradoxus
- Increased respiratory rate

Complications
- Acute respiratory failure
- Arrhythmias
- Cor pulmonale
- Peptic ulcer and gastroesophageal reflux
- Pneumonia
- Polycythemia

- Auscultate the lungs for diminished breath sounds, which may indicate a pleural effusion.
- Auscultate the lungs for wheezes, which may indicate asthma.
- Assess the extremities for edema, a sign of fluid overload.
- Examine your patient's chest for a barrel shape, a sign of COPD.
- Assess your patient for jugular vein distention or an S_3, S_4 gallop, signs of pulmonary edema associated with heart failure and cardiac compromise.

Possible causes
- *Pulmonary edema and heart failure.* When a patient with heart failure lies down flat, interstitial fluid from the legs and the lung bases accumulates around the lungs. Consequently, the patient typically feels more comfortable if he elevates his upper body on several pillows to sleep. If he falls asleep in a flat position, the respiratory compromise from fluid accumulated around the lungs often awakens him.

- *COPD.* Secretions pooling in the throat and airways can cause a patient with COPD to awaken at night with shortness of breath.
- *Cardiac disease.* Compromised cardiac pumping function causes congestion in the pulmonary vasculature system, which can awaken the patient with shortness of breath.

Wheezing

If your patient complains of wheezing, investigate the symptom further by asking him the following questions:
- When did you first notice the wheezing?
- Have you had wheezing in the past?
- Does anything seem to bring on the wheezing, such as exercise or cold?
- Do you have any associated symptoms, such as fever, chills, cough, or shortness of breath?
- Have you ever been evaluated for wheezing before and, if so, did you receive any treatment?

Focusing your assessment

When a patient complains of wheezing, focus your assessment as follows:
- Observe your patient for signs of respiratory distress. He may be having an asthma attack, or he may have an obstructed airway. (See ⏰ *Responding to Airway Obstruction,* p. 206.)
- Assess for signs of cyanosis in the nail beds and mucous membranes. Check the patient's pulse oximetry. If the patient is hypoxic, the physician may order oxygen.
- Check your patient's vital signs. A tachypnic patient may need oxygen, even if the pulse oximetry reading is within a normal range.
- Auscultate the lungs. Wheezes on expiration may indicate asthma. Wheezes on inspiration may indicate bronchitis. Crackles are a sign of pulmonary edema.
- Assess for a cough with sputum production. Clear or yellow sputum may indicate asthma. Purulent sputum may indicate pneumonia.

Possible causes

- *Asthma.* Inflammation of the bronchioles accompanied by bronchiole constriction characterizes an asthma episode. Wheezing accompanied by respiratory distress (tachypnea, use of accessory breathing muscles) may occur suddenly or gradually after exposure to an allergen. The patient also may complain of a cough with clear or yellow sputum. The peak flow and FEV_1 will be decreased (See 🖼 *Asthma,* p. 207.)
- *Pulmonary edema.* Fluid overload may produce wheezing. Other signs include pedal edema, jugular vein distention, or S_3, S_4 gallop.
- *Pneumonia.* Secretions blocking the upper airways may result in wheezes.
- *Reaction to medications.* A common example of this would be an allergic reaction to penicillin.

ACTION STAT

RESPONDING TO AIRWAY OBSTRUCTION

Airway obstruction may result from a wide variety of objects, including an aspirated foreign body, a mucus plug, or, in some cases, the patient's tongue. Whatever its cause, airway obstruction must be corrected quickly. Maintaining a patent airway is the single most important nursing intervention you can perform for your patient. How you respond to acute airway obstruction depends on whether you know the cause of the obstruction and whether your patient is conscious.

What to look for
Clinical findings may include:
- Distressed, panicked appearance on your patient's face
- Inability to speak
- Wheezing, stridor, noisy respirations, sonorous wheezing over large airways
- Nasal flaring or use of accessory breathing muscles
- Decreased or absent breath sounds
- Excessive secretions (mucus or blood) around the mouth
- Cardiac arrhythmias
- Cyanosis
- Hypoxemia

What to do immediately
If your patient develops an airway obstruction, first call for assistance, and then follow these measures:
- Rapidly try to determine the probable cause of the obstruction, possibly a foreign body or food, excessive pulmonary secretions, or mechanical obstruction, such as the patient's tongue.
- If the patient is conscious and the airway is obstructed by a foreign body, such as food or an object, perform the Heimlich maneuver. You may have to modify your technique to perform abdominal thrusts if your patient is supine in bed or if he's upright in a bed or chair.
- If your patient is unconscious, immediately open his airway using the head-tilt or chin-lift method. This will pull your patient's tongue away from his oropharynx and open his airway. If he's in bed, raise the head of his bed to semi-Fowler's position.
- If changing the patient's airway position does not relieve the obstruction, use a gloved finger to perform a tongue sweep to check for a foreign body.
- Prepare to follow the American Heart Association's basic life support recommendations, which include rescue breathing and cardiac compressions.
- If indicated, prepare to suction the anterior and posterior portion of your patient's mouth, his oropharynx, trachea, and mainstem bronchus.

What to do next
Once your patient has been stabilized and the airway is patent, you'll need to:
- Maintain airway patency. Use an appropriate airway device, such as an oropharyngeal or nasopharyngeal airway, as necessary.
- Obtain additional emergency respiratory equipment, such as endotracheal intubation or tracheostomy supplies and supplemental oxygen, as indicated.
- Obtain arterial blood gas levels, if ordered, to further assess the patient's oxygenation.
- Administer oxygen as prescribed.
- Maintain the patient in a comfortable position that promotes airway clearance, with the head of his bed elevated.

Lumps or lesions
If your patient has a lump or lesion on the chest, back, or breast, investigate the symptom further by asking him the following questions:
- When did you first notice the lesion or lump?
- Is it getting worse or larger?

DISORDER CLOSE-UP

ASTHMA

Asthma is a chronic lung disorder characterized by reversible airway obstruction, inflamed airways, and an increased responsiveness of the airways to certain stimuli. During an asthma attack, airways sensitized by allergens become reactive to bronchospastic or inflammatory triggers. Bronchospastic triggers include cold air, exercise, emotional upset, variations in temperature and humidity, and exposure to irritants, such as cigarette smoke. Most episodes of this type are preceded by a severe respiratory tract infection. Inflammatory triggers include such allergens as pollen, animal dander, house dust, mold, and food additives. Patients with allergic asthma may respond to both types of triggers.

Contact with a trigger causes bronchoconstriction. Histamine and related substances are released and initiate contraction of smooth muscle in the bronchi, edema of bronchial mucous membranes, and secretion of copious mucus in the bronchi. This activity causes epithelial injury and edema, changes in mucociliary function, reduced clearance of respiratory tract secretions, and increased airway responsiveness. Expiratory airflow decreases and gas is trapped in the airways, causing alveolar hyperinflation. The increased airway resistance initiates labored breathing.

Health history
- History of allergic reactions
- History of other atopic diseases, such as allergic rhinitis or eczema
- Family history of atopic diseases
- Exposure to allergen
- Sudden onset of dyspnea
- Complaints of chest tightness and feeling of suffocation
- Cough

Characteristic findings

Expect your physical examination findings to vary among patients with asthma, depending on the extent and severity of the disease. Use the information that follows to help distinguish between expected and unexpected findings.

Inspection
- Prolonged expiration
- Pursed-lip breathing
- Perspiration
- Ability to speak only a few words before stopping to catch breath
- Use of accessory muscles to breathe
- Chest muscle retractions
- Increased anterior-posterior thoracic diameter
- Cyanosis
- Confusion
- Lethargy

Palpation
- Vocal fremitus

Percussion
- Hyperresonance
- Decreased diaphragmatic excursion

Auscultation
- Hyperinflated lungs
- Prolonged expiration
- Inspiratory and expiratory high-pitched wheezes throughout lung
- Diminished breath sounds

Vital signs
- Tachycardia
- Tachypnea
- Mild systolic hypertension
- Pulsus paradoxus (danger sign)

Complications
- Respiratory acidosis
- Hypoxemia
- Status asthmaticus
- Respiratory failure

- Has the color or shape changed?
- Do you have any pain or discharge?
- Have you any other lesions or lumps elsewhere on your body?
- Have you had a recent fever or night sweats?

Focusing your assessment

When a patient complains of lumps or lesions, focus your assessment as follows:

- Perform a full breast examination, including the axillae. Check both nipples for discharge. Lumps or lesions on the breasts can indicate breast cancer in both females and males. Use the opportunity to educate the female patient on the technique and importance of performing a monthly breast self-examination.
- Inspect the lesion and note any drainage or scabbing.
- Note the location and size of the lesion.
- For a sacral or iliac lesion, note any sacral edema that could compromise blood supply and delay healing.
- When assessing lumps under the skin, palpate them to determine if they're hard or soft and if they're movable or attached to an underlying structure.

Possible causes

- *Breast cancer.* Occurring most often in females, breast cancer has a good prognosis when diagnosed early. Most lesions are found in the upper outer quadrant of the breast and the axillary region. A nipple discharge may indicate intraductal carcinoma.
- *Shingles.* Caused by a herpes zoster virus, shingles appears after reactivation of the dormant virus in the cerebral ganglia or the ganglia of posterior nerve roots. The patient usually complains of a 2- or 3-day history of fever and malaise. Painful, fluid-filled vesicles develop along the dermatome. They typically dry and form scabs after about 10 days.
- *Hodgkin's disease.* Characterized by painless, progressive enlargement of the lymph nodes, spleen, and other lymphoid tissue, Hodgkin's disease results from proliferation of lymphocytes, histiocytes, eosinophils, and Reed-Sternberg cells. Common early signs include swelling in a cervical, axillary, or groin lymph node and fever, often accompanied by night sweats.
- *Malignant nevi.* Nevi (moles) begin to grow in childhood and increase in number in young adulthood. Up to 70% of malignant melanomas occur from existing nevi that undergo changes in color, size, shape, or texture. They may ulcerate, bleed, or itch. Melanomas commonly occur on the backs of persons exposed to the sun.

EXAMINING THE UPPER EXTREMITIES

People use their upper extremities every waking hour of every day, with little understanding of how important this area of the body is to their quality of life. Only when they suffer an injury, such as a broken arm, or a condition, such as rheumatoid arthritis, do they realize how vital their hands, arms, and shoulders are to their ability to function. As a nurse, however, you can take nothing for granted. Your examination of the upper extremities must be as thorough and effective as your examination of every other part of the body.

To examine the upper extremities properly, you'll need to perform an integrated, systematic assessment of various aspects of the musculoskeletal, neurologic, and vascular systems, as well as the skin. This requires a clear understanding of the anatomy of the upper extremities, including supporting bones and muscles, their vascular and lymphatic supply, and the relationship between these parts of the body and the neurologic system. (See ▮ *Structures of the Upper Extremities,* pp. 210 to 213.)

In addition, you'll need to palpate pulses, lymph nodes, and muscles, evaluate muscle strength, and test your patient's deep tendon reflexes (DTRs), sensory ability, and range of motion (ROM).

This chapter will give you the knowledge and skills you need to perform an accurate, focused assessment of the upper extremities.

(Text continues on p. 214.)

ANATOMY REVIEW

STRUCTURES OF THE UPPER EXTREMITIES

Before you can examine a patient's upper extremities effectively, you must have a working knowledge of the anatomic structures involved. The illustrations presented here provide an overview of the bones, lymph vessels, muscles, and blood vessels of the upper extremities.

SKELETAL STRUCTURES

LYMPH VESSELS

Anterior view

- Clavicle
- Scapula
- Humerus
- Ulna
- Radius
- Carpal
- Metacarpal
- Phalanges

Anterior view

- Brachial (axillary) n
- Brachial collecting duct
- Epitrochlear node
- Radial collecting duct
- Ulnar collecting duct
- Median collecting duct

MUSCLES

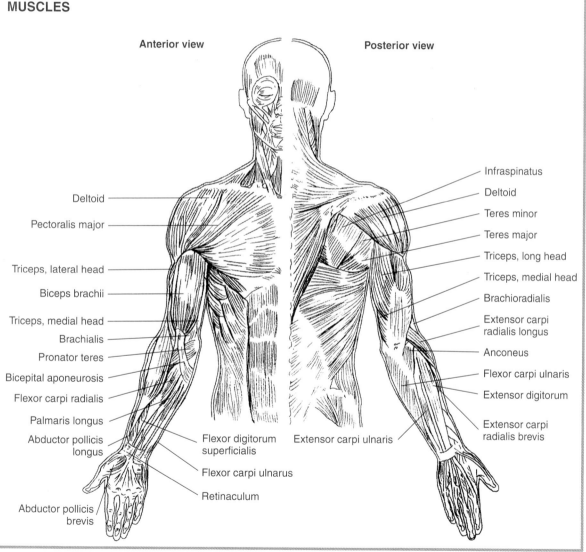

Anterior view

Posterior view

Deltoid

Pectoralis major

Triceps, lateral head

Biceps brachii

Triceps, medial head

Brachialis

Pronator teres

Bicepital aponeurosis

Flexor carpi radialis

Palmaris longus

Abductor pollicis
longus

Abductor pollicis
brevis

Flexor digitorum
superficialis

Flexor carpi ulnarus

Retinaculum

Extensor carpi ulnaris

Infraspinatus

Deltoid

Teres minor

Teres major

Triceps, long head

Triceps, medial head

Brachioradialis

Extensor carpi
radialis longus

Anconeus

Flexor carpi ulnaris

Extensor digitorum

Extensor carpi
radialis brevis

Continued

STRUCTURES OF THE UPPER EXTREMITIES—cont'd

BLOOD VESSELS: ARTERIES   Anterior view

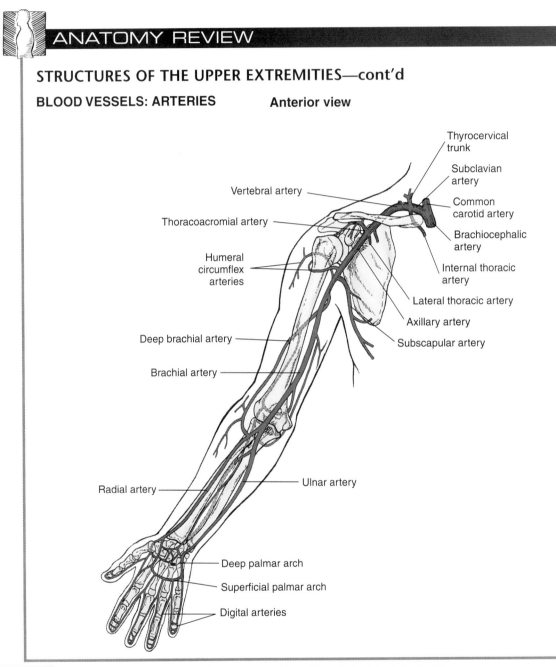

Thyrocervical trunk

Subclavian artery

Vertebral artery

Common carotid artery

Thoracoacromial artery

Brachiocephalic artery

Humeral circumflex arteries

Internal thoracic artery

Lateral thoracic artery

Axillary artery

Deep brachial artery

Subscapular artery

Brachial artery

Radial artery

Ulnar artery

Deep palmar arch

Superficial palmar arch

Digital arteries

From Thibodeau, G. & Patton, K. (2003). *Anatomy and Physiology* (5th ed.). St. Louis: Mosby.

BLOOD VESSELS: VEINS

Anterior view

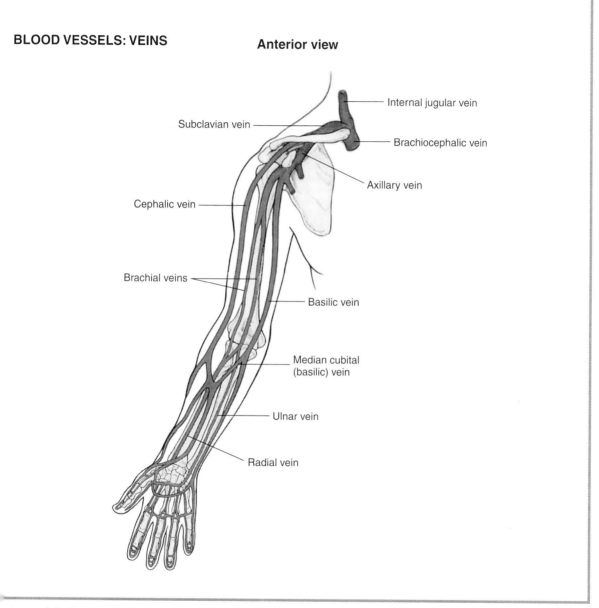

Internal jugular vein

Subclavian vein

Brachiocephalic vein

Axillary vein

Cephalic vein

Brachial veins

Basilic vein

Median cubital
(basilic) vein

Ulnar vein

Radial vein

From Thibodeau, G. & Patton, K. (2003). *Anatomy and Physiology* (5th ed.). St. Louis: Mosby.

EXAMINATION STEPS AND FINDINGS

When examining the upper extremities, you'll rely primarily on your skills of inspection and palpation. For expediency, you can perform these steps simultaneously. (See 🗒 *Key Examination Steps for the Upper Extremities.*)

Before beginning your examination, make sure the room is well lit and warm enough to keep your patient comfortable. Also, have the following equipment readily available: a stethoscope, tape measure, reflex hammer, piece of cotton, cotton-tipped swab or paper clip or both, and low-frequency tuning fork.

If the patient has a complaint involving one extremity, examine the unaffected one first. Doing so will give you a better idea of the normal appearance and function of the patient's extremities. It will also allow your patient to relax while you begin your examination.

Inspection

Inspect the skin of the upper extremities for ecchymosis, abnormal markings, changes in color, and swelling. In addition, note any unusual bruises or marks, such as needle injection sites or track marks. If your patient has an IV catheter in one arm, inspect the insertion site for evidence of infection and inflammation, including redness, swelling, tenderness, heat, drainage, or red streaks along the course of the vein.

Look for scratch marks and other evidence of pruritus, which may offer clues to possible liver disease, diabetes mellitus, kidney disease, or thyroid disorders.

PRIORITY CHECKLIST

KEY EXAMINATION STEPS FOR THE UPPER EXTREMITIES

Use this checklist to make sure you cover the most important steps when examining the upper extremities.

- ❑ Inspect for color and any obvious deformities.
- ❑ Palpate for temperature and moisture.
- ❑ Check palpable lesions.
- ❑ Palpate radial, ulnar, and brachial pulses for rate, rhythm, and contour.
- ❑ Check nail bed refill.
- ❑ Test tactile sensation, vibration, and proprioception.

- ❑ Assess range of motion for shoulders, elbows, wrists, and hands.
- ❑ Listen for joint crepitation as extremities flex and extend.
- ❑ Assess strength of shoulders, upper arms, elbows, wrists, and hands.
- ❑ Test hand-grip strength and compare bilaterally.
- ❑ Palpate infraclavicular and epitrochlear lymph nodes. Test deep tendon reflexes (DTRs).

Examine the color and shape of your patient's nails, looking for pallor, cyanosis, hemorrhages, and clubbing.

Compare the size of your patient's arms for bilateral symmetry. Note any unilateral or bilateral edema. If you suspect asymmetry or your patient has obvious edema in one arm, measure and record arm circumference. Be sure to note the measurement site in your notes so you can compare arm circumference measurements later, using the same location.

Inspect the shoulder joints at all angles. Carefully observe their anterior, posterior, and lateral aspects. Note any swelling, deformity, or surrounding muscle atrophy. Also, inspect all remaining joints, including the elbows, wrists, and interphalangeal joints.

Inspect the upper extremity muscles, looking for obvious deformity, asymmetry, gross hypertrophy or atrophy, and obvious spasms.

Evaluating reflexes

To evaluate your patient's motor reflexes and sensory pathways, you'll use a reflex hammer to elicit DTRs. When testing reflexes, position the patient's extremity so the tendon is slightly stretched. Typically, you can accomplish this by deviating the joint (elbow or wrist) away from you.

To use the reflex hammer properly, swing it briskly downward to strike the tendon. Then quickly snap your wrist back. Be sure to hold the handle of the hammer loosely between your thumb and index finger so you can achieve a full swinging motion.

Test the biceps, triceps, and brachioradialis (supinator) reflexes. (See *Testing Reflexes in the Upper Extremities,* p. 216.)

Be sure to compare the response with the corresponding reflex on the opposite side of the body.

You can record your patient's reflex response several different ways, but many nurses use the following scale:

++++	Brisk, hyperactive, clonus of tendon associated with disease
+++	More brisk than normal, but not necessarily associated with disease
++	Normal
+	Low normal, slightly diminished response
0	No response

To increase the speed with which you record your patient's reflex responses, consider using a stick-figure diagram. Write each reflex result, in plus signs, at the proper location on the stick figure. This method not only spares you from writing down all the reflex names and locations, but it also gives you an easy visual comparison of reflex response at various body locations and testing times.

If you suspect hepatic disease, especially hepatic encephalopathy, ask your patient to hold her arms in front of her with her wrists hyper-extended, as though she were trying to stop traffic. Ask her to hold this

(Text continues on p. 218.)

EXAMINATION TIP

TESTING REFLEXES IN THE UPPER EXTREMITIES

The following directions explain how to accurately test deep tendon reflexes of the upper extremities and also the grasp reflex.

Biceps reflex

With your patient's arm bent 45 degrees at the elbow, place your finger on the inside of the elbow over the tendon of the biceps muscle. Now tap your finger. The biceps should contract and the forearm should flex at the elbow. The biceps reflex, present at birth, is mediated by the spinal cord at the C5-C6 segmental level.

Testing biceps reflex in a sitting patient.

Testing biceps reflex in a recumbent patient.

Triceps reflex

With your patient's arm bent 90 degrees at the elbow, tap the short tendon of the triceps muscle close to its insertion near the tip of the elbow. The muscle should contract in response and the forearm should extend. This reflex is mediated by the spinal cord at the C7-C8 segmental level. It is present 6 weeks after birth.

Testing triceps reflex in a sitting patient.

Testing triceps reflex in a recumbent patient.

If you have trouble eliciting the triceps reflex, try this alternative method. With your patient sitting up, hold her upper arm away from her body and ask her to let her forearm hang limp. Now test the reflex again with the arm in this position.

Brachioradialis reflex

To elicit this reflex (also called the supinator reflex), tap about 2 inches (5 cm) from the styloid process of the radius. In a normal response, the patient's arm flexes at the elbow and the forearm pronates. This reflex is mediated by the spinal cord at the C5-C6 segmental level.

Testing brachioradialis reflex in a sitting patient.

Testing brachioradialis reflex in a recumbent patient.

Grasp reflex

A normal reflex in infants up to about age 8 months, the grasp reflex is also an important test for patients who are unconscious or have weakened upper extremities. To test the grasp reflex, place your index and middle fingers in your patient's palm, between the thumb and index finger. Gently withdraw your fingers, pulling them across the skin of your patient's palm. If your patient's hand tightens to grasp your fingers, she has a positive grasp reflex. In an adult, this reflex indicates widespread brain damage or cortical lesions, especially in the frontal lobe area.

Testing grasp reflex by dragging index and middle fingers across the patient's palm.

A positive response occurs if your patient grasps your hand.

TRACKING THE SOURCE OF SENSORY LOSS

Peripheral nerve damage causes sensory deficits in consistent and predictable locations on the upper extremities, as shown here in the shaded areas.

If your patient has an area of sensory loss, you may be able to use its location to determine which peripheral nerve is involved. Use this illustration as a key to helping track sources of sensory loss.

To track sensory loss, ask your patient to close her eyes. Then, using the stick end of a cotton-tipped swab and warm and cool objects, touch the patient in random areas and ask her to identify each sensation.

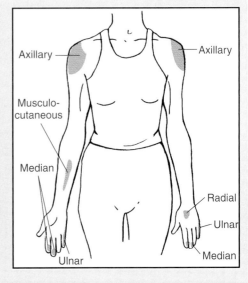

position for at least 1 minute. If abnormal movements appear, the patient may have hepatic disease.

Sensory testing

After testing and documenting your patient's reflexes, turn to the sensory examination. This is a subjective test used to evaluate tactile sensation (superficial pain), vibration, and proprioception.

Peripheral nerve damage causes sensory deficits in consistent and predictable locations on the upper extremities. To refresh your memory, look at a dermatome chart to locate the approximate body areas innervated by the sensory portion of each spinal nerve. That way, if you detect a deficit, or your patient complains of sensory changes, you can determine which spinal nerve might be involved by comparing sensory test results in each extremity. (See *Tracking the Source of Sensory Loss.*)

While performing the sensory portion of your examination, you'll want your patient's eyes to be closed so she responds only to what she feels. To reassure her, first tell her that you're going to perform some painless tests of feeling in her arms. Then ask her to close her eyes.

To assess tactile sensation, ask the patient to tell you when and where she feels you touching her. Then touch a cotton wisp to corresponding areas of each extremity. Compare the sensitivity of both arms, and compare the sensitivity of proximal and distal parts of each arm.

Because pain and temperature sensations are transmitted together in the lateral part of the spinal cord, usually you won't have to test temperature recognition. If you decide to test it anyway, systematically touch cool and warm objects to your patient's arms, and record her responses to temperature identification. Try using test tubes filled with cold and warm water for this part of the examination.

Assess your patient's ability to recognize superficial pain by touching various locations on her arms with the sharp and rounded ends of a paper clip or with the sharp and dull ends of a cotton-tipped swab that's been snapped in two. While your patient's eyes are closed, ask her to tell you whether you're touching her with something sharp or something dull. Be sure to apply the same amount of pressure each time and compare pain sensations between arms.

Vibration and proprioception sensations are transmitted together in the posterior segment of the spinal cord. To test vibration sensation, you can use a low-frequency tuning fork. Place the handle of the vibrating fork against the most distal bony prominence, such as the interphalangeal joint, and ask your patient to tell you when she feels vibration and when it stops vibrating. If your patient doesn't feel any vibrations, move the tuning fork proximally until she does. As with all measurements of sensation, compare each extremity.

LIFESPAN CONSIDERATIONS

Older adults can sometimes have a diminished sense of superficial pain, vibration, and proprioception. Plan to use a stronger stimulus with these individuals.

To test position sense, tell your patient that you're going to move some of her fingers so they point up or down. Show her what you mean. Then ask her to close her eyes. Take one of her fingers or thumbs and move it so it is pointing up or down. Ask the patient to tell you which direction the finger is pointing. Repeat this test several times, on each side.

Normal findings

- Skin color uniform, with fingernails of equal thickness. With age, skin becomes thinner and drier, and nails take on a yellowish overtone.
- Fine, bright red, irregularly shaped blood vessels known as telangiectasis visible through the skin. As the dermis thins, these small blood vessels dilate and sometimes burst. The resulting marks may be called broken blood vessels, venous stars, spider bursts, or angioids.
- Flat, tan-to-brown maculae on the dorsal surface of the hands and other areas of sun-exposed skin. Common in the middle-aged and elderly, these lesions are usually actinic keratoses or senile lentigo, also called liver spots. Most are benign, although actinic keratoses may be premalignant.

- Bright red, soft, dome-shaped lesions with a diameter of 1 mm or greater. They're called cherry angiomas, and they result from proliferation and dilation of superficial skin capillaries. Trauma resulting in extravasation from the capillaries or clotting in the vessels may cause the lesions to appear black. Although cherry angiomas may be observed in early adulthood, they're most numerous after age 40. They're benign.
- Arms symmetrical in length, circumference, and alignment.
- Muscle mass symmetrical, with good tone.

LIFESPAN CONSIDERATIONS

Symmetrical loss of muscle strength occurs normally with aging. Also, bilateral, symmetrical loss of muscle mass can occur and is easily observed in the bone spaces of the dorsal surface of the hands.

- Joints equal in size and shape bilaterally, without obvious deformity or lesions.
- DTRs equal bilaterally. Absence of finger flexor response bilaterally.
- Sensory abilities allowing detection of light touch, vibration, and position. The patient can differentiate between sharp and dull sensations.

Abnormal findings

- Pruritus or itching, a common symptom of dry skin. Be alert for systemic diseases associated with pruritus, such as liver disease, diabetes mellitus, kidney disease, and thyroid disorders.
- Trauma to the skin, including abrasions, incised wounds (incisions), puncture wounds, lacerations, and burns.
- Joint swelling, especially if normal bony landmarks are obscured, indicating excess fluid.
- Joint deformity, possibly resulting from contracture (shortening of surrounding joint structures), subluxation (partial separation of joint surfaces), or disruption of structures surrounding the joint.
- Joint weakness or disruption of joint-supporting structures, possibly resulting in a joint that's too weak to function as designed. It may require external supporting devices.
- Thickened sheath on the palmar surface of the wrist, possibly indicating carpal tunnel syndrome. Thickening of the flexor tendon sheath of the median nerve can lead to numbness and paresthesia. Sustained palmar flexion produces symptoms of numbness and paresthesia over the palmar surface of the hand, the first three fingers, and part of the fourth finger (called Phalen's sign).

- Edema, possibly resulting from an injury, cellulitis, lymphedema, venous obstruction (as might occur with thrombophlebitis, an inflammation of the walls of the veins), or heart failure.
- Flattening of the anterior aspect of the shoulder, possibly indicating dislocation.
- Intermittent pallor and cyanosis of the skin on the hands and fingers, possibly caused by episodic constriction of peripheral small arteries or arterioles characteristic of Raynaud's disease or Raynaud's phenomenon. After an episode of constriction, hyperemia may produce a red color (rubor).
- Ischemic changes and gangrene of the hands and fingers, possibly accompanying Buerger's disease (thromboangiitis obliterans), an occlusive vascular condition affecting the medium-sized arteries and medium-sized, mostly superficial, veins of the extremities. Distal pulses are often diminished.
- Streaky redness, tenderness, and warmth along the course of a vein, possibly resulting from thrombophlebitis.
- Limited ROM, possibly resulting from an injury or arthritis.
- Hyporeflexia (diminished reflexes) on one side, possibly indicating a lower motor neuron disorder, such as poliomyelitis. Tendon reflexes are diminished in muscular dystrophy and polymyositis in proportion to the loss of muscle strength. DTRs are diminished or absent with loss of sensation or damage to the spinal cord. Loss of sensation in an extremity, coupled with loss of reflexes, suggests lesions in the sensory arc, as seen with neurosyphilis.
- Hyperreflexia (increased reflexes) on one side, occurring with upper motor neuron diseases, such as cerebrovascular accident (CVA) or the initial stages of amyotrophic lateral sclerosis (ALS).
- Impaired sensory testing, possibly indicating several neurologic disorders. Loss of position sense may suggest a spinal cord lesion when associated with other neurologic complaints. Vibration is the first sense to be lost in peripheral neuropathies such as diabetes mellitus. This loss also occurs with alcoholism, tertiary syphilis, and vitamin B_{12} deficiency.
- Nonrhythmic flapping of the wrists and hands, with arms extended and wrists hyperflexed, called asterixis. Sometimes termed a liver flap, this is associated with such disorders as hepatic encephalopathy, uremia, and respiratory acidosis. (See ▧ *Three Ways to Check for Asterixis,* p. 222.)

Palpation

Palpate the skin of the upper extremities for temperature, moisture, and lesions or nodules. Compare between arms, noting differences and similarities, as needed. Then move on to test the patient's pulses, lymph nodes, muscles, and ROM.

EXAMINATION TIP

THREE WAYS TO CHECK FOR ASTERIXIS

An excessive involuntary flapping tremor, asterixis is most commonly seen in the wrists and fingers. This sign may be elicited when the patient is asked to sustain a fixed position or posture. Then, brief, irregular relaxation of the muscles used to sustain the position cause the affected body part to display a flapping tremor. Although the exact underlying mechanism of this loss of muscle tone is unknown, asterixis is believed to be the result of a build-up of metabolic toxins, such as ammonia, in the brain. These toxins may cause cerebral metabolic changes that affect the motor neurons in the brain. To confirm asterixis, use one of the following assessment techniques. Your ability to elicit asterixis will depend on your patient's level of consciousness because she'll need to be alert enough to sustain a fixed position.

- If your patient is awake and alert, instruct her to stretch her arms out in front of her, maintaining dorsiflexion of both wrists. Look for intermittent relaxation of the wrists and flapping of the hands.
- If her level of consciousness is diminished, lift one of her legs off of the bed and dorsiflex her foot at the ankle. Look for intermittent relaxation of the ankle and flapping of the foot.
- If she's lethargic and weak but can follow commands, ask her to squeeze your fingers. Look for involuntary clenching and unclenching of her fist.

Palpating pulses

Important circulatory structures and pulse locations are present on your patient's upper extremities. The axillary artery is the major arterial structure of the upper extremity. It's a continuation of the subclavian. As it passes into the shoulder area and begins traveling downward, it becomes the brachial artery. The brachial artery sends branches to the humerus, the muscles, and the skin of the area. About 1 cm below the bend of the elbow, the brachial splits off and becomes the radial and ulnar arteries. The radial artery continues down the lateral aspect of the forearm, but it's smaller in caliber than the ulnar. The ulnar artery is the larger of the two and courses down the medial aspect of the forearm and the wrist.

Palpate the brachial, radial, and ulnar pulses for rate, strength, contour, and amplitude. (See *Performing Allen's Test.*)

Document pulse amplitude using the following scale:

+4	Bounding, hyperkinetic pulse
+3	Normal pulse
+2	Diminished pulse
+1	Weak, thready, hypokinetic pulse
0	Absent pulse

Test the compliance of vein walls by compressing prominent veins with the pads of your fingers. Note resilience, texture, and the presence of valves.

EXAMINATION TIP

PERFORMING ALLEN'S TEST

Before your patient undergoes arterial blood gas sampling or insertion of an arterial catheter, you'll need to check the patency of her radial and ulnar arteries by performing Allen's test.

Ask your patient to open her hand into a relaxed, slightly flexed position. Then ask her to make a tight fist while you use both hands to occlude her radial and ulnar arteries, as shown in the first illustration.

Now have your patient open her hand, as shown in the second illustration. Because of the temporary lack of blood supply, it will look blanched. Be sure your patient doesn't spread her fingers too widely or forcefully, because this may compress the palmar arches between the fascial planes and give a false-positive result.

Now release the pressure over one artery. Most nurses release the ulnar artery first, as shown in the third illustration, but the sequence isn't important. Within 3 to 5 seconds after you release the artery, your patient's palm should flush with color as it fills with blood. This result means that the patient's ulnar artery is patent.

After several minutes, repeat the test, but release the radial artery this time. The results should be the same, indicating that the patient's radial artery is patent.

If you release an artery and your patient's hand is not infused with color within 5 to 10 seconds, the artery or one of its distal branches is occluded. Consequently, you shouldn't puncture either artery.

If your patient is unconscious or anesthetized and can't make a clenched fist, you can still perform Allen's test. Just use an elastic bandage to blanch the hand.

Compress both arteries while the patient makes a clenched fist.

Ask your patient to open the fist. The palm should be blanched.

Release one artery and wait for the patient's palm to flush within a few seconds.

If you haven't done so earlier in the examination, check capillary refill time by pressing on a nail bed for several seconds. Then release the pressure, and note how long it takes for the nail to regain its normal color.

Palpating lymph nodes

To detect possible infection, you'll want to palpate the lymph nodes (the axillary and epitrochlear nodes) for size, consistency, and tenderness. The axillary nodes are located along the chest wall, high in the axilla and midway between the anterior and posterior axillary folds. The epitrochlear nodes are located superficially on the medial side of the elbow.

Palpating muscles

When palpating the muscles of the upper extremities, focus on their bulk (or mass), tone, and strength. Ask your patient to tell you if she feels pain or other abnormal sensations at any time while you're palpating her limbs. Be sure to document it if your patient reports any of these feelings.

Muscle bulk can be determined by bilateral examination of the upper extremities. Remember that your patient's dominant side may tend to have a larger muscle mass than the nondominant side. Examine upper extremity muscles for gross hypertrophy or atrophy. This may be difficult if your patient is markedly obese. Remember that muscle mass declines normally with age.

Upper extremity strength can be evaluated in various ways, based on your patient's age, sex, and level of muscular training. To perform a quick test of muscular strength, ask your patient to move her upper extremities through their full ROM without applying any resistance beyond what's already provided by gravity. For example, ask your patient to fully extend her elbows and place her arms, palms up, in front of her. Ask her to hold this position for about 10 seconds. Watch to see whether one of her extremities drifts or falls and whether she begins to pronate her wrists, which indicates weakness.

Another way to test muscle strength is with resistance. First, ask your patient to flex her elbow and curl her arm toward herself as you apply resistance by trying to pull her forearm toward you. This exercise tests her biceps. Then, with your patient's elbow still flexed, ask her to extend her arm while you try to keep it in the flexed position. This exercise tests the triceps.

You can test wrist extension by having your patient make a fist and then resist your attempts to pull it down.

Evaluate finger abduction by having your patient place her palms down and spread her fingers apart. Ask the patient to resist you as you try to push her fingers back together. Test the thumb by asking your patient to touch her thumb to the tip of her little finger.

To test hand-grip strength, have your patient grasp both of your hands and squeeze them as hard as she can. Note bilateral strength. Remember, however, that your patient's dominant hand may be slightly stronger than

EXAMINATION TIP

ASSESSING HAND-GRIP STRENGTH SAFELY

When testing your patient's hand-grip strength, you can help prevent pain or injury to your hands and fingers by following these suggestions:

- Remove any rings or hand jewelry that could pinch or compress your fingers.
- Cross your index and middle fingers, and ask your patient to squeeze only these fingers, as shown in the photograph. This technique will prevent your fingers from being painfully squeezed together, but you'll still be able to assess the patient's bilateral hand-grip strength.

the nondominant hand. To avoid confusion, cross your arms so that the patient's right hand grips your right hand, and her left hand grips your left hand. (See *Assessing Hand-Grip Strength Safely*.)

Testing for range of motion

Evaluate ROM in the patient's shoulder by asking her to perform three simple maneuvers. First, ask her to raise both arms to a vertical position at the sides of her head. Next, ask her to place both hands behind her neck, with elbows out to the sides. This movement demonstrates external rotation and abduction. Finally, ask your patient to place both hands behind the small of her back. This tests internal rotation.

To test elbow ROM, ask her to bend and straighten her elbow. Now ask her to place her arms at her sides with elbows flexed. Then have your patient supinate and pronate her arms. Finally, ask her to flex and extend her arms at the elbows.

To test wrist ROM, ask your patient to flex and hyperextend her wrists. Also ask her to bend her wrists to the radial side, then to the ulnar side. As she performs these maneuvers, palpate the wrist with both of your thumbs on the wrist dorsum and your fingers underneath. Note any swelling, bogginess, or tenderness.

To test ROM for the hand joints, ask your patient to make a fist with each hand and then extend and spread her fingers. Note any decreased mobility or pain on movement.

Palpation during ROM tests gives you information about joint integrity. A normal joint moves easily through its ROM. A snap or a crack may indicate that a ligament is slipping over a bony prominence. That's why it's important to palpate the joints while checking ROM.

To assess for tenderness, palpate the shoulder in the sternoclavicular joint, acromioclavicular joint, subacromial area, and bicipital groove. Palpate the tendons of the teres minor and infraspinatus muscles (sometimes called the rotator cuff) for swelling, nodes, tears, and pain. To do so, ask your patient to adduct her arm by bringing it over her chest. Facing your patient, place your thumb on the anterior surface of the joint, and the tips of your fingers on the posterior surface. Ask your patient to move the humerus backward about 20 degrees. Now move behind her, and, with your fingertips over the head of the humerus and your other hand between the scapulae, ask your patient to move her arm behind her body, with the dorsum of the hand resting on the small of the back (internal rotation).

To palpate the elbow, flex your patient's arm about 70 degrees and support it in that position with your nondominant hand. If the joint is swollen, you'll probably be able to palpate the swelling in the medial groove. With your dominant hand, palpate the joint with your fingertips while applying pressure with your thumb on the opposite side.

Gently palpate the interphalangeal, metacarpophalangeal, and wrist joints between your thumb and fingers, noting any swelling, bogginess, or tenderness. Assess for nodule formation, which accompanies rheumatoid arthritis, gout, rheumatic fever, and osteoarthritis.

Palpate the brachial pulse, and check for an enlarged epitrochlear lymph node in the depression above and behind the medial condyle of the humerus.

Grading muscle strength and range of motion

You can grade muscle strength and ROM on a numerical scale from 0 to 5. Use the following key to grade muscle strength accurately:

0   Complete paralysis. No visible or palpable muscle contraction or movement of the extremity.

1   Very severe weakness. Weak muscle contraction visible, but the extremity does not move.

2   Severe weakness. Patient can roll the extremity but cannot lift it. Patient can perform full ROM, but not against gravity.

3   Moderate weakness. Patient can perform full ROM against gravity, but not against resistance.

4   Slight weakness. Patient can perform full ROM against gravity and slight resistance.

5   Normal muscle strength. Patient can perform full ROM against gravity and resistance

Normal findings

- Skin temperature cool to warm, with minimal moisture and a smooth, even texture. Stimulation of the sympathetic nervous system, as when the patient is embarrassed or anxious, causes diaphoresis and moist skin.
- Pulses strong and equal bilaterally.
- Joints with no obvious deformity, tenderness, or swelling. No crepitus is heard.
- Muscle strength equal bilaterally, with full movement against resistance.
- Veins soft and pliable.
- Capillary refill brisk, less than 4 seconds.
- Thrill on palpation or a bruit on auscultation over renal shunt or fistula. These findings reflect turbulent blood flow in the area and are considered normal. (See ⬛ *What to Expect When Examining the Upper Extremities.*)

Abnormal findings

- Abnormal bony growths on the distal interphalangeal joints (Heberden's nodes) or the proximal interphalangeal joints

NORMAL FINDINGS

WHAT TO EXPECT WHEN EXAMINING THE UPPER EXTREMITIES

Use this quick review to confirm normal findings when examining the upper extremities.

- ❏ Skin color of upper extremities matches skin color of rest of body, except in areas routinely exposed to sunlight.
- ❏ No edema or any obvious deformities.
- ❏ Skin warm and smooth, with minimal moisture.
- ❏ Radial, ulnar, and brachial pulses easily palpated and bilaterally equal in strength and amplitude.
- ❏ Capillary refill time less than 2 seconds.
- ❏ Full range of motion in all joints, without pain.

- ❏ Symmetrical upper extremities.
- ❏ Shoulder muscle strength equal bilaterally.
- ❏ Hand-grip strength equal bilaterally.
- ❏ Brachioradialis, biceps, triceps, and deep tendon reflexes ++ bilaterally.
- ❏ Subclavian and epitrochlear lymph nodes either nonpalpable or small, soft, mobile, and nontender.
- ❏ Superficial touch and pain sensations normal bilaterally, with intact vibratory and position senses.

(Bouchard's nodes), indicating osteoarthritic joint changes. These growths are firm and usually nontender.

- Subcutaneous nodules (rheumatoid nodules) over bony prominences or along the extensor surface of the ulna, indicating rheumatoid arthritis. These nodules are firm, mobile, and nontender. They may accompany other symptoms of rheumatoid arthritis, such as morning stiffness, pain on motion, or tenderness and swelling in at least one joint.
- Firm, erythematous, painful nodules (tophi). These form over joints during acute flare-ups of gout and, if ulcerated, leak a white, chalky substance composed of uric acid crystals.
- Crepitus (an audible creaking sound as the joint moves through its ROM), possibly indicating pain or limitation of movement. Crepitation may be benign or associated with such joint diseases as arthritis or inflamed tendon sheaths.
- Pulselessness, pallor, pain, or paresthesias of the distal upper extremities, indicating arterial occlusion.
- Arterial compression, occurring with compartment syndrome and possibly resulting from casts, tight dressings, and infiltrated IV fluids. If arterial compression is left untreated, the patient may lose limb function and mobility.
- Swelling of the extremity, along with pallor or cyanosis and dilation of superficial veins, warning of thrombosis of the axillary or subclavian veins. Diminished or absent pulses may occur as well, from associated arterial spasm. The patient also may have moderate-to-severe pain in the arm and shoulder, diffuse pain through the involved extremity, and fever.
- Swelling or bogginess felt over the joint, especially the elbow, possibly accompanied by tenderness and erythema. This indicates an effusion, sometimes called water on the elbow, which is caused by synovitis, an inflammation of the synovial membrane resulting from trauma.
- Decreased joint mobility and ROM, indicating arthritis, trauma, tendinitis, or bursitis. Decreased joint mobility and ROM arise as a complication of immobility or as a normal variant of aging.
- Extreme pain on movement of the wrist, elbow, and shoulder, along with joint heat, redness, or inflammation related to tenosynovitis— an inflammation of the tendon sheath and the enclosed tendons that primarily affects the wrist, shoulder, and ankle.
- Muscle atrophy and weakness, possibly related to malnutrition or disuse, as seen with paralysis and prolonged periods of immobility. Muscles appear flattened or concave when atrophy has affected the extremity. Tremors or fasciculations also may be observed in the atrophic limb. Fasciculations indicate lower motor neuron damage as the cause of the atrophy.
- Paralysis, possibly resulting from such conditions as Guillain-Barré syndrome, spinal cord injury, CVA, diabetic neuropathy, multiple sclerosis, and poliomyelitis.

- Inflamed lymphatic vessels, possibly resulting from bacterial infection. When this occurs in superficial vessels, painful reddish streaks appear beneath the skin (lymphangitis), and are typically followed by an inflammation of the lymph nodes (lymphadenitis). Affected nodes become enlarged and tender.
- Veins that feel hard and cordlike, possibly indicating sclerosis. They may also feel tortuous, with prominent, beadlike valves palpable through the skin.
- Delayed capillary refill, characterized by blanching of the nail beds for more than 4 seconds after being released from pressure. This is usually a warning of compromised circulation, as in diminished cardiac output, hypotension, or arterial occlusion.
- Loss of a palpable thrill or an audible bruit over an arteriovenous fistula, possibly indicating thrombosis or clotting of the fistula.

EXPLORING CHIEF COMPLAINTS

When examining your patient's upper extremities, your first task is to determine her chief complaint. Doing so will help you set your assessment priorities and allow you to focus your assessment appropriately.

Help your patient describe her chief complaint by asking open-ended questions and listening carefully to her answers. Allow her to describe her problem in her own words. Based on your patient's answers, you can focus on areas that need further assessment.

The rest of this chapter lists common complaints involving the upper extremities and outlines your assessment goals and the conditions you should consider as possible causes of the patient's problem.

Muscle stiffness or spasm

If your patient complains of muscle stiffness or spasm, investigate the symptom further by asking her the following questions:
- When did your symptoms start? How long do they usually last?
- Does the stiffness or spasm tend to start after you've been performing certain activities or when you've been sitting, sleeping, or standing in certain positions?
- If the muscle stiffness or spasm occurs at night, does it ever wake you from sleep? If you wake up with it in the morning, what position were you sleeping in?
- How would you describe the stiffness or spasm? Is it sharp, dull, aching, stabbing, or throbbing?
- Did the stiffness or spasm start after an injury or after doing anything unusual?
- Does it tend to worsen with weather changes, especially when conditions become cold and damp or hot and humid?
- Does a fever, headache, or chest pain accompany the stiffness or spasm?

Focusing your assessment

When examining a patient who complains of muscle stiffness or spasm, focus your assessment as follows:

- Look for muscle atrophy in the major muscle groups of the arms. Compare them bilaterally.
- Assess muscle tone and strength by testing each major muscle group with resistance.
- Test the patient's DTRs.

Possible causes

- *Muscle fatigue.* Painful muscle contractions, or spasms, typically are the result of muscle fatigue. Spasms are usually relieved by rest or stretching. They can be found in neurologic disorders and electrolyte imbalances.
- *Muscle rigidity.* Rigidity is seen with such disorders as Parkinson's disease. Symptoms may progress and affect movement.
- *Muscle sprain.* Sprain follows unusual or prolonged exercise or injury. Symptoms improve with rest.
- *Hypocalcemic tetany.* This condition produces frequent spasms in many muscles and is accompanied by paresthesias in the hands and feet. If you suspect this condition, check for Trousseau's and Chvostek's sign (See 🖾 *Detecting Trousseau's and Chvostek's Signs.*)
- *Cervical nerve root compression.* This condition follows injury or strain to the neck. Muscular pain may be accompanied by pain that follows the distribution of the involved nerve root. The patient's DTRs may be diminished.
- *Upper motor neuron disorders.* An example of an upper motor neuron disorder is CVA, in which the patient has increased muscle tone, spasticity, and increased DTRs.
- *Lower motor neuron disorders.* An example is ALS, in which the patient has decreased muscle tone and strength, and decreased DTRs.

Joint pain or stiffness

If your patient complains of joint stiffness or pain, investigate the symptom further by asking her the following questions:

- When are your joints stiff and painful? How long do they stay that way? Does the problem tend to occur more in the morning, during the day, or at night?
- How would you describe the stiffness or pain? Is it sharp, dull, aching, stabbing, or throbbing?
- Did the stiffness or pain start after you were injured or you had done something unusual?
- Do you (the patient who is African-American or of Mediterranean descent) have a history of sickle cell disease?

EXAMINATION TIP

DETECTING TROUSSEAU'S AND CHVOSTEK'S SIGNS

Low serum calcium (and sometimes magnesium) levels can result in tetany, a life-threatening condition characterized by twitching, cramps, seizures, and sharp wrist and ankle flexion. If you suspect either disorder, evaluate your patient for the classic signs: Trousseau's and Chvostek's signs.

Here's how to test for them:

Trousseau's sign
- Place a blood pressure cuff on your patient's upper arm, and inflate the cuff to a point above her systolic blood pressure. Then watch her hand.
- If within 4 minutes she experiences a carpopedal spasm with ventral contraction of the thumb and fingers, the sign is positive.

Chvostek's sign
- Tap the patient's cheek over the facial nerve, just in front of her ear.
- Watch for abnormal contraction of the facial muscles, twitching of the lips, or possible contraction of all the muscles on one side of the face. If any of these occur, the sign is positive.

From Mosby. (1999). *Expert Rapid Response*. St. Louis: Mosby.

- Do you have a family or personal history of rheumatoid or degenerative arthritis or heart disease?
- Does a fever accompany the stiffness or pain?
- Does your skin change color, or do you get a rash before, during, or after the symptoms?
- Do you remember receiving any insect bites, especially tick bites, in the past 7 months or so?
- Have you had any surgery in the affected area (particularly a joint replacement)?

Focusing your assessment
When examining a patient who complains of joint stiffness or pain, focus your assessment as follows:
- Inspect the joints for swelling, ecchymosis, or deformity. Are both arms symmetrical?
- Find out if the joints are tender to the touch.
- Is there pain with ROM? Or is ROM restricted due to pain?
- Take the patient's temperature to see if she has a fever.
- Assess the skin for insect bites or rashes.
- Investigate whether the pain might be referred, such as from the chest. If necessary, obtain electrocardiogram (ECG) tracings to look for patterns of ischemia or infarction.

Possible causes
- *Rheumatoid arthritis.* Patients with rheumatoid arthritis typically have morning stiffness, joint tenderness, swelling in at least two joint groups, and subcutaneous nodules over bony prominences. (See *Rheumatoid Arthritis,* p. 234.)
- *Osteoarthritis.* Also called degenerative joint disease, osteoarthritis becomes more common with age. Characterized by joint pain that worsens throughout the day, it's aggravated by exercise. Onset is gradual and usually involves only a few joints.
- *Fracture.* Your patient will most likely feel intense pain at a fracture site. Pain may radiate through the arm and will be aggravated by movement.
- *Tendinitis.* This condition produces intense localized pain, aggravated by movement and relieved by rest.
- *Septic arthritis.* An acute bacterial infection of a joint, septic arthritis usually results from contamination during surgery or from bacterial migration from an infection elsewhere in the body. It's characterized by acute pain, redness, swelling, fever, and immobility of the joint.
- *Bursitis.* Symptoms of this disorder may develop after unusually vigorous exercise or strain. The patient will complain of pain, localized tenderness, and limitation of movement.

- *Sickle cell anemia.* A form of hemolytic anemia, sickle cell anemia is marked by chronic fatigue and painful, swollen joints. This disease commonly affects people of African-American or Mediterranean descent.
- *Lyme disease.* This is an infectious disease caused by a spirochete transmitted through tick bites. The insect bite initially produces a red mark that eventually forms a pink or red rash resembling a bull's-eye. Complications are far-reaching and range from meningitis to pericarditis. At least half the victims suffer from joint pain and swelling.
- *Angina or myocardial infarction.* Both of these conditions can refer pain to the shoulder and arm. Your patient may have chest pain as well.

Paresthesia or numbness

If your patient complains of paresthesia or numbness, investigate the symptom further by asking her the following questions:
- When did your symptoms begin? Did they follow after any type of trauma or strenuous activity?
- What is the exact location of the paresthesia or numbness? Is it the same in both arms, or do you have it only in one arm?
- Is this the first time you've experienced this problem?
- If this is a recurrence, did anything seem to provoke or start up the symptoms this time?
- How long do the symptoms last? Does anything seem to make them better or worse?
- How would you describe the paresthesia or numbness? What does it feel like? Do you have a heavy, achy, or sharp feeling? If so, does it radiate?
- Do you have any associated conditions, such as long-term alcohol or substance abuse, diabetes mellitus, chronic anemia, sickle cell disease, a recent viral syndrome, a recent immunization or injection, a recent animal bite or scratch, or a recent insect bite (especially ticks)?
- Do you have any associated symptoms, such as temperature change, altered color, swelling, slurred speech, dizziness, fever, headache, respiratory distress (particularly tachypnea), loss of motor control, or chest pain?
- Have you ever experienced anything like this before?

Focusing your assessment

When examining a patient who complains of paresthesia or numbness, focus your assessment as follows:
- Evaluate the sensory system, including your patient's sensitivity to pain, temperature, position, vibration, and light touch, in conjunction with evaluating the motor system (muscle tone, muscle strength, and DTRs).

DISORDER CLOSE-UP

RHEUMATOID ARTHRITIS

A chronic, systemic inflammatory disorder, rheumatoid arthritis is characterized by persistent synovitis of multiple joints. It's found worldwide and affects about 1% of the population. It strikes females three times more often than males.

No one knows what causes rheumatoid arthritis, but researchers have identified genetic and environmental factors that probably play a role in its development. They're also investigating whether the Epstein-Barr virus might help initiate the immune response.

Rheumatoid arthritis is known by its persistent immunologic activity. T lymphocytes infiltrate the synovial membrane of the joint and proliferate, initiating an immune response. The release of cytokines further stimulates macrophage activity, and B cells produce autoantibodies to immunoglobulin G. These antibodies, called rheumatoid factors, are found in nearly all patients who have the disease.

An antigen-antibody reaction sparks formation of immune complexes that generate lysosomal enzymes, which can destroy joint tissue. Vasodilation from the immune response causes tissues to become warm and erythematous. Increased capillary permeability produces swelling of the affected area. Joints are destroyed by the extensive network of new blood vessels (vascular granulation tissue called pannus) in the synovial membrane. Pannus erodes the cartilage and bone of affected joints and invades surrounding tissues, including ligaments and tendons.

Health history
- Insidious onset of nonspecific symptoms
- Fatigue, malaise
- Anorexia, weight loss
- Persistent low-grade fever
- Bilateral and symmetrical stiffening of joints, beginning in the fingers and possibly extending to the wrists, elbows, knees, and ankles
- Stiffening after inactivity, especially on arising
- Tender and painful joints, initially on movement but eventually at rest
- Paresthesias of the fingers or toes
- Stiff, weak, or painful muscles
- Shortness of breath (with pulmonary nodules or fibrosis)
- Neck pain (with cervical vertebral involvement)

Characteristic findings
Expect your physical examination findings to vary among patients with rheumatoid arthritis, depending on the extent and severity of the disease. Use the information that follows to help distinguish between expected and unexpected findings.

Inspection
- Ulnar deviation of the fingers and subluxation at the metacarpophalangeal joints
- Boutonnière deformities (flexion deformity of the proximal interphalangeal joint with extension of distal joint)

Possible causes
- *Fracture, tumor, or swelling.* This can compress a nerve, resulting in numbness or paresthesia.
- *Occlusive vascular diseases.* Raynaud's or Buerger's diseases may cause sensory changes, such as numbness or tingling.
- *Neurologic disorders.* Disorders such as multiple sclerosis and ALS cause paresthesia.

- Swan-neck deformities (hyper-extension of the proximal interphalangeal joint with compensatory flexion of the distal joint)
- Limited range of movement (ROM) in affected joints
- Flexion contractures of the elbows
- Joint swelling and redness

Palpation
- Rheumatoid nodules (firm granulomatous lesions, either fixed or mobile) in subcutaneous tissue of areas subject to pressure
- Joints warm or hot to touch
- Muscle weakness (with spinal cord involvement)
- Positive Babinski's sign (with spinal cord involvement)

Auscultation
- Pericardial friction rub (with pericarditis)

Complications
- Fibrous or bony ankylosis
- Soft-tissue contractures
- Joint deformities
- Vasculitis
- Pleural disease
- Pericarditis
- Episcleritis or scleritis

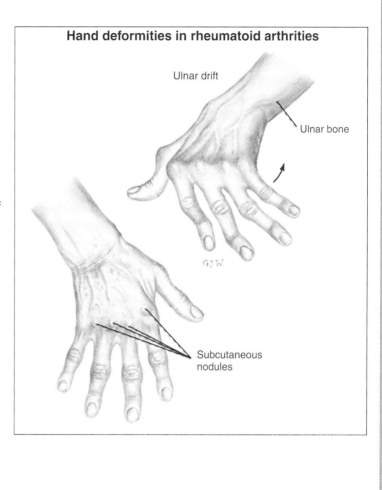

Hand deformities in rheumatoid arthrities

Ulnar drift

Ulnar bone

Subcutaneous nodules

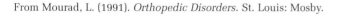

From Mourad, L. (1991). *Orthopedic Disorders*. St. Louis: Mosby.

- *Neuropathy.* Degeneration of peripheral nerves can result from many systemic diseases, such as diabetes mellitus, chronic alcoholism, and lead poisoning. Paresthesia often leads to diminished or absent sensation in the most distal parts of the extremities.
- *Vitamin B_6 deficiency.* Pyridoxine (vitamin B_6) deficiency produces symptoms similar to neuropathy.

- *Hyperventilation.* This condition commonly causes a pins-and-needles sensation because of hypocapnia.
- *Carpal tunnel syndrome.* An occupation-related condition caused by repetitive wrist flexure, this disorder is characterized by paresthesia in the hand and pain in the wrist joint, palm, and sometimes the forearm. The patient may have a sensory deficit in the first three fingers and weakness in the thumb.

Paralysis or weakness

If your patient complains of paralysis or weakness, investigate the symptom further by asking her the following questions:
- When did the problem first occur? Did it follow an event or an injury?
- Have you ever experienced anything like this before?
- Is the paralysis or weakness associated with a specific area of your arm, such as the shoulder or elbow joint, wrist, or fingers?
- Does it affect both of your arms or just one?
- If the paralysis or weakness is a transient occurrence, how long does it usually last?
- Does the paralysis or weakness tend to occur after certain activities, such as a sport? Does it tend to occur in the morning, after sleeping in a certain position?
- If the problem occurs more at night, does it ever wake you?
- What are the characteristics of the paralysis or weakness? Do you have a heavy or achy feeling associated with it, and, if so, does the feeling radiate?
- Does it tend to get worse with temperature changes either indoors or outdoors? Examples include a severe decrease or increase in temperature or when the weather becomes wet or 'humid.
- Do you have any other symptoms associated with the paralysis or weakness, such as swelling, slurred speech, dizziness, fever, headache, or chest pain?

Focusing your assessment

When examining a patient who complains of paralysis or weakness, focus your assessment as follows:
- Look for muscle atrophy in the major muscle groups of the arms. Compare side to side.
- Assess muscle tone and strength by testing each major muscle group against resistance. This evaluates both the musculoskeletal and neurologic systems.
- Test DTRs. Absent or decreased muscle tone and strength and absent or decreased DTRs are observed in such lower motor neuron disorders as ALS Guillain-Barré syndrome. In upper motor neuron disorders, expect increased muscle tone, spasticity, and increased DTRs.

Possible causes
- *Systemic disorder.* Extremity weakness may be caused by many systemic disorders, such as hypokalemia, hypothyroidism, dehydration, vascular disorders, and B-complex vitamin deficiencies. Paralysis can also result from a number of conditions, including Guillain-Barré syndrome, spinal cord injury, CVA, diabetic neuropathy, multiple sclerosis, or poliomyelitis. (See *Cerebrovascular Accident,* p. 238.)
- *Transient ischemia.* Transient or temporary weakness in an extremity or body part may result from temporary interruption of blood supply to the brain, as seen with transient ischemic attacks (TIAs). Other symptoms include blurred vision, aphasia, and dizziness.

Swelling
If your patient complains of swelling, investigate the symptom further by asking her the following questions:
- When did you first notice the swelling or any change in your arm?
- How did it first start? Did it occur in one location and spread? Or did your arm become swollen at one time?
- Has this swelling happened before? How long ago? How long did it last? If it recurs, how often, and what provokes it?
- Does anything make the swelling better or worse?
- Do you have any associated symptoms, such as pain, fever, numbness, or tingling?
- Do you have a history of trauma, a clotting disorder, leukemia or another neoplasm? Have you had recent exposure to an infection or had an IV or any type of puncture (including insect and animal bites)?

Focusing your assessment
When examining a patient who complains of swelling, focus your assessment as follows:
- Palpate the swollen area for temperature and tenderness.
- Determine whether the edema is pitting or nonpitting, unilateral or bilateral.
- Record the size of the swollen area by measuring the circumference of the extremity at the point of swelling.
- If a joint is involved, assess its ROM for limitation and pain on movement.

Possible causes
- *Injury.* Fracture, sprain, or strain may cause swelling, which is typically relieved by elevation. Other associated signs and symptoms include deformity, localized ecchymosis or bleeding, pain,

DISORDER CLOSE-UP

CEREBROVASCULAR ACCIDENT

During a cerebrovascular accident (CVA)—commonly called a stroke—decreased blood flow in one or more cerebral blood vessels results in infarcted brain tissue and permanent neurologic deficit. This decreased blood flow can result when a thrombus or embolism occludes a cerebral blood vessel. It also can result from a ruptured cerebral blood vessel, in which hemorrhage causes cellular ischemia and necrosis.

When cerebral blood flow declines or stops, oxygenation does, too. Within 4 or 5 minutes, pathophysiologic changes begin at the cellular level. Metabolism ceases when glucose, glycogen, and adenosine triphosphate are depleted, and the sodium-potassium pump fails. Cells swell as sodium draws water into them. Cerebral blood vessel walls swell, further decreasing blood flow. Even if circulation is restored, vasospasm and increased blood viscosity can continue to impede blood flow. Severe or prolonged ischemia leads to cellular death and loss of consciousness. Other neurologic deficits vary greatly according to the severity, location, and duration of ischemia.

The neurologic deficits caused by a CVA vary with the area involved and the duration of reduced or halted blood flow. Symptoms may become slightly less severe a few days after the CVA, when brain swelling subsides. When assessing the neurologic deficits and sensory motor functions that result from a CVA, remember that they occur on the side of the body opposite the side of the brain that was damaged.

Health history
- Personal or family history of CVAs
- Obesity
- Sedentary lifestyle
- History of hypertension, diabetes mellitus, atherosclerosis, hyperlipidemia, or atrial fibrillation
- Oral contraception use
- Complaints of motor deficits, such as gait changes, weakness, paralysis, or spasticity
- Speech problems
- Sudden onset of hemiparesis or hemiplegia
- Gradual onset of dizziness, mental disturbance, or seizures
- Complaints of numbness or tingling

Characteristic findings
Expect your physical examination findings to vary among CVA patients, depending on the extent and severity of the disease. Use the information that follows to help distinguish between expected and unexpected findings.

Inspection
- Altered level of consciousness
- Decreased attention span
- Anxiety
- Mobility and communication difficulties
- Possible incontinence
- Agnosia
- Apraxia

immobility, or paresthesia. Joint swelling indicates synovial inflammation or increased synovial fluid.
- *Infiltrated IV fluids.* This is indicated by swelling, coolness, tenderness, and redness at and above the IV catheter insertion site. (See 🖱 *Responding to IV Fluid Extravasation,* p. 240.)
- *Insect bites or stings.* These cause localized swelling that ranges from mild to severe, depending on your patient's reaction to the venom.

- Emotional lability
- Motor deficits
- Visual field deficits

Palpation
- Diminished muscle strength
- Diminished deep tendon reflexes (initially)
- Sensory losses ranging from slight impairment of touch to inability to perceive position and motion of body parts

Auscultation
- Diminished breath sounds

Vital signs
- Hyperthermia
- Unstable blood pressure
- Irregular respiratory rhythm
- Irregular pulse and heart rhythm

Complications
- Fluid imbalances
- Pulmonary embolism
- Malnutrition
- Aspiration
- Sensory impairment
- Contractures
- Encephalitis
- Coma
- Brain abscess
- Pneumonia

- *Infection.* Swelling may be caused by infection, usually bacterial, resulting from injury, surgery, or even IV catheters. The infected tissue may be superficial or deep. It may extend to the bone and result in osteomyelitis. Other symptoms include pain, redness, and decreased function or mobility. Fever also usually occurs.
- *Lymphedema.* An accumulation of lymph in the soft tissue of the extremity, lymphedema commonly results from surgical removal of lymph nodes. It also may result from obstructed lymph channels.

RESPONDING TO IV FLUID EXTRAVASATION

When an IV catheter slips out of a vein or passes through a vein, fluids infusing through the catheter enter surrounding tissues rather than entering the intended blood vessel. Called extravasation or infiltration, this can arise even with the catheter in proper position. In this case, extravasation may occur if fluid passes through the vessel wall or backs up through the insertion site.

The consequences of IV extravasation depend on the substance that's being infused and how long the extravasation continues. Adverse reactions range from mild redness and tenderness to pain and tissue destruction that can cause infection or loss of mobility of the extremity.

Chemotherapeutic agents (such as doxorubicin) are among a group of IV medications known as vesicants because they can cause blistering, tissue destruction, or both. Other agents (such as dopamine) cause vasoconstriction at the site of extravasation, resulting in tissue destruction. Whatever the agent, be sure to follow your institution's policy for treatments and antidotes.

What to look for
Signs and symptoms of IV extravasation include:
- an infusion rate that slows or stops
- swelling, redness, pain, and coolness around and proximal to the catheter insertion site
- decreased pulse distal to the insertion site
- failure of blood to flash back into the tubing when you lower the IV bag below the level of the needle (not always a reliable sign)
- signs of tissue necrosis (with vesicants or vasoconstrictive drugs)

What to do immediately
If you suspect IV fluid has extravasated into the soft tissue of your patient's arm, notify the physician, and follow these measures:
- Immediately stop the infusion. Identify the IV solution and any additives or medications.
- If the infiltrated substance is a vesicant, try aspirating it back through the catheter and prepare to instill an antidote, such as sodium bicarbonate and saline, through the catheter according to your institution's policy. If you can't aspirate the medication, remove the catheter.
- Consult the pharmacist to determine how toxic the additives are to soft tissue.
- If the IV solution contained a potent vasoconstrictor, such as norepinephrine or dopamine, add 5 to 10 mg of phentolamine to 0.9% saline to make 1 ml of solution. Inject it subcutaneously into the extravasation site, as prescribed.
- Remove constrictive clothing or devices (blood pressure cuff, dressings, or tape) distal or proximal to the catheter site within 12 hours. Otherwise, they could obstruct circulation to the area.
- Assess skin color and temperature at the site for early signs of tissue necrosis.
- Measure the circumference of the swollen area, noting the exact point of measurement so you can compare readings later.
- Check vital signs, looking specifically for signs and symptoms of sepsis, such as fever, tachycardia, and hypotension.

What to do next
Once you've completed these steps, you'll need to:
- Restart the infusion at another site, if necessary (preferably not in the same extremity). If you must use the same extremity, choose a site proximal to the site of extravasation.
- Apply warm compresses to the swollen area. If the infiltrated substance is a vesicant, apply cold compresses or ice.
- Continuously assess the extremity for increased pain and redness along the vein (a sign of thrombophlebitis or infection).
- Continuously assess the extremity for evidence of compartment syndrome, including loss of distal pulses, coolness, pale and mottled skin, and paresthesias.
- Photograph the site of extravasation according to policy, especially if the patient has tissue destruction.
- Document your assessment findings and interventions promptly and carefully.

Swelling may affect the extremity or only the most distal portion. Usually, elevation of the arm improves lymph drainage and reduces swelling.

- *Tumor.* Superior vena cava syndrome may be caused by tumor compression of the superior vena cava. This results in swelling, flushing, and venous engorgement of the face, chest, and arms.
- *Thrombophlebitis.* Acute inflammation of a vein, thrombophlebitis is marked by redness and tenderness along the course of a vein, as well as by localized swelling and warmth.

EXAMINING THE ABDOMINAL REGION

The very nature of the abdominal region, its structures, and associated health complaints make assessing this area of the body a challenge. Most people are embarrassed by signs and symptoms related to what they consider "private" matters, such as bowel or bladder dysfunction and gynecologic or urologic disorders. Similarly, many people have an almost irrational fear of cancer, permanent loss of bladder or bowel control, venereal disease, or erectile dysfunction. And what's worse, these fears may trigger feelings of guilt or shame.

Your goal is to create an atmosphere of openness, mutual trust, and compassion and to make your examination of the abdominal region as comfortable for the patient as possible. To do that effectively, you'll need detailed knowledge of the structures involved, including the lower pelvis, rectum, external genitalia, liver, gallbladder, stomach, spleen, intestines, and reproductive organs. (See ▌▌ *Structures of the Abdominal Region,* pp. 244 to 249.)

You'll also need to know how to perform a general examination of the abdominal region, as well as how to assess patients with complaints associated with disorders and conditions that commonly affect this complex body area.

ANATOMY REVIEW

STRUCTURES OF THE ABDOMINAL REGION

The following illustrations present the abdominal structures in their normal positions.

MAJOR STRUCTURES OF THE ABDOMINAL CAVITY

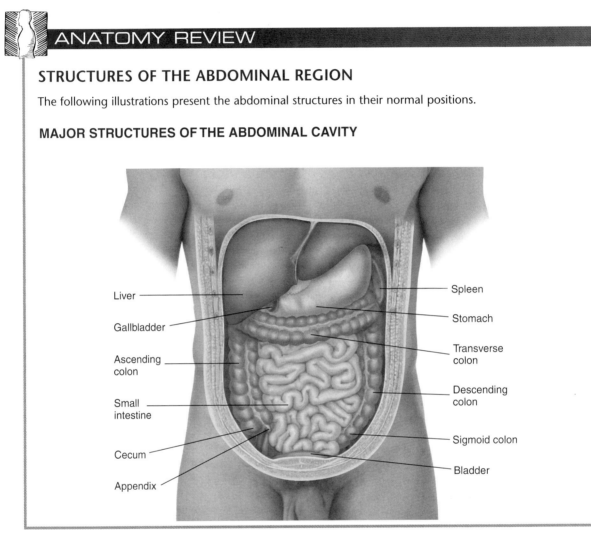

Liver

Gallbladder

Ascending colon

Small intestine

Cecum

Appendix

Spleen

Stomach

Transverse colon

Descending colon

Sigmoid colon

Bladder

From Seidel, H. M., Ball, J. W., Dains, J. E., & Benedict, G. W. (2003). *Mosby's Guide to Physical Examination* (5th ed.). St. Louis: Mosby.

This chapter will show you how to perform an efficient yet thorough examination of the abdominal region, providing you with focused, time-saving assessment steps you'll use when examining patients with common health complaints specific to this area.

EXAMINATION STEPS AND FINDINGS

To perform a deft examination of the abdominal region, you'll need to be adequately prepared. Start by gathering basic assessment equipment,

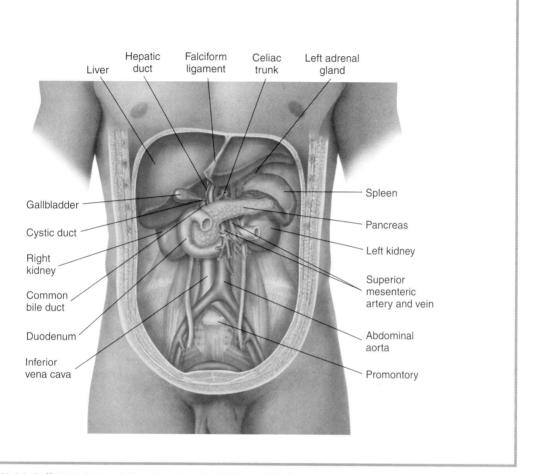

Hepatic duct
Falciform ligament
Celiac trunk
Left adrenal gland
Liver
Spleen
Gallbladder
Pancreas
Cystic duct
Left kidney
Right kidney
Superior mesenteric artery and vein
Common bile duct
Abdominal aorta
Duodenum
Inferior vena cava
Promontory

From Seidel, H. M., Ball, J. W., Dains, J. E., & Benedict, G. W. (2003). *Mosby's Guide to Physical Examination* (5th ed.). St. Louis: Mosby.

(Continued)

including a stethoscope, an examination drape, examination gloves, water-soluble jelly, a flashlight, a Hematest slide and reagent, and an examination light. You'll also need to keep in mind the most important steps to cover when assessing this area. (See 🔲 *Key Examination Steps for the Abdominal Region,* p. 250.)

Before you begin, make sure your examination room provides absolute privacy. You'll need to expose male patients from the chest to the pubis and female patients from below the breasts to the pubis. During auscultation, palpation, and percussion, keep the patient fully draped, except for the areas you're examining. Make sure you have adequate lighting to

STRUCTURES OF THE ABDOMINAL REGION—cont'd

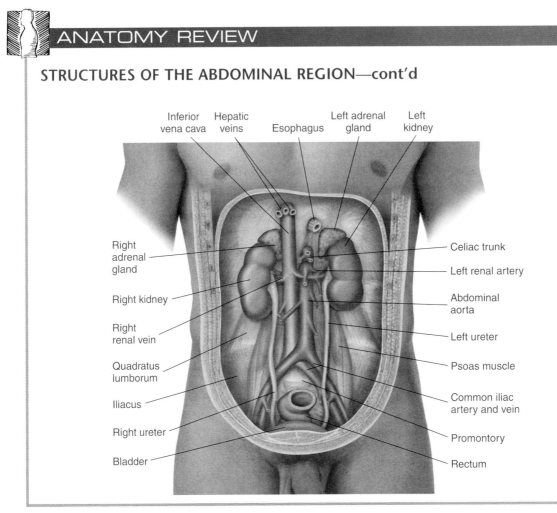

From Seidel, H. M., Ball, J. W., Dains, J. E., & Benedict, G. W. (2003). *Mosby's Guide to Physical Examination* (5th ed.). St. Louis: Mosby.

assess the abdominal wall. Finally, make sure the room is warm and comfortable.

Inspection

Begin your examination with inspection. Place the patient in a supine position to assess abdominal contour. Do this by kneeling at eye level at your patient's side. Note the shape of the abdominal outline. A slender patient will have a flat or slightly concave outline. An obese patient will have a protruding abdomen. Observe for any irregularities in

FEMALE GENITOURINARY SYSTEM

Lateral cross-section view

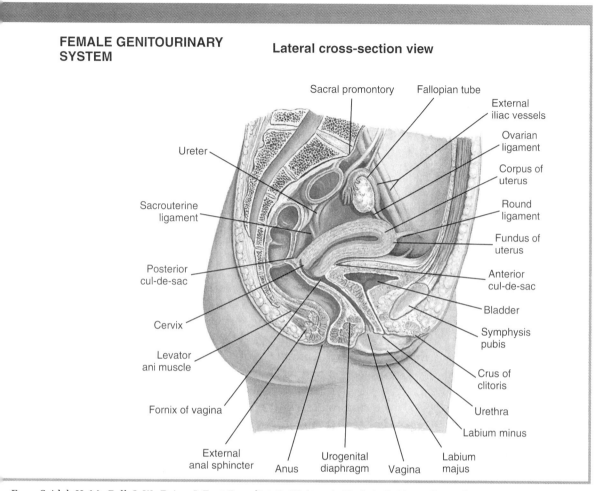

From Seidel, H. M., Ball, J. W., Dains, J. E., & Benedict, G. W. (2003). *Mosby's Guide to Physical Examination* (5th ed.). St. Louis: Mosby.

(Continued)

the outline. Assess abdominal symmetry by standing at the end of the bed.

While performing this first inspection, pay attention to your patient's apparent comfort level. If the patient seems tense or adjusts his position frequently, he may be uncomfortable. If his abdomen is distended, he may have trouble breathing because the abdominal contents are pressing against his diaphragm. To increase this patient's comfort, have him turn

(Text continues on p. 250.)

ANATOMY REVIEW

STRUCTURES OF THE ABDOMINAL REGION—cont'd

FEMALE GENITOURINARY SYSTEM

Inferior view of external genitalia

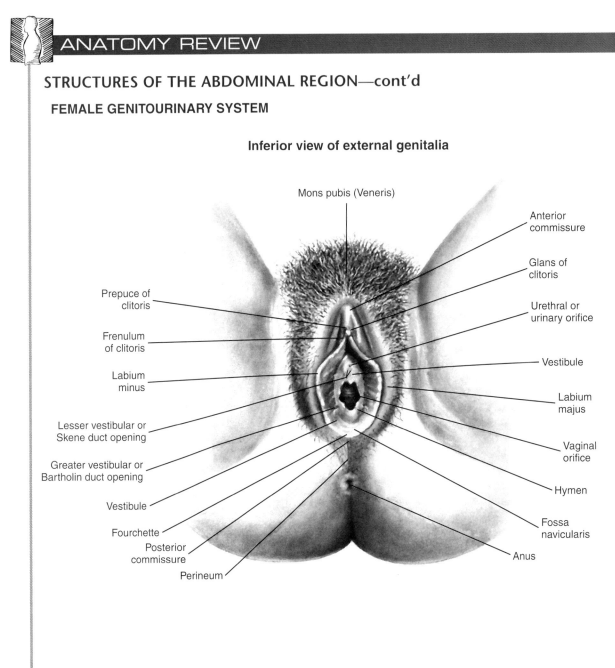

Mons pubis (Veneris)

Anterior commissure

Glans of clitoris

Prepuce of clitoris

Urethral or urinary orifice

Frenulum of clitoris

Vestibule

Labium minus

Labium majus

Lesser vestibular or Skene duct opening

Vaginal orifice

Greater vestibular or Bartholin duct opening

Hymen

Vestibule

Fossa navicularis

Fourchette

Posterior commissure

Anus

Perineum

From Seidel, H. M., Ball, J. W., Dains, J. E., & Benedict, G. W. (2003). *Mosby's Guide to Physical Examination* (5th ed.). St. Louis: Mosby.

MALE GENITOURINARY SYSTEM

Lateral cross-section view

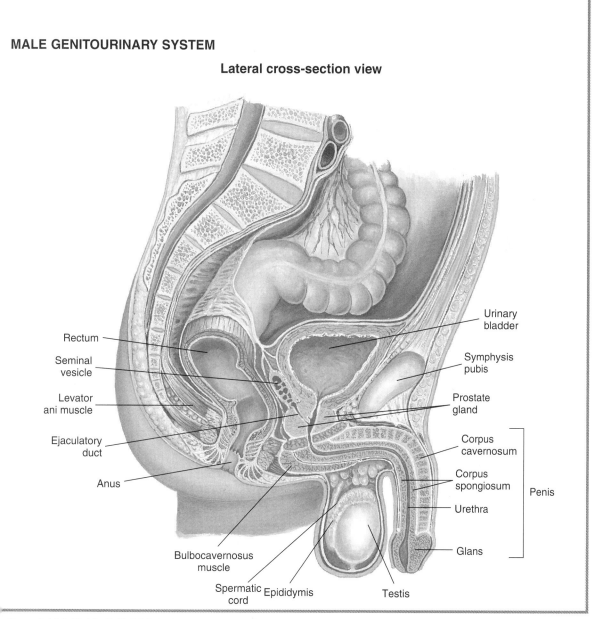

Rectum

Seminal
vesicle

Levator
ani muscle

Ejaculatory
duct

Anus

Bulbocavernosus
muscle

Spermatic
cord Epididymis

Testis

Urinary
bladder

Symphysis
pubis

Prostate
gland

Corpus
cavernosum

Corpus
spongiosum Penis

Urethra

Glans

From Seidel, H. M., Ball, J. W., Dains, J. E., & Benedict, G. W. (2003). *Mosby's Guide to Physical Examination* (5th ed.).
St. Louis: Mosby.

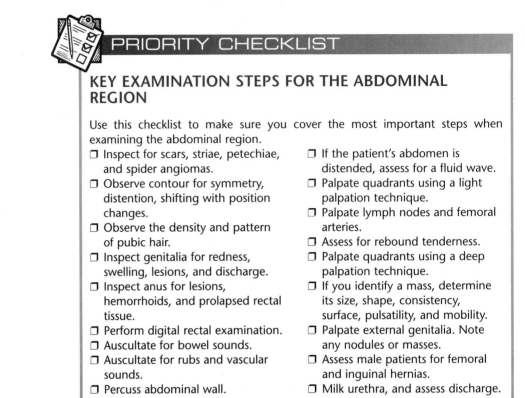

PRIORITY CHECKLIST

KEY EXAMINATION STEPS FOR THE ABDOMINAL REGION

Use this checklist to make sure you cover the most important steps when examining the abdominal region.

❐ Inspect for scars, striae, petechiae, and spider angiomas.

❐ Observe contour for symmetry, distention, shifting with position changes.

❐ Observe the density and pattern of pubic hair.

❐ Inspect genitalia for redness, swelling, lesions, and discharge.

❐ Inspect anus for lesions, hemorrhoids, and prolapsed rectal tissue.

❐ Perform digital rectal examination.

❐ Auscultate for bowel sounds.

❐ Auscultate for rubs and vascular sounds.

❐ Percuss abdominal wall.

❐ If the patient's abdomen is distended, assess for a fluid wave.

❐ Palpate quadrants using a light palpation technique.

❐ Palpate lymph nodes and femoral arteries.

❐ Assess for rebound tenderness.

❐ Palpate quadrants using a deep palpation technique.

❐ If you identify a mass, determine its size, shape, consistency, surface, pulsatility, and mobility.

❐ Palpate external genitalia. Note any nodules or masses.

❐ Assess male patients for femoral and inguinal hernias.

❐ Milk urethra, and assess discharge.

from the supine position to a lateral one, and assess abdominal contour by looking down.

Now observe the contour of the skin and any peristaltic movement or pulsations. Normally, peristaltic movements aren't visible. Some patients may have visible aortic pulsations. Note any superficial veins, petechiae, spider angiomas, striae, or scars.

Note the shape and location of the umbilicus and the hair density and pattern in the pubic region. To check for an umbilical or incisional hernia, ask your patient to raise his head and shoulders while remaining supine. A true hernia will protrude during this maneuver.

To inspect a male patient's genitals, observe the dorsal, lateral, and ventral surfaces of the penis for color, lesions, moles, size, and shape.

CULTURAL CONSIDERATIONS

Umbilical hernias are common in African-American children before the age of 7 and in Caucasian children before the age of 2.

If the patient is uncircumcised, retract the prepuce (foreskin) by grasping the penis behind the glans with your thumb and index finger and moving your fingers in the direction of the penile root. Be sure to replace the foreskin after your examination. The urethral opening (meatus) should be slitlike and have no discharge.

Spread the rugae (wrinkles) of the scrotum between your fingers to inspect the scrotal skin. Inspect the testicles for symmetry. If one testicle is larger than the other, is hard, or has a fluid consistency, you'll need to illuminate the scrotal sac to differentiate fluid from a mass. Darken the room and hold a flashlight close behind the affected testicle. You'll be able to see the light shining through fluid. If the scrotum contains a loop of bowel, indicating intestinal herniation, the light will not shine through, and the area will appear opaque.

To examine a female patient's genitals, spread the labia majora and inspect them and the labia minora. Note any lesions or discharge. Inspect the vestibule, especially the area around Bartholin's and Skene's glands. Look for swelling, redness, lesions, or discharge. Inspect the urethral opening and the vaginal opening.

Now ask your patient, whether male or female, to turn to the side in a lateral position. Watch the abdomen as your patient turns. Note any fluid shifting or abnormal protrusions. Help your patient draw knees to chest and gently spread the buttocks to expose the anus. Observe for lesions. Note any hemorrhoids or prolapsed rectal tissue.

Normal findings
- Abdominal contour flat, scaphoid (concave), or round.
- Abdominal veins barely visible. They may be more prominent in elderly or pregnant patients from a loss of subcutaneous tissue.
- Involuntary undulations under the abdominal skin of a thin adult. These are normal peristaltic waves and usually move downward and to the right.
- Arterial pulsations at the midline over the aorta in thin adults.
- Respirations producing abdominal movement, mostly in male patients.
- Slight abdominal shift when your patient turns from the supine to the lateral position.
- Anal opening puckered and dark, with intact perianal skin.
- In a male patient, a soft but not flabby penile shaft. In an older adult, the penis may be slightly flabby.
- Glans smooth and cone-shaped, without protrusions or induration.
- Glans pink in a Caucasian male, more pigmented in males with darker skin.
- Meatus slitlike and producing no discharge.
- Scrotal skin intact, with rugae (folds and creases). The left side of the scrotum usually hangs lower than the right.

- Pubic hair usually thick, appearing on the mons pubis and inner aspects of the upper thighs in a female patient. In an elderly female, pubic hair will appear thin and sparse. In a prepubescent female, hair will be absent or thin, depending upon the patient's age.
- Labia pink and moist, with no lesions.
- Vestibule and urethral opening free of swelling, redness, lesions, or discharge.
- Vaginal opening a thin vertical slit in a female with an intact hymen, and a larger opening with irregular edges in a female with a perforated hymen.
- Cervical discharge normal in quantity and character. Before ovulation, the discharge will be clear and stringy. After ovulation, it will be white and opaque.
- Striae marks, which may be visible in patients who are now or were obese or pregnant or in those with ascites or abdominal tumor.

Abnormal findings
- Abdominal contour indrawn (indicating high muscular tension), distended, asymmetrical, or bulging at the flanks when supine, or hollow (indicating malnutrition).
- Bulges on the abdominal wall or groin area or a grossly distended testicle, indicating an intestinal hernia.
- Fluid shifting or unusual protrusions when the patient changes position from supine to lateral. Gravity causes fluid in the abdominal cavity to shift when the patient changes position, altering abdominal contour. Fluid accumulation in the gastrointestinal (GI) tract also may cause some shifting but not to the same degree. Accumulated air does not shift when your patient changes position.
- Diastasis recti, an abnormal separation of abdominal rectus muscles. You may notice this first as abdominal distention. To confirm it, have your patient raise his head from the bed, and watch to see if the rectus muscle separates.

CULTURAL CONSIDERATIONS

Diastasis recti is a common finding in African-American children, but it usually disappears by age 4 or 5.

- Visible, active peristaltic waves in normal adults, possibly indicating hyperactive bowel activity and impending bowel obstruction.
- Bluish discoloration around the umbilicus (Cullen's sign) or along the lower abdomen and flanks (Grey Turner's sign), possibly indicating a retroperitoneal bleed. The color may be a shade of

blue-red, blue-purple, or green-brown, depending on the stage of hemoglobin breakdown.

- Tense, shiny abdominal skin, possibly resulting from ascites or edema.
- Jaundice (yellow color) of the abdominal wall, caused by staining of tissue with bile pigments and usually seen with liver dysfunction.
- Caput medusae (engorged veins around the umbilicus), indicating portal hypertension.
- Scars on the abdominal wall, possibly resulting from surgery or injury.
- Visible pulsations, possibly a sign of an aneurysm. This will require further assessment with auscultation and light palpation.
- Abdominal respirations in the female patient, possibly indicating respiratory distress.
- Umbilical fistula, possibly draining pus, urine, or feces, depending upon where the tract formed.
- Umbilical calculus (a hard mass of dirt and desquamated epithelium in the umbilicus causing inflammation and resulting from poor hygiene).
- Hemorrhoids (reddish protrusions from the anus containing distended veins).
- Prolapsed rectal mucosa (reddish velvety tissue projecting from the anus).
- Organisms attached to the pubic hair, indicating infestation by the *Pediculus pubis* louse or its nits (small, white lice eggs).
- Discharge from the meatus or urethra, with or without compression, indicating infection.
- Penile lesions, possibly indicating a sexually transmitted disease.
- Phimosis (an abnormal tightness of the prepuce preventing its retraction over the glans).
- Paraphimosis (a strangulation of the glans caused by a prepuce that will not retract over the glans).
- Epispadias (a congenital defect in which the urethral meatus opens on the dorsal surface of the penis).
- Hypospadias (a congenital defect in which the urethral meatus opens on the ventral surface of the penis).
- Absence of pubic hair in a postpubescent adult or bald spots in the pubic hair, possibly indicating a vascular or hormonal problem.
- Enlarged testicle, possibly indicating hernia (if bowel loops appear on illumination) or a cyst (if fluid is present).
- Hypertrophic, indurated, soft or hard tissue of the labia majora.
- Varicosities (distended superficial vessels) on the labia, possibly a sign of increased pressure in the pelvic region. This problem occurs with increased uterine size, as in pregnancy or uterine cancer.
- Lesions, possibly indicating genital infection.

- Edema of the mons pubis, labia majora, labia minora, urethral orifice, vaginal introitus, or surrounding skin, possibly indicating vaginal infection or infestation.
- Purulent vaginal discharge, which may be green, gray, yellow, or white, indicating infection.

Auscultation

The next step in your examination, auscultation, allows you to assess the function of your patient's GI tract. Always auscultate the abdomen before percussing or palpating it because manipulating the abdominal wall may increase bowel sounds or produce sounds that usually aren't present.

Before you begin, make sure the room, your hands, and your stethoscope are warm. Placing cold hands or a cold stethoscope on your patient's abdomen could make the muscles contract. If your patient has a nasogastric tube attached to low suction, turn the suction off, or clamp the tube during auscultation to keep it from producing misleading sounds or interfering with your ability to hear.

Begin by mentally dividing the patient's abdomen into four quadrants, and systematically auscultate all four. You'll probably want to develop a routine to use each time you examine a patient's abdomen. That way, you'll be sure not to miss a quadrant.

Use the diaphragm of your stethoscope to auscultate high-pitched bowel sounds. Normal bowel sounds are not constant, so you'll want to listen for about a minute over each quadrant. You must listen for 3 to 5 minutes before concluding a patient has no bowel sounds.

Remember that the thickness of the abdominal wall may affect what you can hear. Bowel sounds are more difficult to auscultate in obese patients. Also, remember not to drag your stethoscope across the patient's abdominal wall because doing so could increase irritation and cause muscle spasm.

After auscultating bowel sounds, use the bell of your stethoscope to auscultate vascular sounds, bruits, or friction rubs. To assess the abdominal vascular system, auscultate over the aortic site and the iliac, femoral, and renal arteries. (See ▨ *Identifying Vascular Sounds in the Abdomen*.)

Normal findings

- Peristaltic sounds, or high-pitched, gurgling noises heard about every 5 to 15 seconds in an irregular pattern. They may be loud when your patient is hungry or has missed a meal.
- Continuous sounds over the ileocecal valve if it has been more than 4 hours since the patient last ate.

Abnormal findings

- Absent or infrequent bowel sounds, possibly indicating peritonitis, ileus, or late bowel obstruction.

IDENTIFYING VASCULAR SOUNDS IN THE ABDOMEN

You can detect abdominal vascular problems by auscultating your patient's abdomen with the bell of your stethoscope.

Listen for bruits over major abdominal blood vessels, including the aorta, renal arteries, iliac arteries, and femoral arteries.

Listen for venous hums in the umbilical and epigastric regions. Venous hums are generally softer than aortic bruits.

Finally, listen for a grating or scratching noise above and below the right and left costal borders. These sounds, known as friction rubs, may indicate inflammation of the kidneys or spleen.

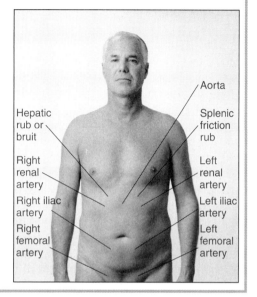

Hepatic rub or bruit · Right renal artery · Right iliac artery · Right femoral artery · Aorta · Splenic friction rub · Left renal artery · Left iliac artery · Left femoral artery

- Frequent, loud, rushing, high-pitched sounds, possibly indicating early mechanical obstruction or GI hypermotility. You may see peristaltic waves on the surface of the patient's abdomen.
- Borborygmus (loud intestinal rumbling). This is abnormal, except when the patient is hungry. Borborygmi signal passage of flatus through the large intestine.
- Bruits, resulting from narrowing of an artery or turbulent blood flow. They are described as blowing sounds and may indicate an aneurysm or a constricted vessel. If you auscultate a midline abdominal bruit, the patient may have an aortic aneurysm. Do not perform deep palpation.
- Friction rubs, possibly sounding like a grating noise or like two pieces of leather being rubbed together. A peritoneal friction rub may indicate peritoneal inflammation. A friction rub over the liver may indicate inflammation of the organ surface.
- Venous hum (a continuous soft sound heard in both systole and diastole), indicating collateral circulation between the portal and systemic venous systems and usually heard over the epigastric region and umbilicus.

Percussion

You'll use percussion to determine the size and density of structures and organs inside your patient's abdominal cavity and to detect the presence of fluid or air. You may use direct or indirect percussion, but indirect percussion provides better patient comfort. It's also easier to use over a large area. To perform indirect percussion, you'll rest one hand on the abdominal wall and sharply tap your middle finger with the index finger of the other hand.

Most patients tolerate abdominal percussion if you explain what you'll be doing and provide reassurance before you begin. Remember that percussion is contraindicated in patients with suspected abdominal aortic aneurysm or those who have received abdominal organ transplants. Use caution when percussing the abdomen of a patient who might have appendicitis.

As in auscultation, begin by mentally dividing the abdomen into four quadrants, and proceed to systematically percuss all four. As you address each quadrant, keep a mental image of the abdominal structures beneath your fingers. Percussion sounds will change, depending on the structure involved. Solid structures, such as the liver, produce dull sounds. So do fluid-filled structures, such as a full urinary bladder. Air-filled structures, such as the stomach, produce tympanic sounds.

Once you've percussed all four abdominal quadrants, go back and percuss the liver and spleen, noting their size and position. To percuss the liver and determine its size, begin on the right side, at the midclavicular line, just above the patient's right nipple. Percuss downward until the sound becomes dull. This spot is the liver's upper margin. Usually, you'll find it between the fifth and seventh intercostal spaces (ICSs). If you need to, mark the location to help you remember it. To find the liver's lower margin, begin percussing at a point in the abdomen where you hear tympanic sounds. Work upward along the midclavicular line until the sound becomes dull. This spot is the liver's lower margin. Usually, you'll find it at the costal margin. Mark this spot as well, and measure the distance between the two marks. Record the measurement in centimeters. Keep in mind that excess air in the large intestine will produce a tympanic sound that may obscure the dullness of the liver.

The spleen is more difficult to percuss. Beginning on the left side, posterior to the midaxillary line, percuss toward the umbilicus at a level between the sixth and tenth ribs. Percussion sounds should change from resonance (over the left lung) to dullness (indicating the spleen).

If your patient has a distended abdomen, check for excess fluid accumulation by percussing for a fluid wave. You'll need an assistant to perform this procedure. (See ◪ *Percussing for a Fluid Wave.*)

Normal findings
- Tympany over the stomach, epigastric area, and upper midline.
- Dullness over the liver, a full bladder, a pregnant uterus, and the left lower quadrant over the sigmoid colon (shortly before a bowel movement).

EXAMINATION TIP

PERCUSSING FOR A FLUID WAVE

If you want to find out whether your patient's abdominal distention results from fluid or air, percuss his abdomen for a fluid wave. This procedure requires three hands, so you'll have to ask a colleague for help.

To perform the procedure, place the patient in a supine position, and ask your colleague to place her arm and hand along the midline of the patient's abdomen, as shown in the photograph. Your colleague should press her arm gently but firmly against the patient's abdomen to prevent transmission of fat waves.

Next, place your fingertips along the sides of your patient's lower abdomen, in the lumbar region. Keeping your nondominant hand in place, use the fingertips of your dominant hand to thrust quickly into the patient's side, as shown here. Do you feel a wave with your nondominant hand? If so, your

patient's abdominal distention probably results from excess fluid.

By contrast, if your patient's distention is caused by air, you won't feel a wave.

- Upper and lower liver margins about 6 to 12 cm apart.
- Spleen, if located, percussed in the area between the sixth and tenth ribs.

Abnormal findings
- Flat percussion sounds over the abdominal cavity, possibly indicating a tumor.
- Fluid wave, indicating accumulated fluid in the abdominal cavity.
- More than 12 cm between the upper and lower margins of the liver, indicating hepatomegaly.
- Large area of dullness in the left upper quadrant, indicating splenomegaly.
- High-pitched tympany sound in association with abdominal distention, indicating air in the bowel.
- Dull sounds in the flank area, present with ascites.
- Tenderness with percussion, possibly indicating peritoneal inflammation.

Palpation

Abdominal palpation should include both light and deep methods. Be aware that your patient may feel anxious about abdominal palpation, which can increase tension in the abdominal muscles and make your job more difficult. To help keep your patient relaxed during the examination, keep him draped for privacy in areas where you aren't working. Make sure your hands are warm; wash them in hot water, if necessary, before palpating. Explain the examination before you begin, and talk to the patient soothingly and quietly throughout.

Positioning also can help in keeping your patient's abdominal muscles relaxed. If possible, place the patient in a supine position with a pillow under his head and his knees slightly bent. Put his arms at his sides rather than over his head. Ask him to breathe through his mouth during the examination. Also ask him not to talk or raise his head during the examination.

Sometimes you may want your patient in positions other than supine. For example, a lateral position may help you locate abdominal masses that you can't find with the patient supine. A standing position may help you identify hernias. If your patient is uncomfortable in a supine position, you may be forced to choose another position. For example, if your patient is prone to respiratory distress when supine, raise the backrest. If the patient has kyphosis, try elevating his head and shoulders for comfort.

Your positioning in relation to your patient depends on which of your hands is dominant. If you're right-handed, stand on your patient's right side for palpation. Keep your fingers close together, with the palmar surface down.

EXAMINATION TIP

If your patient is ticklish, have him place his hand on top of yours as you palpate. Alternatively, try distracting the patient by pressing on the lower half of his sternum with your nondominant hand.

As in the other abdominal assessment techniques, you'll want to divide the patient's abdomen into quadrants and palpate all four. Use the same pattern as you did with auscultation to avoid missing an area. If the patient complains of abdominal pain, begin with quadrants that aren't painful, saving painful areas for last. If your patient tightens his abdominal muscles or becomes uncomfortable, proceed more slowly, or switch to another assessment technique and come back to palpation.

Begin your examination with a light touch, pressing only $\frac{1}{4}$ to $\frac{1}{2}$ inches (0.5 to 1 cm) into the patient's abdomen. Light palpation is used to determine characteristics of skin and subcutaneous tissue and to note temperature, tenderness, and large masses. Move your fingers in a circular motion. Proceed slowly and gently. Avoid any sudden movements. As you move over the femoral area, note the femoral pulse, and palpate the inguinal lymph nodes. (See *Locating the Inguinal Lymph Nodes.*)

LOCATING THE INGUINAL LYMPH NODES

Located on both sides of the pubic region, along the inguinal canal, the inguinal lymph nodes consist of two discrete chains: the superficial superior chain and the superficial inferior chain.

Palpating your patient's inguinal lymph nodes can provide clues to infectious processes in his abdominal and genital areas. Use this illustration as a guide in locating these nodes.

If you feel any nodes during palpation, make sure that you note their size and consistency and whether or not they are tender.

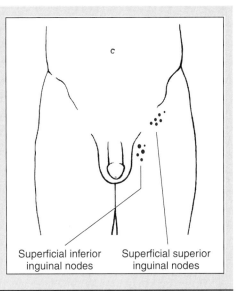

Superficial inferior inguinal nodes   Superficial superior inguinal nodes

Watch your patient's face for grimacing during light palpation. If you identify any tenderness with light palpation, remember to reassess the area when you get to the deep palpation part of your examination.

LIFESPAN CONSIDERATIONS

Don't assume that an older adult doesn't have an abdominal condition, such as appendicitis, if he doesn't complain of pain or have a fever. That's because older adults can have a diminished sense of pain and a blunted febrile response.

If you find that your patient's abdominal muscles are contracted, you'll want to determine whether the contraction is voluntary or involuntary. Do this by correlating the contraction with the patient's respirations. If the muscles are contracted during both inspiration and expiration, the condition probably is involuntary, indicating an underlying abdominal problem. If the muscles contract more strongly during inspiration and less strongly during expiration, the condition probably is voluntary and related to your patient's anxiety level.

Once you've lightly palpated the entire abdomen, begin deep palpation. This method is used to locate normal structures, identify masses, and assess for tenderness. Do not perform deep palpation if the patient has a suspected abdominal aortic aneurysm or appendicitis, a tender spleen, a kidney transplantation, or polycystic kidneys.

During deep palpation, you're going to be pressing 1½ to 2 inches (3 to 4 cm) into the patient's abdomen. You can do so using one hand alone or with one hand on top of the other. Many nurses prefer the two-handed method because it allows you to add pressure with the nonexamining hand while the muscles of your examining hand remain relatively passive.

As you palpate the abdomen, keep in mind you probably won't be able to feel abdominal organs in an obese but otherwise healthy individual. In a relatively thin person, you may feel the muscular structures of the abdomen, such as the rectus muscle, the bowel (which is soft, unless filled with feces), and aortic pulsations.

To palpate the liver, feel deeply beneath the costal margin as your patient takes a deep breath. During inspiration the liver will descend, and you may be able to feel its edge move against your hand. Usually it's firm and rubbery. Alternatively, you can try hooking the liver by standing near your patient's head and, as he takes a deep breath, curling your fingers over the costal margin.

To palpate the kidneys, place your nondominant hand beneath your patient's right flank as you press downward against the right outer edge of the abdomen, attempting to sandwich the kidney between your hands. Normally it feels firm and smooth. Repeat this procedure on the left flank, keeping in mind that the left kidney is usually nonpalpable because of its position beneath the bowel. In fact, usually all remaining abdominal structures, including the spleen (beneath the left costal margin) and the gallbladder (beneath the liver's margin), are nonpalpable, unless they're enlarged.

If you find a mass during abdominal palpation, you'll need to document its size, shape, consistency (solid or soft), surface (smooth or irregular), tenderness, pulsatility, and mobility. If the mass is small, you can make these determinations by grasping it between your thumb and index finger. If the mass is large, you'll need to perform bimanual palpation to assess it fully. (See ▨ *Performing Bimanual Palpation*.)

To determine if the mass is mobile, press suddenly and deeply into the region. A mobile mass will bound upward and touch the fingers of your examining hand.

To check for rebound tenderness, have your patient flex his knees to relax his abdominal muscles. Now place your hands lightly on the abdominal wall, midway between the umbilicus and the anterior-superior iliac spine (at McBurney's point). Press your fingers slowly and deeply into the abdomen; then release the pressure in a quick, smooth motion. If the patient feels pain when you release pressure, he has rebound tenderness, possibly from an inflamed appendix. The pain may radiate to the umbilicus. To minimize the risk of rupturing the appendix, do not repeat this test if you get a positive result.

EXAMINATION TIP

PERFORMING BIMANUAL PALPATION

If you find a large mass in your patient's abdomen, you'll want to perform bimanual palpation to accurately determine its position and size.

To perform bimanual palpation of the upper abdomen, place your patient in the supine position and stand on the side opposite the mass. Now place your nondominant hand on the outside of the patient's rib cage farthest from you, as shown in the illustration. Ask your patient to take a deep breath and, while his rib cage expands, press your dominant hand under the costal margin to probe for the mass. Angle your dominant hand in the direction of your nondominant hand, as shown. Adjust the positions of both hands as needed to fully assess the mass.

You can perform bimanual palpation on the lower abdomen as well. Simply position your nondominant hand on the patient's flank, and use your dominant hand to probe the abdomen, keeping the mass positioned between your two hands.

Another way to check for peritoneal inflammation is to test for tenderness when the heels are jarred. Have your patient stand on his toes with his legs straight. Then ask him to relax suddenly and allow his heels to strike the floor. If this maneuver produces abdominal pain, the patient may have peritoneal inflammation. Some patients with peritoneal inflammation complain of abdominal pain when walking.

EXAMINATION TIP

If your patient can't stand, try to extend the patient's leg and strike his heel with the lateral aspect of your fist while he's supine. If the patient experiences abdominal pain, suspect peritoneal inflammation.

Once you've palpated the patient's abdomen, move on to the genitalia. Again, be aware that your patient may be nervous and embarrassed. Use draping whenever possible, and proceed gently but firmly. Be sure to wear examination gloves.

For a male patient, palpate the bulb of the penis to note consistency and the presence or absence of induration. Use both hands to palpate the penile shaft, working from the base toward the tip to milk the urethra. Watch for urethral discharge at the meatus.

Palpate each testicle for size, shape, symmetry, mobility, and consistency. If you feel a mass, try to press your fingers together above it. If your fingers meet, you can conclude that the mass is confined to the scrotum. If they don't meet, the mass probably started in the abdomen and extends through the inguinal ring and into the scrotal sac.

Next, palpate each epididymis between your index finger and thumb. Locate the spermatic cord near the root of the scrotum and, with gentle pressure, roll the cord between your thumb and finger as you move downward toward the testicle. Be careful not to pinch the skin or the cord because it will cause a sharp pain.

Finally, evaluate the inguinal ring, and palpate for inguinal and femoral hernias.

For a female patient, palpate the labia majora and labia minora. Palpate the area of Bartholin's gland. Moisten your gloved index finger with water. Separate the labia with your other gloved hand, and gently insert your index finger, pad up, about 1¼ inches (3 cm) into the anterior vagina. Press the pad of your finger upward, and pull outward to milk the urethra. Note any pain or discharge.

LIFESPAN CONSIDERATIONS

As estrogen levels diminish after age 40, changes to the female genitalia begin to occur. You may observe a narrowing of the vaginal opening and changes in the vagina, including shortening and narrowing of the vaginal canal and a lack of moisture. If you're not planning to perform a Papanicolaou (Pap) smear or take other samples for testing, use a water-based lubricant when performing a vaginal examination to decrease discomfort.

If you've received special training, perform a full internal pelvic examination.

Normal findings
- No tenderness with light or deep palpation.
- Inguinal lymph nodes small (¼ to ½ inches [0.5 to 1 cm] in diameter), smooth, and mobile.
- In a thin patient, palpable pulsatile mass at the midline of the upper abdomen, reflecting aortic pulsations.
- In a male patient, testicles mobile and tender under pressure. If your patient is older, the testes may be softer and smaller in size. Your fingers should meet when palpating the skin at the root of the scrotum.

- Epididymis firm and rubbery.
- Spermatic cord round, cordlike, smooth, and firm with resilience.
- Inguinal ring that exerts a slight pulsation against your finger.
- In the female patient, labia free of nodules or masses.
- Bartholin's glands nonpalpable.
- Urethra producing no pain or discharge. (See 🖼 *What to Expect When Examining the Abdomen.*)

Abnormal findings
- Rebound tenderness, indicating peritoneal inflammation.
- Voluntary rigidity of abdominal muscles during palpation, possibly resulting from peritoneal irritation or your patient's anxiety.
- Involuntary contraction of the abdominal wall (commonly described as a "boardlike" abdomen), indicating peritonitis.
- Abdominal tenderness elicited by heel jarring, indicating peritoneal inflammation.
- Suprapubic mass, possibly resulting from bladder distention. In a female patient, it may result from an ovarian cyst or a uterine fibroid.
- Decreased or absent femoral pulse, possibly indicating coarctation of the aorta, thrombosis of the iliac artery, or dissecting aortic aneurysm.
- In the male patient, a scrotal mass. If an abdominal mass protrudes into the scrotal sac, your fingers won't be able to approximate above it.
- Discharge from the meatus, indicating infection.

NORMAL FINDINGS

WHAT TO EXPECT WHEN EXAMINING THE ABDOMEN

Use this quick review to confirm normal findings when examining the abdominal region.

Inspection
- Smooth, unbroken skin, relatively pale, with fine venous network.
- No skin legions or nodules.
- Flat, round, or concave abdominal contour that's symmetrical.
- Striae from pregnancy or weight gain.
- Smooth, even abdominal movement in males, costal movement in females, during breathing.
- No peristalsis; thin patients may show slight motion.
- Pulsations of the aorta visible in thin patients.

Palpation
- No masses.
- No tenderness.

Auscultation
- High-pitched bowel sounds at least every 15 seconds.

- Fibrotic thickening, indurations, or protrusions of the penis, possibly indicating venereal disease, such as condyloma.
- Small, palpable nodules in the midline ventral surface of the penis (possibly occluded periurethral glands).
- Small, yellowish, palpable nodules on the scrotal skin (sebaceous cysts caused by blocked sebaceous glands).
- Dilated, tortuous testicular veins, possibly indicating benign, pain-producing varicosities or metastatic cellular proliferation.
- A spindlelike mass on the spermatic cord, possibly indicating hydrocele of the cord.
- A hard, nodular, elongated spermatic cord, possibly indicating varicoceles, varices, or varicose veins.
- The sensation of sliding or bulging during the inguinal ring examination, indicating a hernia.
- In the female patient, reddened or excoriated perineal skin, indicating chronic incontinence, poor hygiene, or recurrent infections (for example, vaginal yeast infections).
- Reddened and inflamed hair follicles, with or without pustules, indicating folliculitis (inflamed hair follicles) or shaving against the direction of hair growth.
- Swollen labia (unilaterally or bilaterally), possibly resulting from injury, inflammation, or infection of the Bartholin's gland. The swollen area may be tender and warm.
- Vaginal discharge that's white, green, or yellow and thin, thick, creamy, or of a consistency like cottage cheese, often indicating vaginal infection.
- Lesions on or around the labia. If they are painful, raised, reddened, and filled with fluid, they may be herpetic vesicles. If they appear as painless, rubbery skin tags, they're probably condylomas. If they appear as discrete ulcers or nontender chancres, they may have been caused by syphilis.
- Bulging of the vaginal wall, probably resulting from internal muscle weakness that may be seen through the vaginal opening. If the bulging occurs anteriorly, it may be due to a cyctocele, or bladder prolapse. A posterior bulging may be related to a rectocele, or prolapse of the rectal wall.

EXPLORING CHIEF COMPLAINTS

In the abdominal region, chief complaints can take many forms and involve a large variety of organs and structures. To explore your patient's chief complaint accurately and quickly, you'll need a sound working knowledge of the structures and functions involved. Be sure to refer to your patient's medical history, family history, previous surgeries (especially abdominal surgeries), previous traumatic injuries to the abdomen, and current medications for clues to the patient's problem. For a female patient, make sure you know the date of her last menses, her typical pattern of menstruation, number of previous pregnancies, and past gynecologic infections. Armed with general knowledge about the abdominal region and specific knowledge about your patient's history, you'll be well equipped to quickly and accurately assess the following chief complaints and more.

Nausea and vomiting

If your patient complains of nausea and vomiting, investigate the symptom further by asking him the following questions:
* Did you experience pain or nausea before or after vomiting?
* Did you vomit once or several times?
* Describe the episode of vomiting. Did it come out in a forceful stream? Did you retch without actually vomiting? Did you regurgitate burning fluid? Food?
* Was there blood in your vomit?
* Did you vomit after you ate? What had you eaten?
* What characteristics did the vomit display?
* What have you eaten in the last 24 hours?
* When was your last bowel movement?
* Have you lost weight recently?
* What medications are you currently taking?

Focusing your assessment

When you examine a patient who complains of nausea and vomiting, focus your assessment as follows:
* Inspect your patient's skin turgor. Poor turgor indicates dehydration, probably as a result of vomiting.
* Check your patient's vital signs. Increased heart rate and low blood pressure are signs of dehydration. Fever is a sign of infection, as in gastroenteritis or pelvic inflammatory disease.
* Inspect the abdomen for distention or visible peristaltic waves. Abdominal distention may suggest intestinal obstruction, paralytic ileus, or constipation. Visible peristaltic waves may occur early in intestinal obstruction and gastroenteritis.
* Auscultate for bowel sounds, listening for changes in their normal frequency and pitch. (See ▩ *Assessing Bowel Sounds,* p. 266.)
* Assess for abdominal pain. Right lower quadrant pain may indicate appendicitis. Diffuse lower abdominal pain may accompany bowel obstruction or pelvic inflammatory disease.

Possible causes

* *Small intestine obstruction.* This condition is characterized by colicky pain, nausea, vomiting, constipation, and abdominal distention.

INTERPRETING ABNORMAL FINDINGS

ASSESSING BOWEL SOUNDS

Bowel sounds reflect the activity of underlying intestines and offer information about intestinal health and function. Normally, the bowel produces soft clicks and gurgles every 5 to 15 seconds. Because bowel sounds are usually irregular, listen for a full minute in all four quadrants using the diaphragm of your stethoscope. Changes in the frequency and pitch of your patient's bowel sounds may indicate a problem. Use this table to help pinpoint the cause of abnormal bowel sounds.

Bowel sound	Probable mechanism	Probable causes
Hyperactive sounds not related to hunger	Abnormally rapid passage of air and fluid through the intestine	• Diarrhea • Early intestinal obstruction
Hypoactive or absent sounds	Inactivity of smooth muscle in the bowel	• Paralytic ileus • Peritonitis • Decreased bowel motility
High-pitched rushing sounds	Intestinal straining to push fluid and air past an obstruction	• Intestinal obstruction
High-pitched tinkling sounds	Intestinal fluid and air under tension	• Dilated bowel loops • Fecal impaction

The vomitus begins as gastric juice and bile. Eventually, it contains ileal fecal contents.

- *Gastroenteritis.* This condition is characterized by nausea and vomiting accompanied by diarrhea and abdominal discomfort. Other signs include fever, malaise, and hyperactive bowel sounds.
- *Peptic ulcer disease.* Ulcers in the stomach and duodenum may result in bloody vomitus.
- *Esophageal varices.* A large volume of bright red blood in the vomit may result from ruptured esophageal varices and constitutes a life-threatening medical emergency. (See 🕐 *Responding to GI Bleeding.*)
- *Paralytic ileus.* A physiologic intestinal obstruction usually affects the small bowel and occurs most commonly after abdominal surgery or use of anticholinergic medications. Signs include severe abdominal distention and vomiting.
- *Constipation.* This condition may occur with narcotic use, poor dietary habits, or sluggish bowel function. Nausea and vomiting begin after several days.
- *Pregnancy.* From early in pregnancy until about week 16, nausea and vomiting may occur, most often in the morning (morning sickness).

Abdominal pain

If your patient complains of abdominal pain, investigate the symptom further by asking him the following questions:

- Where is the pain located?

ACTION STAT

RESPONDING TO GI BLEEDING

Gastrointestinal (GI) bleeding, which you'll usually observe coming from a patient's mouth, anus, or both, can result from various conditions. Blood that appears in vomitus could signal a gastric ulcer, life-threatening esophageal varices, or other upper GI problems. Blood that exits your patient's anus may be bright red or tarry black and could warn of a disorder as simple as hemorrhoids or as serious as gastric or colon cancer.

All cases of GI bleeding deserve prompt attention. However, bleeding that occurs unchecked and in large amounts requires immediate intervention in order to protect the patient against hypovolemic shock, ischemia, and possible death.

What to look for
Clinical findings vary, depending upon the location of the bleeding, but may include:
- Vomiting of bright red blood or brownish-black granular material that looks like coffee grounds, indicating old blood and gastric juices from a slow bleed
- Passing of bright red blood via the anus, indicating lower GI bleeding
- Passing of black, tarry stools, indicating upper GI bleeding
- Pale, cool skin with delayed capillary refill
- Narrow pulse pressure
- Tachycardia
- Hyperactive bowel sounds
- Positive tilt test (increase in heart rate of more than 20 beats per minute or decrease in blood pressure of more than 10 mm Hg when the patient rises from a lying to a sitting position, suggesting hypovolemic shock)

What to do immediately
If you suspect your patient has acute GI bleeding, notify the physician, then proceed as follows:
- Maintain nothing by mouth status and administer IV fluids (lactated Ringer's or isotonic saline solutions) by large-bore IV catheter, as ordered, to maintain circulatory volume.
- Expect to insert a nasogastric (NG) tube to administer saline lavages to clear blood from

the stomach. In cases of uncontrolled upper GI bleeding, norepinephrine may be added to the saline to constrict the blood vessels.
- If the physician suspects esophageal bleeding or a Mallory-Weiss tear (an esophageal tear associated with prolonged vomiting or retching), an NG tube usually isn't inserted because it could worsen the bleeding. Instead, a chambered-balloon tube (Sengstaken-Blakemore) may be inserted to apply pressure to the bleeding areas.
- Assess vital signs frequently. Monitor the patient for signs of shock, including increased pulse rate, hypotension, and pallor.
- Administer blood transfusions, as ordered, to replace volume. Monitor hemoglobin and hematocrit to assess blood loss and recovery.
- Administer prescribed medications, such as H_2-blockers (cimetidine) or proton-pump inhibitors (omeprazole), to decrease gastric acidity. Antacids may be ordered by mouth or NG tube to neutralize stomach acids. If bleeding results from a peptic ulcer and *Helicobacter pylori* is the cause, antibiotics may be prescribed.
- If the bleeding can't be controlled by saline lavage or medications, prepare your patient for possible surgery, depending on the site and cause of the bleeding. The patient may have a Billroth procedure, for example, or a rectal resection.
- Expect to insert an indwelling urinary catheter to monitor urinary output.

What to do next
Once the patient has been stabilized, you'll need to:
- Maintain and monitor fluid intake and output. Include all vomitus and drainage in your calculation of output. If ice chips are allowed, make sure you include them as intake.
- Continue monitoring hemoglobin and hematocrit. Look for signs of decreased hemoglobin, such as pale mucous membranes and conjunctivae.
- Administer transfusions, as ordered, and watch for signs of adverse transfusion reactions, such as fever, chills, and lower back pain.
- Begin a clear liquid diet when ordered. Watch for any signs of vomiting.

- Does the pain radiate or extend to another part of your body?
- Did it begin gradually or suddenly?
- Can you describe the pain?
- How often have you experienced the pain, and how long has the pain lasted? What is the timing and pattern of your pain?
- Which activities make the pain worse? What makes it better?
- What are you doing when the pain begins? Does it wake you from sleep?
- Are you (female patient) possibly pregnant?
- Where are you (female patient) in your monthly cycle?
- Have you (female patient) noticed any vaginal discharge?

Focusing your assessment

When examining a patient who complains of abdominal pain, focus your assessment as follows:

- Identify the type of pain involved. The three major types include visceral, somatic (also called parietal), and referred. Visceral pain results from stretching or distention of an abdominal viscus and is usually described as diffuse, poorly localized, and cramping or gnawing. Somatic pain emanates from the abdominal wall, peritoneum, mesentery, or diaphragm. It is more intense and localized. Referred pain is experienced at a site removed from the actual source of pain. Usually it is sharp, well localized, and resembles somatic pain. (See *Telltale Signs of Peritonitis*.)
- Identify the area of the abdomen where the pain is occurring. Knowing where your patient's pain is located and where the pain is referred can help you identify the organ involved. (See ▨ *Acute Abdominal Pain*, pp. 270 and 271.)

TELLTALE SIGNS OF PERITONITIS

An acute localized or generalized inflammation of the peritoneal layer of the abdominal cavity, peritonitis results from bacterial contamination after perforation of an abdominal organ, such as the large bowel, or the release of irritating chemicals, such as pancreatic enzymes.

If you suspect your patient has peritonitis, notify the physician immediately. Peritonitis requires rapid intervention, including administration of antibiotics and surgery.

Clinical findings associated with peritonitis can vary, depending on the severity of the infection, but may include the following:

- Acute, diffuse, abdominal pain with rebound tenderness and abdominal rigidity
- Pain that eventually localizes to the source of infection
- Referred pain to the shoulder, at times accompanied by hiccups caused by diaphragmatic irritation
- Elevated temperature, often as high as 103° F (39.4° C), along with chills, nausea, and vomiting
- Abdominal distention
- Diminished or absent bowel sounds
- Elevated white blood cell counts with high neutrophil count.

- Inspect the abdomen for distention, a sign of intestinal obstruction.
- Inspect the perineal area of a female patient for vaginal discharge.
- Check your patient's temperature. Abdominal pain with a fever may indicate appendicitis or gastroenteritis.
- Auscultate for vascular sounds. A bruit heard over the abdominal aorta may indicate an abdominal aortic aneurysm.
- Auscultate for bowel sounds. Absent or hypoactive bowel sounds may indicate peritonitis. Hyperactive bowel sounds may suggest Crohn's disease or ulcerative colitis.
- Check for rebound tenderness and heel-jarring tenderness, signs of appendicitis and peritonitis.

Possible causes
- *Peritonitis.* Sudden, diffuse abdominal pain usually is most intense over the area of the underlying problem. The patient will also have weakness, pallor, sweating, and cold skin from loss of fluids and electrolytes. As bacterial toxins invade the intestinal muscles, intestinal motility decreases, and paralytic ileus develops.
- *Intestinal obstruction.* This condition is characterized by colicky pain, nausea, vomiting, constipation, and abdominal distention. Your patient may also complain of drowsiness, intense thirst, malaise, and aching. Bowel sounds are hyperactive with a rushing sound.
- *Pancreatitis.* Steady epigastric pain centers close to the umbilicus and radiates between the tenth thoracic and sixth lumbar vertebrae. The pain is unrelieved by vomiting. Severe attacks produce extreme pain, persistent vomiting, and abdominal rigidity.
- *Diverticulitis.* Recurrent left lower quadrant pain is accompanied by alternating constipation and diarrhea. The pain usually abates after defecation or passage of flatus. The patient may have mild nausea and a low-grade fever.
- *Peptic ulcer.* This condition is characterized by localized midepigastric pain with heartburn that develops 2 hours or more after meals, when the stomach is empty. Eating may relieve the pain. Acidic liquids, such as orange juice or coffee, may aggravate the pain. (See *Peptic Ulcer Disease,* p. 272.)
- *Crohn's disease.* This condition produces steady, colicky pain in the right lower quadrant, with cramping, tenderness, flatulence, nausea, fever, and diarrhea. The patient may have bloody stools and complain of weight loss, weakness, and fatigue.
- *Appendicitis.* Beginning as right upper quadrant abdominal pain, the pain later localizes in the right lower quadrant. Palpation reveals a rigid, "boardlike" abdominal wall and rebound tenderness. Diarrhea, fever, and tachycardia develop later.
- *Cholecystitis.* This condition produces acute abdominal pain in the right upper quadrant, occasionally radiating to the back. The pain

INTERPRETING ABNORMAL FINDINGS

ACUTE ABDOMINAL PAIN

Acute abdominal pain is a common complaint that can have many causes. When thinking of the source of the pain, it helps to mentally divide the abdomen into four quadrants, upper and lower right and upper and lower left. Then remember the organs that lie within these quadrants. As you proceed with the physical examination, watch the patient's facial expression for grimacing and other signs of pain. Prepare to intervene quickly if the cause is one of the serious disorders listed in this chart.

Characteristics	Location	Possible findings	Probable cause
• Sudden and severe • Colicky	• Generalized • May refer to shoulder	• Nausea, vomiting • Constipation • Abdominal distention • Visible peristalsis • High-pitched, hyperactive bowel sounds or absent bowel sounds • Hiccups • Signs of shock, such as hypotension, with bowel ischemia or infarction • Lactic acidosis (with bowel infarction)	• Intestinal obstruction
• Severe and acute • Rebound tenderness	• Diffuse, may localize to the source of infection • Referred to shoulder	• Fever • Nausea, vomiting, anorexia • Guarding, boardlike abdomen, abdominal distention • Diminished or absent bowel sounds • Leukocytosis	• Peritonitis
• Steady, with episodes of severe, extreme pain	• Epigastric, close to umbilicus • May involve flanks and left upper quadrant • Radiates to area between 10th thoracic and 6th lumbar vertebrae, left shoulder, groin	• Vomiting • Abdominal tenderness and rigidity • Cullen's sign (periumbilical ecchymosis) • Grey Turner's sign (ecchymosis of flanks) • Elevated lipase and amylase levels • Leukocytosis	• Pancreatitis
• Sharp or colicky	• Periumbilical and generalized • Localized in right lower quadrant or McBurney's point	• Fever • Nausea, vomiting, anorexia • Guarding, boardlike abdomen • Pain with flexion of the right leg at the knee and hip to 90 degrees • Rebound tenderness • Diarrhea • Leukocytosis	• Appendicitis

usually develops after a meal rich in fats. It may occur at night, awakening the patient from sleep. The patient also may complain of belching, gassiness, sweating, vomiting, and clay-colored stools (if a stone obstructs the common bile duct). Jaundice will occur if the bile duct is blocked. (See 🖥 *Cholecystitis*, p. 273.)

Characteristics	Location	Possible findings	Probable cause
• Severe and acute • Often nocturnal and precipitated by rich foods	• Right upper quadrant or epigastric • May radiate to the back in the subscapular area	• Flatulence • Diaphoresis • Nausea and vomiting • Jaundice or clay-colored stool (with biliary obstruction)	• Cholecystitis
• Colicky	• Usually left lower quadrant or epigastric radiating to left side or back	• Abdominal tenderness • Low-grade fever • Alternating constipation and diarrhea • Flatulence • Nausea • High-pitched, hyperactive bowel sounds	• Diverticulitis
• Severe and sudden	• Lower quadrants • Referred to shoulder (especially left shoulder)	• Symptoms of pregnancy, including amenorrhea or irregular menstruation • Abdominal tenderness and distention • Palpable mass • Signs of shock, such as hypotension	• Ruptured ectopic pregnancy
• Progressively severe	• Lower quadrant	• Cervical and adnexal tenderness • Abdominal guarding and rebound tenderness • Vaginal discharge, often purulent • Fever • Dyspareunia	• Pelvic inflammatory disease
• Deep, boring, steady, occasional, relieved by change of position	• Lower quadrants • Lumbosacral region	• Wide aortic pulsation • Abdominal bruit • Nausea and vomiting • Possible tenderness • Signs of shock and loss of distal pulses with rupture	• Abdominal aortic aneurysm
• Severe, may worsen with feet elevation	• Left upper quadrant • Radiates to left shoulder	• Hypothermia • Signs of shock, such as hypotension • Abdominal trauma • Mononucleosis	• Ruptured spleen

• *Renal calculi.* A calculus traveling down the ureter may cause severe abdominal and flank pain. Nausea and vomiting usually are also present.

(Text continues on p. 274.)

PEPTIC ULCER DISEASE

A common and potentially serious problem, peptic ulcer disease affects about one American adult in ten. A peptic ulcer can develop in any area of the gastrointestinal (GI) tract exposed to acid-pepsin secretions, including the esophagus, stomach, and duodenum. A defect develops in the GI mucosa when the mucosal barrier fails to protect the mucosa from damage by hydrochloric acid and pepsin, the gastric digestive juices.

For many years, most experts believed this failure resulted from the patient's lifestyle and stress level. Not so anymore. Researchers have discovered that the bacterium *Helicobacter pylori* plays a major role in the formation of duodenal ulcers, although still incidence is falling because recent treatment has targeted the bacterium. The organism most likely damages the mucosa by producing urease, an enzyme that splits urea into ammonia, carbon dioxide, and bicarbonate. The ammonia erodes the mucosa.

Nonsteroidal antiinflammatory drug use is a common cause of gastric ulcers. Other factors can aggravate the problem, including smoking and excessive alcohol use.

Another cause of peptic ulcer disease is increased production of, or susceptibility to, gastric acid. With duodenal ulcers, increased hydrochloric acid production by the stomach's parietal cells and faster emptying of stomach contents means the duodenum receives more acid more quickly. Gastric ulcers are accompanied by normal or reduced acid secretion. However, the mucosa seems more permeable to damaging acid backflow.

Health history
- Gnawing or burning epigastric pain
- Pain occurring 2 hours or so after meals and at night, usually relieved by food (duodenal ulcer)
- Pain of varying pattern that may be relieved or aggravated by food (gastric ulcer)
- History of analgesic use, especially aspirin, ibuprofen, or naproxen
- History of smoking
- Recent loss of weight or appetite (gastric ulcer)
- Feelings of fullness or distention

Characteristic findings
Expect your physical examination findings to vary among patients with peptic ulcer disease, depending on the extent and severity of the disease. Use the information that follows to help distinguish between expected and unexpected findings.

Inspection
- Pallor (if anemic from blood loss)

Auscultation
- Hyperactive bowel sounds (possible)

Palpation
- Epigastric tenderness

Complications
- GI hemorrhage
- Hypovolemic shock
- Perforation
- Obstruction
- Intestinal infarction
- Penetration to adjacent structures, such as the pancreas, biliary tract, liver, or gastrohepatic omentum

DISORDER CLOSE-UP

CHOLECYSTITIS

An inflammation of the gallbladder, cholecystitis usually results from the obstructing presence of gallstones in the cystic or common bile ducts.

Gallstones develop in the gallbladder when such factors as age, obesity, and estrogen imbalance cause the liver to secrete bile abnormally high in cholesterol or lacking in the proper concentration of bile salts. Excessive water and bile salts are reabsorbed, making the bile less soluble. Cholesterol, calcium, and bilirubin then precipitate into gallstones.

Usually, cholecystitis develops after a high-fat meal. Fat entering the duodenum causes the intestinal mucosa to secrete cholecystokinin, a hormone that prompts the gallbladder to contract and empty its bile. If the gallbladder contains stones, this strong contraction can force one or more of them to lodge in the cystic duct, the common bile duct, or other locations. The obstruction prevents bile from flowing into the duodenum and causes bilirubin to be absorbed into the blood.

Biliary stasis and ischemia of tissues around the calculus may irritate and inflame the common bile duct. This inflammation can progress up the biliary tree and lead to infection of any of the bile ducts, causing scar tissue, edema, cirrhosis, portal hypertension, and variceal hemorrhage.

Health history
- Asymptomatic
- Sudden onset of severe, steady or aching pain in the midepigastric region or right upper abdominal quadrant that radiates to the back, between the shoulder blades, or over the right shoulder or shoulder blade
- Recent ingestion of a large or fatty meal, especially after fasting
- Nausea and vomiting
- Chills
- History of mild upper gastrointestinal symptoms, such as indigestion, vague abdominal discomfort, belching, and flatulence after high-fat meals or snacks

Characteristic findings
Expect your physical examination findings to vary among patients with cholecystitis, depending on the extent and severity of the disease. Use the information that follows to help distinguish between expected and unexpected findings.

Inspection
- Pallor
- Diaphoresis
- Exhaustion
- Abdominal muscle guarding
- Jaundice of sclerae and mucous membranes (chronic)
- Dark-colored urine (chronic)
- Clay-colored stools (chronic)

Palpation
- Rebound tenderness over gallbladder area, increasing with inspiration
- Abdominal rigidity, with peritoneal involvement
- Painless, sausage-like mass in the abdomen (calculus-filled gallbladder without obstruction)

Auscultation
- Hypoactive bowel sounds

Vital signs
- Fever
- Tachycardia

Complications
- Empyema, hydrops, mucocele, or gangrene of gallbladder
- Perforation
- Peritonitis
- Fistula formation
- Pancreatitis
- Chronic cholecystitis
- Cholangitis

- *Pyelonephritis.* Resulting from an infection (usually with *Escherichia coli*), this condition affects the renal pelvis and parenchyma. Your patient will complain of severe flank pain. Other symptoms include shaking chills, elevated temperature, tachycardia, hematuria, nausea, vomiting, and costovertebral angle (CVA) tenderness.
- *Pelvic inflammatory disease.* This condition affects females and results from infection by anaerobic or aerobic organisms, most commonly *Neisseria gonorrhoeae* and *Chlamydia trachomatis*. Fever and a purulent vaginal discharge usually are present.
- *Ruptured ectopic pregnancy.* This condition is characterized by a rapid onset of sharp, lower abdominal pain, occasionally radiating to the shoulders and neck. Commonly, the pain begins after an activity that increases abdominal pressure, such as a bowel movement. Vaginal bleeding may or may not be present.
- *Endometriosis.* Characterized by constant pain in the lower abdomen, vagina, posterior pelvis, and back, this condition usually begins 5 to 7 days before menses peaks and lasts for 2 to 3 days.

Abdominal distention

If your patient complains of abdominal distention, investigate the symptom further by asking him the following questions:
- When did you first notice an increase in the size of your abdomen?
- Are you having any difficulty breathing?
- Do you have a feeling of fullness or pressure?
- When was your last bowel movement?
- Have you noticed any change in your bowel or bladder habits?
- Could you (female patient) possibly be pregnant?
- What medications are you currently taking?

Focusing your assessment

When examining a patient who complains of abdominal distention, focus your assessment as follows:
- Examine your patient's sclerae and mucous membranes for signs of jaundice. Jaundice and abdominal distention caused by ascitic fluid are signs of liver disease.
- Inspect the abdomen for signs of asymmetry. Asymmetrical distention may result from tumor, cysts, or bowel obstruction. A lump in the abdominal wall may be a section of herniated intestine. If the patient is female, and distention appears between the umbilicus and symphysis pubis, suspect bladder distention, pregnancy, or ovarian tumor. Distention of the upper half of the abdomen may indicate gastric dilation or a pancreatic cyst or tumor. Ascites appears as a single curve from the xiphoid process to the pubic symphysis when viewed from the side. In the supine position, a patient with ascites will appear to have bulging flanks.

- Inspect the umbilicus to determine if it is inverted or everted. Symmetrical distention with an inverted umbilicus suggests obesity or recent fluid or gas pressure within the hollow intestines. An everted umbilicus suggests ascites or an underlying tumor.
- Inspect the abdominal wall for enlarged superficial abdominal veins, a sign of portal congestion.
- Auscultate the abdomen for bowel sounds or venous hum. Absent or hypoactive bowel sounds may indicate a paralytic ileus. Hyperactive bowel sounds may indicate an intestinal obstruction. A venous hum may indicate portal congestion from liver disease.
- Palpate the abdomen for an enlarged liver (a sign of cirrhosis), or palpable feces (a sign of fecal impaction or large bowel obstruction).
- Assess the abdomen for a fluid wave, which indicates ascites. Ascites is found in cirrhosis, peritonitis, metastatic carcinoma, ovarian carcinoma, and pancreatitis.

Possible causes

- *Cirrhosis.* Ascites from portal congestion may cause abdominal distention severe enough to impair breathing. A late symptom, abdominal distention accompanies jaundice, lethargy, mental status changes, asterixis, coagulopathies, pruritus, dependent edema, and enlarged superficial abdominal veins.
- *Ovarian cancer.* Abdominal distention from ascites occurs in advanced disease. Your patient may also complain of dyspepsia, urinary frequency, constipation, pelvic discomfort, and weight loss.
- *Pregnancy.* Abdominal distention and weight gain typically begin in the thirteenth week of pregnancy. Suspect pregnancy in a woman of child-bearing age who reports irregularities in menses. Other early signs include urinary frequency, nausea and vomiting in the morning, and breast swelling and tenderness.
- *Intestinal obstruction.* Abdominal distention is accompanied by hyperactive bowel sounds. Your patient also may complain of nausea, vomiting, or diarrhea. (See 🕐 *Responding to Acute Intestinal Obstruction,* p. 276.)
- *Paralytic ileus.* Abdominal distention is accompanied by absent or hypoactive bowel sounds. Symptoms occasionally include nausea and vomiting.
- *Fecal impaction.* Abdominal distention is accompanied by high-pitched tinkling bowel sounds. Diarrhea may develop from liquid stool being forced around the fecal blockage.
- *Hernia.* A protrusion of intestine through the abdominal wall, a hernia may disappear momentarily when pressed back into the abdominal wall. If the section of intestine becomes strangulated, your patient will complain of pain and may experience anorexia and vomiting.

ACTION STAT

RESPONDING TO ACUTE INTESTINAL OBSTRUCTION

Abdominal distention is a hallmark of acute intestinal obstruction, a common but potentially life-threatening disorder. When left untreated, an intestinal obstruction can lead to peritonitis, septicemia, bowel ischemia, perforation, or necrosis. These conditions, in turn, may lead to septic or hypovolemic shock and eventually death.

If you discover abdominal distention during your inspection, quickly assess your patient for a possible intestinal obstruction.

What to look for
Clinical findings vary, depending on the location of the obstruction, but may include:
- Sudden, severe, colicky epigastric or periumbilical pain
- Vomiting
- Visible peristalsis
- Hiccups
- Localized tenderness
- Minimal rigidity and rebound tenderness
- Absent bowel sounds (nonmechanical obstruction, such as paralytic ileus)
- Hyperactive, high-pitched borborygmi, with rushes coinciding with cramps (from mechanical obstruction caused by fecal impaction or a tumor, for example)

What to do immediately
If you suspect that your patient has an acute intestinal obstruction, notify the physician and follow these measures:
- Maintain nothing by mouth status until bowel sounds return or the obstruction is resolved through decompression or surgical intervention.
- Administer IV fluids (lactated Ringer's or isotonic saline solutions), as prescribed, to maintain fluid and electrolyte balance.
- Expect to insert a nasogastric tube and attach it to low, intermittent suction to help remove fluids from the gastrointestinal system,

relieve abdominal distention, and stop the vomiting.
- If a long intestinal tube (such as a Cantor, Harris, or Miller-Abbott) is indicated, assist with insertion. After insertion, reposition the patient from side to side to help advance the tube. Check the tube periodically to make sure it's advancing.
- Assess vital signs frequently. If you suspect a strangulating obstruction, monitor the patient for signs of shock (increased pulse rate, hypotension, and pallor).
- Administer prescribed medications, such as analgesics, antiemetics, and broad-spectrum antibiotics. Analgesics may be withheld until a diagnosis is confirmed because they can mask other signs and symptoms and decrease intestinal motility. Broad-spectrum antibiotics may be prescribed if the patient has a strangulating obstruction.
- Expect to insert a catheter to monitor urinary output.

What to do next
Once your patient has been stabilized, you'll need to:
- Maintain and monitor fluid intake and output. Include all vomitus and tube drainage as output. If ice chips are allowed, make sure you include them as intake.
- Monitor fluid and electrolyte status. Monitor serum electrolyte, blood urea nitrogen, and creatinine levels. Look for signs of dehydration, such as poor skin turgor, dry skin, parched tongue, dry mucous membranes, and decreased urinary output. Monitor daily weights.
- Administer rectal enemas, as prescribed, to relieve partial obstruction.
- Keep the patient in semi-Fowler's or Fowler's position to alleviate respiratory distress from abdominal distention and to promote optimal pulmonary ventilation.
- Measure abdominal girth every 8 hours to monitor the patient's condition.

- *Obesity.* A uniformly rounded abdomen is accompanied by an umbilicus buried deeply in the abdominal wall and excessive fat in other body areas.
- *Aerophagia.* Swallowing air can cause an excess of air in the GI tract (tympanites), resulting in abdominal distention. Some patients swallow air when they're anxious, in pain, or nauseated. Ingestion of gas-forming foods, such as cabbage, turnips, and onions, and drinking fluids through a straw are other possible causes. Your patient will have a large area of tympany on percussion, with voluntary or involuntary muscle spasm of the abdominal wall.

Fecal incontinence

If your patient complains of fecal incontinence, investigate the symptom further by asking him the following questions:
- When does the fecal incontinence occur?
- Is it associated with activity, such as exercise or walking? Or does it occur during periods of rest?
- Does it occur in the morning?
- How long has it been occurring?
- What is your normal pattern of bowel elimination?
- Do you ever find fecal matter on your underwear?
- Do you ever engage in anal sex?

Focusing your assessment

When examining a patient who complains of fecal incontinence, focus your assessment as follows:
- Use a gloved and lubricated index finger to assess anal sphincter tone, and inspect any stool found in the rectum. Blood or mucus in the stool or rectum could indicate colorectal cancer. Poor sphincter tone may be the result of sphincter trauma.
- Inspect the anus for rectal prolapse or signs of trauma.
- Assess lower extremity strength. Lower extremity weakness may be a sign of spinal cord compression.

Possible causes

- *Colorectal cancer.* Signs include loss of sphincter control or an urgent need to defecate upon arising in the morning, blood or mucus in the stool, and a sense of incomplete evacuation.
- *Sphincter trauma.* Injury can cause loss of sphincter control and lead to incontinence.
- *Rectal prolapse.* This condition is evidenced by protrusion of the rectal mucosa through the anus. The patient may also complain of a persistent sensation of rectal fullness, bloody diarrhea, and pain in the lower abdomen from ulceration.
- *Spinal cord compression.* Compression affecting the lumbar or sacral area may cause loss of bowel control.

Urinary incontinence

If your patient complains of urinary incontinence, investigate the symptom further by asking him the following questions:
- When does the urinary incontinence occur?
- Is it associated with activity, such as exercise, lifting, coughing, or laughing? Or does it occur during periods of rest?
- How long has this been occurring? Did it start gradually or suddenly?
- What is your normal pattern of bladder elimination?
- Have you noticed any changes in the color or odor of your urine?
- Do you have urinary hesitancy or urgency?
- Describe your fluid intake during a typical day.
- What medications are you currently taking?
- Might you (female patient) be pregnant?

Focusing your assessment

When examining a patient who complains of urinary incontinence, focus your assessment as follows:
- Inspect the abdomen for distention. Abdominal distention may indicate urinary retention or pregnancy.
- Ask your patient to void into a specimen cup, and inspect the urine. Cloudy or foul-smelling urine suggests infection.
- Inspect the vulva or penis for purulent discharge or redness and swelling, signs of gonorrhea.

Possible causes

- *Muscle weakness.* Urine leakage results from physical strain, such as sneezing, coughing, or quick movements (stress incontinence). Elderly females and females who have given birth vaginally are candidates for this type of incontinence.
- *Pregnancy.* Incontinence in pregnancy is a form of stress incontinence arising from pressure on the bladder by the enlarging uterus.
- *Urinary retention.* Retention causes dribbling because the distended bladder can't contract strongly enough to force a urine stream (overflow incontinence). The bladder will be distended upon palpation.
- *Diuretic medications.* These medications can cause bladder distention, which may result in incontinence from overflow or from weak muscles unaccustomed to a full bladder.
- *Gonorrhea.* Urinary incontinence accompanies purulent vaginal or penile discharge and dysuria.
- *Cognitive impairment.* Your patient may be unaware of the need to urinate.

Constipation

If your patient complains of constipation, investigate the symptom further by asking him the following questions:
- What is your usual pattern of bowel movement?

- Do you take anything on a regular basis to assist with bowel movement?
- When was your last bowel movement?
- How is your appetite? Do you feel full more easily than you used to?
- Have you changed your diet recently?
- Have you lost weight recently?
- Has the shape, color, or consistency of your stool changed recently?
- What medications are you currently taking?

Focusing your assessment

When examining a patient who complains of constipation, focus your assessment as follows:

- Inspect the abdomen for distention.
- Assess the abdomen for symmetry. An asymmetrical contour may indicate tumor, hernia, or bowel obstruction.
- Auscultate for bowel sounds. Absence of bowel sounds may indicate a paralytic ileus.
- Palpate the abdomen. Masses may be tumors or distended sections of intestine. A palpable colon may be a sign of inactive colon or large bowel obstruction.
- Use a gloved and lubricated index finger to examine rectal contents. Stool is found in the lower portion of the rectum with inactive colon.

Possible causes

- *Large intestine obstruction.* Constipation may be the only early sign. After several days, your patient may complain of colicky abdominal pain with spasms. The abdomen will be distended, and loops of large bowel may become visible on the abdominal wall.
- *Colorectal cancer.* A tumor can occlude the lumen of the descending colon. If so, your patient probably will report a history of pencil-shaped or ribbon-shaped stools.
- *Narcotic use.* Narcotics slow bowel motility, possibly causing fecal material to block the large intestine.
- *Inactive colon.* This condition is characterized by chronic constipation. Causes include low dietary fiber, chronic laxative or enema use, poor hydration, and a sedentary lifestyle. Your patient will complain of mild abdominal discomfort and of having to strain to produce hard, dry stool.

LIFESPAN CONSIDERATIONS

Constipation and fecal impaction occur more commonly in older adults because intestinal motility declines with age.

Diarrhea

If your patient complains of diarrhea, investigate the symptom further by asking him the following questions:

- How long have you had the diarrhea? (If less than 3 weeks, it's considered an acute episode. If more than 3 weeks, it's considered chronic.)
- How often do you have episodes of diarrhea?
- What are the consistency and volume of your stool?
- What color is the stool?
- Is eating meals followed by diarrhea?
- Do you have any abdominal pain?
- Have you traveled recently out of the state or out of the country?
- What prescription and over-the-counter medications are you currently taking?
- Have you participated recently in anal sex?

Focusing your assessment

When examining a patient who complains of diarrhea, focus your assessment as follows:

- Assess hydration by checking your patient's skin turgor and mucous membrane moisture. Diarrhea can lead to dehydration.
- Check your patient's vital signs. Low blood pressure is a sign of dehydration.
- Inspect the abdomen for distention or peristaltic waves, which may indicate bowel obstruction or fecal impaction.
- Auscultate for bowel sounds. Hyperactive sounds may indicate gastroenteritis.
- Assess the color, amount, and odor of any stools passed.

Possible causes

- *Gastroenteritis.* This condition is characterized by diarrhea with nausea, vomiting, and abdominal discomfort. Other symptoms include fever, malaise, and hyperactive bowel sounds.
- *Ulcerative colitis.* Recurrent bloody diarrhea, commonly contains mucus. Patients with ulcerative colitis experience intermittent asymptomatic remissions. The intensity of the attacks varies with the extent of the inflammation. Other symptoms include spastic rectum and anus, abdominal pain, irritability, weight loss, weakness, anorexia, nausea, and vomiting.
- *Acquired immunodeficiency syndrome (AIDS) or its treatment.* A common problem for AIDS patients, diarrhea may result from opportunistic infection in the GI tract, Kaposi's sarcoma (KS), drug therapy, chemotherapy, or radiation therapy. (See 🔲 *AIDS.*)
- *Crohn's disease.* This condition is characterized by diarrhea accompanied by colicky abdominal pain in the right lower quadrant, cramping, tenderness, flatulence, and fever.

(Text continues on p. 284.)

AIDS

An infectious disease syndrome that destroys the body's immune system, acquired immunodeficiency syndrome (AIDS) can result in death by overwhelming opportunistic infection. The syndrome originates with infection by the human immunodeficiency virus (HIV).

HIV spreads through contact with infected blood or body fluids. Most often, transmission occurs from blood or blood products transfusion, sexual contact, needle sharing among intravenous drug users, perinatal exposure (including through breast milk), and occupational exposure (such as through needle-stick injuries). The virus is not spread by casual contact or by insects.

A retrovirus that carries its genetic material in ribonucleic acid (RNA) rather than deoxyribonucleic acid (DNA), HIV cannot replicate until it invades host cells. The invasion process begins when the virus attaches to $CD4^+$ receptors on the surface of cells, including:

- Lymphocytes
- Macrophages
- Colorectal cells
- Glial cells (central nervous system)
- Langerhans' cells
- Follicular dendritic cells

Because of this variety in host cells, the virus can express itself in many ways, producing a wide variety of symptoms that mimic other diseases.

Once HIV binds to a $CD4^+$ receptor site, it enters the cell and injects its genetic material into the host cell's cytoplasm. There, reverse transcriptase (an enzyme) transcribes DNA from viral RNA. Because this transcription process is faulty, mutations occur that prevent antiviral drugs from having a consistent and long-term effect.

This newly formed DNA invades the host cell's nucleus and is transcribed back into RNA. Now, every time the cell divides, it spreads the HIV infection. Transcribed RNA is translated into long protein chains and enzymes. A viral enzyme called protease cuts the long chains and incorporates them into new virus particles. New HIV particles can then bud away to infect other cells.

The body's immune system produces antibodies in an attempt to fight the HIV infection. However, by selectively infecting immune system cells, and by mutating regularly, the virus ultimately destroys the body's defense against infection, leaving the person vulnerable to opportunistic infections. These opportunistic infections account for 90% of AIDS-related deaths.

Health history

- Exposure to HIV-infected blood or body fluids
- History of flulike symptoms, including fever, sweats, sore throat, malaise, myalgia, arthralgia, photophobia, diarrhea, anorexia, nausea, vomiting, or headache
- Weight loss
- Increasing incidence and severity of infections
- Chest pain, as in *Pneumocystis carinii* pneumonia (PCP)
- Cough and increased sputum production (PCP)
- Mood, motor, behavioral, or cognitive changes (AIDS dementia)
- Visual changes, such as blurring or loss of vision
- Stiff neck (cryptococcal meningitis)

Characteristic findings

Expect your physical findings to vary among patients with AIDS, depending on the extent and severity of the disease, the stage of the disease, and the AIDS-related conditions present. Use the information that follows to help distinguish between expected and unexpected findings.

Inspection

- Diaphoresis
- Transient maculopapular rashes on chest and extremities
- Hairy leukoplakia of the oral mucosa
- Pink, red, or purple nodules or plaques, as in Kaposi's sarcoma (KS)
- Tachypnea (PCP)
- Flat affect and apathy (AIDS dementia)
- Unsteady gait and incoordination
- Confusion, staring, disorientation, and delirium (advanced stages)

(Continued)

DISORDER CLOSE-UP

AIDS—cont'd

- Retinitis, as in cytomegalovirus (CMV), with granular areas, perivascular exudates, and hemorrhages at the optic fundus
- Candidiasis of mouth, esophagus, or vagina
- Loss of more than 10 pounds or 10% of body weight

Palpation
- Firm, nontender nodules or plaques on the skin (KS)

- Generalized lymphadenopathy (lymph nodes larger than ½ inches (1 cm) in diameter in two or more extrainguinal sites for more than 3 months)
- Hepatomegaly
- Splenomegaly

Auscultation
- Hyperactive bowel sounds (cryptosporidiosis)
- Normal breath sounds or coarse breath sounds (PCP)

Host Sites for HIV Infection

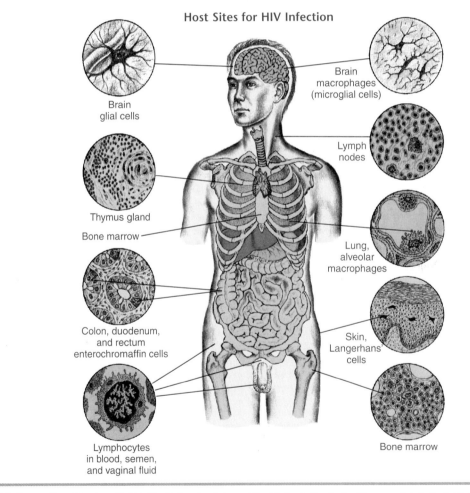

Brain
glial cells

Brain
macrophages
(microglial cells)

Lymph
nodes

Thymus gland

Bone marrow

Lung,
alveolar
macrophages

Colon, duodenum,
and rectum
enterochromaffin cells

Skin,
Langerhans'
cells

Lymphocytes
in blood, semen,
and vaginal fluid

Bone marrow

From McCance, K. & Huether, S. (2002). *Pathophysiology: The Biologic Basis for Disease of Adults & Children* (4th ed.). St. Louis: Mosby.

Vital signs
- Fever
- Increased respiratory rate

Complications
- Repeated overwhelming opportunistic infections of the respiratory and gastrointestinal tracts, central nervous system involvement, and KS
- Gingival erosion and loss of teeth from oral candidiasis
- Night blindness and loss of peripheral vision from CMV retinitis
- Anemia and neutropenia
- Dermatologic problems, such as folliculitis, molluscum contagiosum, and dermatitis
- Neuropathy
- Wasting syndrome
- Respiratory failure, typically related to PCP

Categories of HIV Infection
Experts at the Centers for Disease Control and Prevention have identified three category systems of HIV infection based on clinical symptoms (A, B, and C), and three categories based on CD4+ cell count (1, 2, and 3).

Clinical symptoms
A = The patient is infected with HIV, but has no symptoms other than those produced by the initial seroconversion. These flulike symptoms and persistent generalized lymphadenopathy can last up to 3 months. Symptoms then resolve, and the infection becomes latent, sometimes for 10 years or more.

B = The patient has symptoms of impaired cell-mediated immunity but no AIDS indicator conditions. Symptoms can include weight loss, thrush, cervical dysplasia, fever, diarrhea lasting more than a month, peripheral neuropathy, and pelvic inflammatory disease.

C = The patient has one or more AIDS indicator conditions. AIDS indicator conditions are characterized by the development of tumors and opportunistic infections, such as, PCP, cryptococcal meningitis, toxoplasmosis, cryptosporidiosis, herpes simplex infection, CMV, tuberculosis, HIV-related encephalopathy, Mycobacterium avium complex (MAC), KS, non-Hodgkin's lymphoma.

CD4+ cell count categories
A patient's CD4+ cell count normal is 800 to 1,500/mm^3, depending on the laboratory values used.
1 = Greater than 500mm^3
2 = 200 to 499/mm^3
3 = Less than 200 mm^3
Combining both systems, the CDC uses nine separate categories to further define the progression of the disease. Keep in mind that patients in categories A3, B3, and C1 to C3 are categorized as having acquired immunodeficiency syndrome (AIDS). The categories are as follows:

CD4+ Cell Count Categories	Clinical Categories		
	A	B	C
1	A1	B1	C1
2	A2	B2	C2
3	A3	B3	C3

- *Fecal impaction.* Diarrhea may result from liquid stool being forced around a fecal blockage. Your patient may have high-pitched, tinkling bowel sounds and a distended abdomen.
- *Partial or early small bowel obstruction.* Diarrhea results from hyper-motility of the intestinal tract as it attempts to move material past the obstruction.

Frequent urination

If your patient complains of urinary frequency, investigate the symptom further by asking him the following questions:

- Have you recently increased the amount of fluid you drink?
- Have you been outside in the heat recently?
- How many cups of coffee or tea do you drink a day?
- Have you recently had an episode of vomiting, diarrhea, or nausea?
- Do you have diabetes? Does anyone in your immediate family have diabetes?
- Do you wake up in the night to urinate? Is that your usual pattern or something new?
- What medications do you take?
- Is your urine dark or light?
- What volume of urine do you pass each time?
- Do you have any pain during or after urination?

Focusing your assessment

When examining a patient who complains of frequent urination, focus your assessment as follows:

- Assess skin turgor. Dehydration may accompany urinary frequency caused by diabetes mellitus or diuretic use.
- Palpate the abdomen. Bladder distention may be present with urethral obstruction or urinary retention.
- Ask your patient to void in a specimen cup, and inspect the urine for color and odor. Cloudy or hazy urine or urine with a foul odor may indicate an infection of the urinary tract or prostate.
- For a male patient, perform a digital rectal examination and palpate the prostate. A tender, indurated, swollen, firm prostate is a sign of prostatitis.

Possible causes

- *Urinary tract infection.* Infection increases urinary frequency and decreases the amount voided each time. Other symptoms include dysuria, cramps or spasm of the bladder, nocturia, and a feeling of warmth during urination. Urine typically will be cloudy or may have a foul odor. In older people, confusion may be the first sign of a urinary tract infection.
- *Urinary tract obstruction.* Obstruction increases urinary frequency and decreases the amount voided each time.

- *Prostatitis.* This condition causes frequent, urgent urination. Other symptoms include dysuria, nocturia, fever, chills, low-back pain, and myalgia.
- *Urinary retention with incomplete emptying of the bladder.* A high residual volume in the bladder does not require much extra volume to produce the urge to urinate.
- *Excessive fluid intake.* Consider diabetes in patients who have high fluid intake and complain of thirst.
- *Alcohol or caffeine consumption.* These substances may cause polyuria.
- *Diabetes mellitus.* Diabetes usually increases urine excretion. Glucose spilling into the urine acts as an osmotic diuretic.
- *Diabetes insipidus.* This form of diabetes results from inadequate antidiuretic hormone and can be caused by a neurologic disorder or a primary renal disorder.
- *Bladder calculi and bladder cancer.* The typical patient experiences pain when the bladder is full and so urinates more often to avoid the pain.

Difficult or painful urination

If your patient complains of difficult or painful urination (dysuria), investigate the symptom further by asking him the following questions:
- Do you have difficulty starting the urine stream (hesitancy)?
- Do you have difficulty maintaining the urine stream?
- Does pain occur with urination or after urination?
- What is your normal daily fluid intake?

Focusing your assessment

When examining a patient who complains of difficult or painful urination, focus your assessment as follows:
- Ask your patient to void in a specimen cup, and inspect the urine. Cloudy, hazy, or foul-smelling urine is a sign of infection.
- Palpate the abdomen for bladder distention, a sign of urethral obstruction.
- For a male patient, perform a digital rectal examination and palpate the prostate. A tender, indurated, swollen, and firm prostate is a sign of prostatitis.

Possible causes

- *Urinary tract infection.* Infection produces pain during urination. Other signs include fever, urinary frequency, and cloudy, hazy, or foul-smelling urine. In older adults, confusion (linked to the effects of infection) may be the first sign of a urinary tract infection.
- *Urethral obstruction.* Obstruction may cause pain during urination. The bladder may be distended.

- *Bladder calculi.* Pain occurs after urination because stones in the bladder cause pain when the bladder is empty. Causes of calculi include dehydration, infection, and urinary stasis.
- *Prostatitis.* This condition causes dysuria and urinary frequency and urgency. Other symptoms include fever, malaise, chills, low-back pain, and myalgia.
- *Benign prostatic hyperplasia.* Symptoms include urinary frequency and hesitancy with postvoid dribbling, a diminished force of urinary stream, urgency, dysuria, and nocturia. Upon palpation, the prostate gland feels symmetrically enlarged but smooth and somewhat rubbery.

LIFESPAN CONSIDERATIONS

Benign prostatic hyperplasia commonly begins after age 50, and nearly 80% of males have the disorder by age 80. This disorder occurs because of gradual, progressive enlargement of the prostate gland.

Hematuria

If your patient complains of frank blood in the urine or tea-colored urine, investigate the symptom further by asking him the following questions:

- Does the blood appear at the beginning of urination, at the end, or throughout?
- Have you noticed any new bruises or bleeding from your gums?
- What medications are you currently taking?
- Do you smoke cigarettes?
- What is your exercise pattern?
- Have you had any recent abdominal trauma?
- Have you had a recent infection or sore throat?

Focusing your assessment

When examining a patient who complains of hematuria, focus your assessment as follows:

- Assess the skin for signs of bruising or petechiae.
- Assess the abdominal wall for signs of recent trauma.
- Palpate the abdomen for an abdominal mass. Hematuria may be the first sign of renal cell carcinoma.

Possible causes

- *Renal cell carcinoma.* This condition accounts for 85% of all renal tumors. Your patient also may complain of colicky abdominal pain and have a palpable abdominal mass. Smoking increases the risk of renal cell carcinoma.

- *Trauma or injury to the kidneys.* Hematuria caused by bleeding from the kidneys is continuous during urination.
- *Thrombocytopenia.* Low platelet counts can cause bleeding from the kidney, bladder, or urethra. Bleeding usually is continuous during urination.
- *Bladder infection.* Infection can cause irritation and bleeding of the bladder wall. Your patient will complain of bleeding at the end of urination. Caffeine intake can contribute to bladder irritation.
- *Renal calculi.* Calculi cause bleeding by irritating the urethral wall. Bleeding usually occurs at the beginning of urination.
- *Glomerulonephritis.* Bleeding from glomerular damage usually is continuous during urination. Your patient probably will have a history of streptococcal infection or sore throat.
- *Anticoagulation medications.* These medications can cause spontaneous bleeding in the urinary tract. However, many patients also have an underlying urinary problem.
- *Smoking.* Smoking may cause hematuria without any underlying pathology.
- *Strenuous exercise.* Vigorous exercise may cause hematuria for unknown reasons.

Abnormal menses

If your female patient has irregular menses, dysmenorrhea (painful menstruation), menorrhagia (profuse menstruation), metrorrhagia (intermenstrual bleeding), or amenorrhea (absence of menstruation), investigate the problem further by asking her the following questions:
- At what age did you begin your menstrual cycles?
- How often do you menstruate?
- Are your menstrual cycles regular?
- How many days does your menses usually last?
- How would you characterize your flow?
- Do you have pain at any time during your cycle? When?
- What was the first day of your last cycle?
- Do you have any trouble tolerating heat or cold?
- Do you have any trouble sleeping?
- Have you gained or lost weight recently?
- Do you exercise excessively?
- Have you noticed any change in your sexual habits?

Focusing your assessment

When examining a patient who complains of abnormal menses, focus your assessment as follows:
- Assess your patient for abdominal pain. The pain of dysmenorrhea is sharp, intermittent, and cramping. It occurs in the lower abdomen and radiates to the back, thighs, groin, and vulva. The pain of

endometriosis is constant. It usually begins 5 to 7 days before menses peaks and lasts for 2 to 3 days. Ectopic pregnancy is associated with sharp, lower abdominal pain that radiates to the shoulders and neck.

- Assess the skin for thinness, dryness, or flakiness, a sign of hypothyroidism.
- Palpate the neck for an enlarged thyroid gland, a sign of hyperthyroidism.

Possible causes

- *Premenstrual syndrome.* For most patients, dysmenorrhea begins just before the menstrual flow and peaks within 24 hours. Other symptoms include urinary frequency, nausea, vomiting, diarrhea, headache, chills, abdominal bloating, painful breasts, and irritability.
- *Hypothyroidism.* This condition is associated with menorrhagia and amenorrhea. Symptoms include fatigue, cold sensitivity, weight gain, constipation, dry or flaky skin, a puffy face, and hoarseness.
- *Endometriosis.* Associated with menorrhagia and metrorrhagia, this condition produces constant pain in the lower abdomen.
- *Threatened abortion.* Your patient may experience a pink or scant brown discharge for several weeks before the onset of cramps and increased vaginal bleeding, signaling an abortion.
- *Ectopic pregnancy.* This condition is associated with amenorrhea or abnormal menstruation. Early symptoms mimic those of intrauterine pregnancy. As the pregnancy progresses, abdominal pain develops.
- *Neoplasms.* Tumors involving the uterus, cervix, or ovaries can cause abnormal menstruation.
- *Pelvic inflammatory disease.* This condition is characterized by bleeding between periods and a purulent vaginal discharge accompanied by abdominal pain, malaise, and fever.
- *Hypopituitarism.* This abnormality is associated with amenorrhea, lethargy, cold intolerance, anorexia, and abdominal pain.
- *Hyperthyroidism.* In addition to amenorrhea, this condition can cause an enlarged thyroid, nervousness, heat intolerance, weight loss with increased appetite, sweating, and diarrhea.
- *Anorexia nervosa.* Symptoms include amenorrhea, fear of being fat, anger, ritualistic behavior, loss of libido, fatigue, sleep alterations, and cold intolerance.
- *Female athletic triad.* If a young female athlete frequently misses a menstrual period or stops menstruating altogether, suspect this condition. In addition to menstrual irregularities, the condition is also marked by abnormal eating habits, such as crash dieting, and excessive exercise. The patient may also develop osteoporosis.

Penile or vaginal discharge or lesions

If your patient complains of a discharge from the penis or vagina, investigate the symptom by asking the following questions:

- What color is the discharge?
- Does the discharge have any odor?
- Do you have any pain or burning with urination?
- Do you (female patient) use vaginal spermicides or douches with intercourse?
- Do you (female patient) use birth control pills?
- Have you recently taken antibiotics?
- Do you wear tight underwear? Or have you recently spent time in a wet bathing suit?
- Do your genitals itch or burn?
- Do you use douches, feminine hygiene sprays, bubble baths, talcum powder, or scented toilet paper?

Focusing your assessment

When examining a patient who complains of penile or vaginal discharge or lesions, focus your assessment as follows:

- Inspect the genital area for any open sores or other lesions. Syphilis produces an open chancre, (a small, fluid-filled lesion).
- Inspect the genital area for redness or swelling, signs of gonorrhea.
- Check your patient's vital signs. Pelvic inflammatory disease typically causes fever.
- Inspect the genital area for the discharge. The color and consistency of the discharge provide clues to the causative organism. (See *Assessing Vaginal Discharge,* p. 290.)
- Palpate the inguinal lymph nodes. Inflamed nodes are found with genital herpes.

Possible causes

- *Syphilis.* Chancres develop on the genitalia and anus. The lesions are painless and have indurated, raised edges and clear bases. They usually disappear in 3 to 6 weeks.
- *Gonorrhea.* Purulent discharge from the penis or vagina is accompanied by dysuria. Redness or swelling may develop at the site of the infection. Your patient may complain of urinary frequency and incontinence. If the vulva is infected, the female patient will complain of burning and pain with occasional itching.
- *Chlamydia.* Mucopurulent discharge occurs with painful urination. Other symptoms include burning on urination and urinary frequency.
- *Genital herpes.* This infection is indicated by fluid-filled vesicles with yellow, oozing centers. Other symptoms include prodromal itching, tingling, redness, and pain at the site of the lesions, and tender inguinal lymph nodes.

INTERPRETING ABNORMAL FINDINGS

ASSESSING VAGINAL DISCHARGE

Does your patient have abnormal vaginal discharge? If so, the character and consistency of the discharge can give you clues to your patient's problem. Use this table to help guide your differential diagnosis.

Discharge characteristics	Other symptoms	Probable causes
• White and thick, resembling cottage cheese • Odorless	• Severe itching • Dyspareunia • Patches on vaginal walls • Inflamed vaginal walls	• *Candida albicans* infection
• Gray-white • Scant amount • Fishy or foul odor	• Itching • Normal mucosa	• *Gardnerella vaginalis* infection
• Green, yellow, or white • May be frothy • Foul smell	• Burning and itching • Dyspareunia • Strawberry spots on cervix	• *Trichomonas vaginalis* infection
• White or pink • Scant amount • Odorless	• Itching • Dyspareunia • Pale, thin, dry mucosa	• Atrophic vaginitis

- *Pelvic inflammatory disease.* Mucopurulent discharge occurs with severe abdominal pain and fever.
- *Urethritis.* This is an infection or inflammation of the urethra. Chemicals from vaginal spermicides or douches can cause urethritis in the female patient. Sexually transmitted diseases, such as gonorrhea and chlamydia, are other causes.
- *Vaginitis.* This inflammation of the vagina causes burning and itching of the labia and vulva. Overgrowth of *Candida albicans, Gardnerella vaginalis,* or *Trichomonas vaginalis* is commonly the cause. Antibiotic use can cause an imbalance of vaginal microorganisms, allowing one to proliferate. Use of vaginal spermicides or douches can change the vaginal lining, allowing bacterial invasion. Wearing underwear with a nylon crotch or wearing a wet bathing suit can create a moist, warm environment favorable for bacteria. Use of talcum powder, bubble baths, feminine hygiene sprays, or scented toilet paper can irritate the vaginal lining. Noninfectious vaginitis from chemical irritation has no discharge but does have intense itching and irritation.

Erectile dysfunction

If your male patient complains of erectile dysfunction, investigate the symptom further by asking him the following questions:
- Are you experiencing stress in your job?
- Are you experiencing stress in any of your relationships?

- Are you afraid of having a heart attack during intercourse?
- How much alcohol do you consume?
- What medications or recreational drugs do you take?

Focusing your assessment
When examining a patient who complains of erectile dysfunction, focus your assessment as follows:
- Check for signs of decreased testosterone, including general muscle weakness, shrinkage of the testicles, softening of the testicular tissues, and decreased amounts of pubic, chest, and axillary hair.

Possible causes
- *Stress.* A leading cause of erectile dysfunction, stress can arise in the workplace, community, or family. Erectile dysfunction caused by stress is usually situational and temporary.
- *Psychogenic factors.* Along with stress, psychogenic factors include fear of intimacy, feelings of inadequacy, previous trauma, and lack of communication.
- *Alcohol use.* Excessive use can cause erectile dysfunction.
- *Medications.* Beta-blockers and steroids commonly cause erectile dysfunction. It usually resolves with discontinuation of the medication.
- *Decreased testosterone.* A result of hypopituitarism, decreased testosterone affects libido and causes erectile dysfunction.

Rectal bleeding
If your patient complains of rectal bleeding, investigate the symptom further by asking him the following questions:
- Is the blood a part of the stool? Or does it appear on the toilet paper after the bowel movement?
- Do you have a strong urge to defecate in the morning?
- Do you have burning or itching in the anal area?
- Do you experience dizziness?
- Do you ever feel that you're not able to empty your rectum when defecating?
- Do you engage in anal intercourse?

Focusing your assessment
When examining a patient who complains of rectal bleeding, focus your assessment as follows:
- Inspect the anus for hemorrhoids, rectal prolapse, fissures, or drainage. Drainage may indicate an anorectal abscess.
- If possible, perform a digital rectal examination, and look for any acute bleeding or rectal polyps. Test any stool for occult blood. Positive stool findings may indicate colorectal cancer or high internal hemorrhoids.

Possible causes

- *Hemorrhoids.* These structures cause intermittent bleeding with defecation. Bleeding from first-degree hemorrhoids appears on stool or toilet paper. Prolapsed, second-degree hemorrhoids usually return to the anal canal spontaneously after defecation. Third-degree hemorrhoids cause constant discomfort and prolapse in response to any increase in intra-abdominal pressure.
- *Rectal prolapse.* This condition is characterized by bloody diarrhea and abdominal pain. Other symptoms include a persistent sensation of rectal fullness.
- *Anorectal abscesses or fissures.* Abscesses and fissures result from abrasions or tears in the lining of the anal canal and subsequent *Escherichia coli* infection. Abrasions may result from treatment of internal hemorrhoids, enema tips, puncture wounds from ingested eggshells or fish bones, anal sex, or insertion of foreign objects.
- *Lower GI bleeding.* This condition is characterized by blood in the stool. Frank blood indicates a lower GI source of bleeding. Black, tarry, guaiac-positive stools indicate a source of bleeding higher in the intestinal tract.
- *Anorectal stricture.* This condition is characterized by excessive straining and the inability to completely evacuate the bowel. Pain, bleeding, and pruritus ani are other signs. Scarring after surgery, inflammation, or laxative abuse may cause anorectal strictures.
- *Rectal polyps.* Polyps high in the rectum leave a streak of blood on the stool. Low rectal polyps bleed freely.
- *Colorectal cancer.* Symptoms include the urgent need to defecate upon arising and blood or mucus in the stool.

EXAMINING
THE LOWER EXTREMITIES

Free and easy use of the lower extremities is critical to your patient's quality of life. The hips, legs, and feet function as a weight-bearing team to support ambulation and other body movements. When problems develop in the lower limbs, they can cause pain and discomfort, as well as disrupt the patient's ability to move at will.

A range of debilitating conditions can affect the lower extremities, including arthritis, gout, thrombophlebitis, and chronic venous insufficiency. That's why you must examine your patient's lower extremities skillfully and thoroughly—especially if your patient has specific complaints.

This chapter reviews information and skills essential for examining the lower extremities accurately. To use this information wisely, you'll need to first recognize that your physical examination will be only as good as your understanding of the structures involved. (See █ *Structures of the Lower Extremities*, pp. 294 to 296.)

In this chapter, you'll learn how to perform a series of important tests, including range of motion (ROM), muscle strength, deep tendon reflexes (DTRs), and sensory ability. In addition to providing an overview of examination procedures, normal findings, and abnormal findings for the lower extremities, the chapter also outlines rapid assessments for a number of chief complaints.

(Text continues on p. 297.)

ANATOMY REVIEW

STRUCTURES OF THE LOWER EXTREMITIES

The lower extremities form a foundation on which physical mobility is built. Use the illustrations here to refresh your memory of the bones, muscles, and blood vessels of the lower extremities.

SKELETAL STRUCTURE

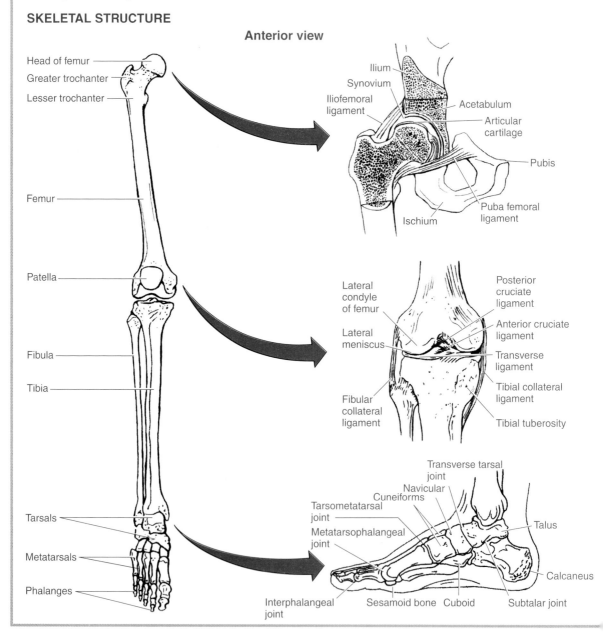

Anterior view

Head of femur

Greater trochanter

Lesser trochanter

Femur

Patella

Fibula

Tibia

Tarsals

Metatarsals

Phalanges

Ilium

Synovium

Iliofemoral ligament

Acetabulum

Articular cartilage

Pubis

Puba femoral ligament

Ischium

Lateral condyle of femur

Lateral meniscus

Posterior cruciate ligament

Anterior cruciate ligament

Transverse ligament

Tibial collateral ligament

Fibular collateral ligament

Tibial tuberosity

Transverse tarsal joint

Navicular

Cuneiforms

Tarsometatarsal joint

Metatarsophalangeal joint

Talus

Calcaneus

Interphalangeal joint

Sesamoid bone

Cuboid

Subtalar joint

MUSCLES

Anterior view

Posterior view

Pectineus

Tensor fasciae latae

Adductor longus

Adductor magnus

Gracilis

Sartorius

Rectus femoris

Vastus medialis

Tendon of rectus femoris

Patella

Patellar ligament

Peroneus longus

Tibialis anterior

Extensor digitorum longus

Gluteus maximus

Semimembranosus

Biceps femoris

Semitendinosus

Iliotibial tract

Semimembranosus

Plantaris

Gastrocnemius

Soleus

Peroneus longus

Peroneus brevis

Flexor hallucis longus

Calcaneal tendon
(Achilles tendon)

(Continued)

From Thibodeau, G. & Patton, K. (2003). *Anatomy and Physiology* (5th ed.). St. Louis: Mosby.

ANATOMY REVIEW

STRUCTURES OF THE LOWER EXTREMITIES—cont'd

BLOOD VESSELS

Arteries

Inferior vena cava

Common iliac artery

External iliac artery

Superior gluteal artery

Inferior gluteal artery

Abdominal aorta

Median sacral artery

Internal iliac artery

Lateral sacral artery

Internal pudendal artery

Obturator artery

Deep femoral artery

Descending branch of lateral circumflex artery

Popliteal artery

Femoral artery

Genicular arteries

Fibular artery

Anterior tibial artery

Posterior tibial artery

Lateral plantar arch

Medial plantar artery

Plantar arch

Dorsalis pedis artery

Digital arteries

Veins

Common iliac vein

Inferior vena cava

Internal iliac vein

Femoral vein

Great saphenous vein

Popliteal vein

Small saphenous vein

Fibular (peroneal) vein

Anterior tibial vein

posterior tibial vein

Great saphenous vein

Dorsal veins of the foot

Dorsal venous arch

Digital vein

From Thibodeau, G. & Patton, K. (2003). *Anatomy and Physiology* (5th ed.). St. Louis: Mosby.

EXAMINATION STEPS AND FINDINGS

As always, review your patient's health history before beginning your examination. Note any important details in the history, and adjust your examination accordingly. For example, if your patient has had a recent hip replacement, you may need to alter some aspects of the typical lower extremity examination to avoid causing your patient discomfort.

Examining the lower extremities starts with the proper tools. Before starting your examination, gather the following equipment: tape measure, skin-marking pen, reflex hammer, cotton-tipped swab, and tuning fork.

For the lower extremities, you'll rely primarily on inspection and palpation when conducting your examination. These two skills, typically used together for greater efficiency, also play a part in further testing for ROM, muscle strength, DTRs, and sensory responses. (See *Key Examination Steps for the Lower Extremities.*)

Inspection

Begin your examination by assessing skin color and integrity. Remember, whether your patient is standing, sitting, or lying down, inspection always depends on good lighting. Note any discoloration, such as erythema, jaundice, or ecchymoses. When assessing skin integrity, note any changes, such as rashes, abrasions, lacerations, ulcers, or hematomas. Check the toenails for color, shape, and thickness. Also look at hair distribution and quantity.

Now inspect the size and symmetry of your patient's legs, joints, and muscle groups. Look at the anterior and posterior aspects of the patient's legs in the standing position. Are the legs of equal length? Is the pelvis level? Do you see any muscle asymmetry or atrophy? Be sure to inspect

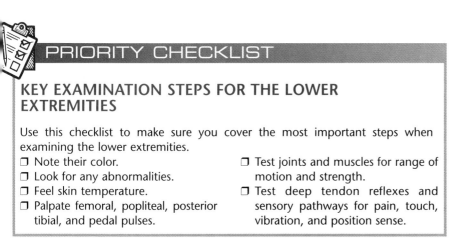

PRIORITY CHECKLIST

KEY EXAMINATION STEPS FOR THE LOWER EXTREMITIES

Use this checklist to make sure you cover the most important steps when examining the lower extremities.

❐ Note their color.
❐ Look for any abnormalities.
❐ Feel skin temperature.
❐ Palpate femoral, popliteal, posterior tibial, and pedal pulses.

❐ Test joints and muscles for range of motion and strength.
❐ Test deep tendon reflexes and sensory pathways for pain, touch, vibration, and position sense.

each joint for erythema, swelling, and deformity. Remember to compare your findings bilaterally, especially if you think you've detected something abnormal.

With your patient still in the standing position, check the legs for varicosities or edema. The standing position accentuates varicosities not visible when your patient is lying down. One way to detect unilateral edema is by measuring the circumference of both legs and comparing your measurements. For example, you could measure both legs just above the ankle, at the widest circumference of the calf, and at midthigh for comparison.

Normal findings
- Skin color ranging from dark brown to light tan, with pink or yellow overtones. Skin color may be darker around the knees. Calloused areas on the feet may appear slightly yellow.
- No obvious gross deformity.
- Leg hair distributed evenly. Elderly patients may have normal variations, including skin that's thinner and drier, leg hair that's more scarce, and pigmentation that's somewhat altered.
- Toenails equal in thickness. In elderly people, the nails thicken and are typically yellow.
- Legs with no varicosities or only superficial varicosities. These are especially likely in patients who are now or were at one time overweight or pregnant.
- No swelling or edema.

Abnormal findings
- Brownish skin coloring and thickened skin, as with lymphedema and advanced venous insufficiency. You may also see brown discoloration around the ankles, with thickened skin and narrowed leg muscles as scarring develops. Skin temperature and pulses will be normal, but pulses will be difficult to palpate through the edema. Usually, the patient complains of little pain or aching pain when the legs are in a dependent position.
- Skin ulcers, possibly indicating trauma, chronic arterial insufficiency, or chronic venous insufficiency. Ulcers develop most often on the toes or feet, but they may form on the shin or other areas of the lower leg after trauma. You may see gangrene if the patient's ulcers result from chronic arterial insufficiency. If you see scars above the patient's ankle from previous leg ulcers, the patient probably has chronic venous insufficiency. (See ⬛ *Chronic Venous Insufficiency.*)
- Skin color normal but cyanotic when the patient stands or sits.
- Edema, possibly resulting from injury; inflammation, as seen with cellulitis; venous obstruction, as seen with thrombosis or

DISORDER CLOSE-UP

CHRONIC VENOUS INSUFFICIENCY

Chronic venous insufficiency refers to stasis of blood in the lower extremities and resulting chronic lower leg edema. Over time, the patient also develops dermatologic changes in the lower leg and foot from prolonged interruption in venous circulation.

These changes typically stem from thrombophlebitis and valvular incompetence. Many patients with chronic venous insufficiency also have varicose veins or tumorous obstructions in the pelvic veins.

When venous valves become incompetent, blood can't progress efficiently from the legs back to the heart. Instead, it collects and stagnates in the lower legs. This increased collection of blood causes venous pressures to rise, distending the thin-walled veins. Unable to close completely, the incompetent veins allow blood to backflow. Over time, the veins become weak, overstretched, and chronically distended from the excessive pressure.

As congestion increases in the lower extremities, peripheral circulation continues to slow down, thus interfering with the body's ability to provide sufficient oxygen and nutrients to the cells. Eventually, cells begin to die. The result is formation of a venous stasis ulcer. Because impaired circulation prevents the body from sending extra nutrients and oxygen to the site to heal the ulcer, it tends to heal very slowly. In fact, it may enlarge and become chronic. Venous congestion also interferes with the normal inflammatory response, predisposing the patient to infection.

Health history
- History of varicose veins
- History of deep vein thrombosis
- Complaints of ankle swelling, legs feeling heavy

- Skin discoloration around the ankle
- Sore on the lower extremity that heals slowly

Characteristic findings

Expect your physical examination findings to vary among patients with chronic venous insufficiency, depending on the extent and severity of the disease. The information that follows will help you distinguish between expected and unexpected findings.

Inspection
- Prominent leg veins, possibly with ropelike and dilated appearance or purplish and spiderlike appearance
- Lower leg edema, possibly extending to the knee of the affected extremity
- Ulcer over the ankle, usually the medial aspect
- Shiny, atrophic, and cyanotic areas around the ulcer
- Brownish skin pigmentation
- Area easily traumatized
- Eczema or stasis dermatitis

Palpation
- Hard subcutaneous tissues
- Pitting edema of lower extremity
- Affected leg area hard and leathery to touch

Vital signs
- Fever, if ulcer is infected

Complications
- Wound infection
- Chronic stasis ulcers
- Amputation

thrombophlebitis; varicosities; congestive heart failure; or other conditions. Be sure to note whether the edema involves one or both legs.
- Joint swelling, possibly resulting from gout, rheumatoid arthritis, or injury.

Palpation

This phase of the examination involves palpating the joints, bones, and surrounding muscles for tenderness, deformity, or crepitus. Have the patient lie supine and start by palpating the hip joint. It is easily palpable by finding the major landmarks of the iliac crest and the greater trochanter of the femur. Then, with one hand on each lateral aspect of the iliac crest, gently rock the pelvis, testing for instability or tenderness.

After palpating the hips, move down to the knees. With your patient in either a sitting or supine position on the examination table, feel the major landmarks of each knee: tibial tuberosity, medial and lateral epicondyles, medial and lateral condyles, the adductor tubercle of the femur, and the patella. Also palpate the popliteal space and the tibiofemoral joint space. Palpation should be performed with the knee flexed and then extended.

While palpating, be sure to notice the temperature of the patient's legs, especially the feet. If they're cool, the patient could have a vascular problem; if they're warm, the patient could have an inflammatory problem.

Now palpate the major landmarks of each ankle, including the medial and lateral malleolus and Achilles tendon. Examine the metatarsal bones by compressing the forefoot between your thumb and forefingers, exerting pressure near the heads of the first and fifth metatarsals. Palpate each metatarsophalangeal joint individually by gently compressing it between your thumb and index finger.

If you noticed during inspection that your patient has dependent edema, be sure to palpate for pitting edema. Do so by pressing your thumb into the skin of the patient's lower leg for about 5 seconds. If the skin remains depressed after you remove your thumb, the patient has pitting edema.

If your patient has pitting edema, you can describe it in one of two ways. The first is to document it as slight, moderate, or marked edema. The second is to use a scale from +1 to +4. In this system, +1 signifies slight pitting edema of the foot or leg, +4 signifies deep pitting with loss of normal foot and leg contours, and +2 and +3 signify conditions in between.

Arterial pulses

An important part of your lower extremity assessment, palpation of arterial pulses gives you information about the patient's vascular system. Comparing one side to the other, you'll palpate the femoral, popliteal, posterior tibial, and pedal pulses. If necessary, you'll also auscultate for abnormal vascular sounds or bruits. (See ▓ *Palpating Difficult Pulses.*)

When checking pulse points, keep in mind that an occlusion can affect any artery. The two most common causes of arterial occlusion are embolism (from the heart, aorta, or large arteries) and thrombus formation (from atherosclerosis or trauma). A diminished or absent peripheral pulse

EXAMINATION TIP

PALPATING DIFFICULT PULSES

If your patient has weak arterial pulses or is obese, you may have difficulty feeling her pulse. For the best results when palpating difficult arterial pulses, follow these examination tips.

- When checking each pulse site, make sure you and your patient are in a comfortable position. An awkward position may interfere with your tactile sensitivity.
- Use the distal pads of your index and middle fingers, and apply firm pressure. Your fingertips are the most sensitive part of your hand for palpating pulses.
- To help find the pulse in a patient's leg, support and relax any nearby joint with your free hand while palpating with your examining hand. If you can't find the pulse, move your fingers in and around the area, varying the pressure you exert with your finger pads.

- Once you locate the pulse, mark the spot with a felt-tipped pen so you can find it easily the next time.
- Make sure you don't confuse your patient's pulse with your own pulsating finger pads. To make sure, palpate your own carotid pulse to determine your heart rate, and then compare it to your patient's. Usually, the heart rates differ. Don't palpate with your thumb because it has strong pulsations easily confused with your patient's.
- Don't press too hard because you could occlude the artery and stop the pulse you're trying to find.
- If you're having difficulty palpating the femoral pulse in an obese patient, apply more pressure to feel through adipose tissue. Use both hands, placing one on top of the other, and apply downward pressure on the hand on the bottom.

may indicate a partial or complete obstruction proximally. Typically, all pulses distal to the occlusion are affected.

To palpate the femoral pulse, place your patient in a supine position, and feel below the inguinal ligament, halfway between the symphysis pubis and the anterior-superior iliac spine. Palpate in the groin crease halfway between the symphysis pubis and the anterior-superior iliac spine. After palpating each femoral pulse, gently place the bell of the stethoscope over the area just examined and listen for any abnormal vascular sounds.

To palpate the popliteal pulse, flex your patient's knee so her foot rests on the examination table. Place one hand on each side of the knee, with your thumbs near the front of the patella. Curl your fingers around the knee, and rest your fingertips in the popliteal fossa. Now gently press your fingers deep into the popliteal fossa. The pulse may be difficult to feel. If it is, try straightening the patient's leg slightly to make the pulse more accessible.

To palpate the posterior tibial pulse, place your fingertips in the groove between the medial malleolus and the Achilles tendon, and feel for the pulse. Sometimes, passive dorsiflexion of the foot will make this pulse easier to palpate.

To palpate the dorsalis pedis pulse, place your fingers between the patient's great and first toes, and slowly move away from the toes between the extensor tendons until you feel the pulse. Plantar flexing the foot slightly makes the pedal pulse easier to palpate. Keep in mind that, in some patients, the pedal pulse may be congenitally absent or branch high up in the ankle.

Lymph nodes

When assessing your patient's lower extremities, don't forget to palpate the superficial lymph nodes. They'll give you important information about immune system activity in the area, such as the presence of a recent or active infection.

If you didn't palpate the inguinal lymph nodes as part of the abdominal examination, you can easily do so now. You should be able to palpate horizontal and vertical chains of inguinal nodes in most patients. To palpate them, first locate the femoral pulse. Then gently press in that area to palpate the nodes. You may even be able to palpate popliteal nodes with the knee slightly flexed. Note the size, consistency, mobility, and any signs of tenderness of all nodes.

Normal findings

- No obvious deformity, tenderness, or swelling.
- Extremities, especially feet, cool to warm with touch.
- Extremities the same temperature bilaterally.
- Skin texture smooth, with minimal moisture.
- No edema or varicose veins.
- Pulses equal and strong bilaterally.
- Superficial inguinal nodes palpable at times but not tender.

Abnormal findings

- Diminished or absent pulses, indicating a partial or complete arterial occlusion. All pulses distal to the occlusion are affected.
- A decreased or absent femoral pulse, suggesting pathology of the aorta. A widened, exaggerated femoral pulse suggests a femoral aneurysm. If pulses are diminished, listen for a bruit to detect arterial narrowing. Remember that pedal pulses may be congenitally absent. But if your patient has always had pedal pulses and now they're absent or diminished, consider arterial occlusive disease if popliteal and femoral pulses are normal. Sudden arterial occlusion causes intense leg pain distal to the occlusion, often with numbness and tingling. The limb becomes cold, pale, and pulseless.
- Cold feet (especially unilateral), suggesting arterial insufficiency. Usually the foot is pale, especially on elevation, and dusky red after

standing or sitting. Skin changes also occur with arterial insufficiency. The skin becomes shiny and thin. Hair becomes thin, and toenails thicken. Usually, the patient has no edema, and pulses are diminished or absent. The patient complains of intermittent calf pain; eventually, it will progress to pain at rest.

Testing range of motion

Before testing ROM, be sure you're thoroughly familiar with the muscle groups involved in the lower extremities. Then check the patient's history to be sure ROM testing is safe. Once you're sure it is, test each major joint and related muscle group for active and passive ROM.

Start with hip flexion. With the patient's knees extended, raise one leg upward. The hip should be able to flex up to 90 degrees. With the knee flexed, raise the leg toward the patient's chest. The hip should be able to flex to 120 degrees.

Now move on to hip extension. With the patient standing or prone, swing the straightened leg out behind the body. The hip should be able to extend up to 30 degrees.

To test hip abduction, place the patient in a supine position with knees extended. Now swing the leg laterally. It should move out to 45 degrees. Then test hip adduction by swinging the leg medially. It should move to about 30 degrees. Lift the leg slightly to allow full movement during this phase of the examination.

To test internal rotation, ask the patient to remain in the supine position and flex her knee. Hold the patient's ankle and gently rotate the leg inward toward the other. The hip should rotate internally up to 40 degrees. To check the external rotation, hold the same ankle, and gently rotate the leg outward toward you. External hip rotation should be up to 45 degrees.

Now check ROM in the patient's knees with the patient either lying down or sitting up. Test knee flexion by asking her to bend the knee; it should have 130-degree flexion. Test knee extension by asking her to straighten the leg and stretch it; it should have full extension and up to 15 degrees of hyperextension.

One additional step you may consider is the ballottement test, which you should perform if the patient has excessive fluid or an effusion in the knee. With the knee extended, apply downward pressure on the suprapatellar pouch with the thumb and fingers of one hand. Then sharply push the patella upward against the femur with the fingers of your other hand. Sudden release of pressure on the patella may cause a tapping sensation against your fingers. This tapping suggests fluid on the knee.

The bulge test also can help you determine if fluid is present. With the patient's knee extended, milk the medial aspect of the knee upward a few times. Then tap the lateral side of the knee; if the patient has excess fluid, this may create a bulge of fluid moving to the medial aspect of the knee.

Test flexion of the tibiotalar joint by instructing your patient to bend her foot downward, a procedure called plantar flexion. She should have 45 to 50 degrees of flexion. Also test hyperextension or dorsiflexion by instructing your patient to bend her foot upward. She should have 20 degrees of flexion.

Inversion is accomplished by asking your patient to point her toes and turn her foot inward. Asking your patient to point her foot outward is called eversion. Both should reach 5 degrees.

Flexing and extending each toe assesses the ROM in that joint. Normally, both flexion and extension will reach 40 degrees.

Normal findings
- Joints with full ROM without pain.
- Joints with equal ROM bilaterally.

Abnormal findings
- Limited ROM, possibly resulting from swelling or pain caused by injury, a flare-up of gout, or arthritis.

Testing muscle strength

When testing muscle strength, remember that strength varies normally with the patient's age, sex, and physical condition. Also remember that the dominant side typically is stronger than the nondominant side.

Test muscle strength by asking your patient to move actively against your resistance. Then, issue a grade based on the 0 to 5 muscle-strength rating system as follows:

0	Flaccid
1	Trace; slight contractility, but no movement
2	Weak; movement possible when gravity is eliminated
3	Fair; movement against gravity, but not against resistance
4	Good; movement against gravity, with some resistance
5	Normal; movement against gravity and resistance

Tests to judge the strength of your patient's muscles include flexion, extension, adduction, and abduction. You'll also perform the Thomas test.

Hip flexion assesses the iliopsoas muscle. Have the patient lie supine. Place your hand on your patient's anterior thigh, and ask her to raise her leg against your resisting hand.

Hip extension tests the gluteus maximus muscle. With your patient in the supine position, place your hand on her posterior thigh, and ask her to push the leg down against your hand as you offer resistance.

Next, test the adductor muscles. Place your hands between your patient's knees, and ask her to press her legs together as your hands offer resistance.

Now test abduction, which allows you to evaluate the gluteus medius and minimus. Place your hands on the outside of your patient's knees, and ask her to spread her legs against your resistance.

Finally, perform the Thomas test to assess flexion contracture of the hip. With your patient in a supine position, ask her to fully extend one leg flat on the examination table while flexing the other leg so that the knee touches her chest. With a hip contracture, the extended leg will lift off the table.

Knee flexion helps you evaluate the hamstrings. With the patient's leg partially flexed, rest your hand on the knee and the other behind the lower leg. With your patient's foot planted on the bed, try to straighten the leg, pushing it down toward the examination table while the patient resists.

Knee extension tests the quadriceps. With the knee in partial flexion, place one hand behind the knee and the other on the anterior lower leg. Then, ask your patient to try to straighten the leg against your hands.

Plantar flexion and dorsiflexion assess the strength of the foot and ankle muscles. To assess plantar flexion, ask your patient to extend her foot against your hand; for dorsiflexion, ask your patient to pull the foot up against your hand.

Normal findings
- Legs symmetrical in length, circumference, and alignment.
- Muscles symmetrical in size bilaterally.
- Muscles with firm tone.

Abnormal findings
- Muscle strength graded below 5. Elderly patients may lose muscle bulk, but those muscles should retain strength. Elderly patients also may have a slight change in ROM, usually because of osteoarthritis.

Testing deep tendon reflexes

DTRs, also called stretch reflexes, depend upon intact sensory and motor nerves, muscle fibers, and an intact spinal cord at the level of the reflex. You'll use a reflex hammer to examine DTRs.

Have your patient sit on the side of the bed, or on a chair with her legs dangling. If your patient can't sit up, she may remain supine, but you'll need to raise and support the extremity you're testing with your hand to gently stretch the tendon. (See ▨ *Testing Reflexes in the Lower Extremities,* pp. 306 and 307.)

One additional point to remember in performing these tests is that the reflex action may be inhibited if your patient is not relaxed. Having your patient focus on another task will help her relax. Have her lock her fingers together and pull one hand against the other, for instance, when you tap the patellar tendon.

(Text continues on p. 308.)

EXAMINATION TIP

TESTING REFLEXES IN THE LOWER EXTREMITIES

Here's how to accurately and thoroughly test deep tendon reflexes (DTRs) in the lower extremities.

Knee reflex

To test the patellar tendon, which is mediated by the spinal cord at the level of L2, L3, and L4, flex the knee to 90 degrees. If your patient is sitting, make sure the upper leg is not resting against the edge of the examination table. Palpate the patellar tendon just below the patella. Then tap the pointed end of a reflex hammer briskly on the tendon, using a quick wrist motion. The normal response is contraction of the quadriceps muscles with knee extension.

Testing the knee reflex in a patient sitting up

Testing the knee reflex in a patient lying down

Ankle reflex

The Achilles reflex is mediated at spinal cord segments S1 and S2. It is usually tested with the foot slightly dorsiflexed and your patient in the sitting position. Alternatively, if your patient is supine, flex the leg at the hip and knee and rotate it externally, placing the foot on its side, resting on the shin of the opposite leg. Strike the Achilles tendon with the pointed end of the reflex hammer. The normal response is plantar flexion of the foot.

Testing the Achilles reflex in a patient sitting up

Testing the Achilles reflex in a patient lying down

Plantar response

The plantar response, often called Babinski's response, is a superficial reflex mediated by spinal cord segments L5 and S1. Using the handle end of the reflex hammer, stroke the lateral aspect of the sole, from the heel to the ball of the foot. The toes should flex inward and downward. If you see dorsiflexion of the great toe, possibly accompanied by fanning of the other toes, Babinski's response may be present. This indicates an abnormality in the pyramidal tract in an adult but is a normal finding in a newborn. Because this finding sometimes is normal, document it by writing "Babinski present" rather than using negative positive.

Testing the plantar response.

Ankle clonus

Test ankle clonus if the other reflexes seem hyperactive. Supporting the knee in a slightly flexed position, plantar flex and dorsiflex the foot several times with your other hand. Then sharply dorsiflex the foot, maintaining that position. Look and feel for rhythmic oscillations. Normally, few clonic oscillations may be seen and felt. But sustained clonus, where the foot plantar flexes and dorsiflexes in rapid succession, indicates upper motor neuron disease.

Testing for ankle clonus.

With that understanding, you may now test the patellar tendon, Achilles tendon, and plantar response, as well as check for ankle clonus. For each reflex you test, compare sides and assign a grade on the following DTR scale:

0	No response
+	Sluggish or diminished response
++	Normal, active or expected response
+++	More brisk than expected; slightly hyperactive, but could be considered normal
++++	Very brisk; hyperactive, with clonus

Normal findings

- DTRs equal bilaterally when testing the patellar, Achilles, and plantar (Babinski) reflexes. Patellar testing causes extension of the lower leg. Achilles testing causes plantar flexion of the foot. Plantar testing causes the toes to flex or curl down.
- A DTR rating (++) that indicates normal reflex responses. Normal variations in the older patient include diminished or absent ankle reflexes. All the reflexes may be slower.

Abnormal findings

- Diminished DTRs and muscle weakness, possibly suggesting such lower motor neuron disorders as amyotrophic lateral sclerosis (ALS) or Guillain-Barré syndrome. Loss of muscle tone and sometimes muscle atrophy will occur.
- Muscle spasticity and hyperactive reflexes, resulting from such upper motor neuron disorders as stroke and paralysis, if the disorder is extensive enough. Usually, you'll find little or no muscle atrophy, but muscle strength may be decreased.

Sensory testing

Sensory testing evaluates the integrity of sensory pathways in the spinal cord and brain responsible for such sensations as light touch, pain, temperature, position, and vibration. Sensory testing is especially important for patients who complain of numbness or tingling. Check a dermatome chart to determine the approximate areas innervated by the sensory portion of each spinal nerve.

When a patient complains of sensory changes, you can determine which spinal nerve might be involved by comparing the reactions to sensory testing in each of the extremities.

To test for light touch, use a wisp of cotton. Ask your patient to close her eyes and tell you when she feels your touch. Lightly touch the cotton to her feet, calves, and thighs, both medially and laterally. Proceed systematically, comparing sides and moving distally to proximally.

To test pain sensation, poke your patient lightly with a sharp object, such as the stick end of a cotton-tipped swab or the end of an unbent paper clip. Take care not to break the skin. Be sure to apply the same amount of pressure to each site while you compare pain sensations. If you suspect peripheral neuropathy, or if your patient is known to have diabetes mellitus, test for sensory loss in the feet using a monofilament device. (See 🖾 *Using a Monofilament Device to Test for Sensory Loss.*)

EXAMINATION TIP

USING A MONOFILAMENT DEVICE TO TEST FOR SENSORY LOSS

To test for sensory loss with the monofilament device, follow these key steps. If your patient can't feel the end of the device in any one spot, suspect sensory loss. As you proceed with the examination, remember to avoid areas that have broken skin or calluses.

- Have your patient close her eyes during the entire examination.

- Place the device in the spots shown in the illustrations. Make sure to use the device on both the dorsal and plantar surfaces of the foot.
- Apply enough pressure to make the filament bend, and keep it there for 1.5 seconds.
- Use a random pattern, and avoid touching a spot more than once.

From Mosby. (1999). *Managing Major Diseases: Diabetes Mellitus and Hypertension.* St. Louis: Mosby.

Sensations of pain and temperature travel along the same spinothalamic tract in the spinal cord. When your patient responds normally to pain sensation, you probably don't need to test for temperature sensation. However, if you decide to check for temperature identification, systematically touch cool and warm objects, such as test tubes filled with cold and warm water, to each leg, and check your patient's response.

To test vibration sensation, strike a tuning fork on the heel of your hand and place it firmly over the interphalangeal joint of the great toe. Ask if your patient can feel the vibration. If she can, no further vibratory testing is needed. If she can't, proceed to more proximal bony prominences, such as the medial malleolus, the patella, and the anterior-superior iliac spine.

Tell your patient that you're going to move some of her toes so they point up or down. Show her what you mean. Then ask her to close her eyes. Grasping the great toe and holding it away from the others, move it up or down, and ask your patient to tell you its position. Repeat this several times on each side.

Normal findings
- Recognition of light touch and pain.
- Vibratory sensation intact when testing the great toe. In the elderly, the vibratory sensation may be absent or diminished.
- Accurate position sense. (See 🖥 *What to Expect When Examining the Lower Extremities.*)

Abnormal findings
- Impaired sensory response, indicating a neurologic disorder. A loss of position sense may suggest a spinal cord lesion when associated with other neurologic complaints. Vibration is the first sense to be lost in peripheral neuropathies, such as diabetes mellitus. It also disappears in alcoholism, tertiary syphilis, and vitamin B_{12} deficiency.

EXPLORING CHIEF COMPLAINTS

Complaints involving the lower extremities are common and wide-ranging. If your patient has one of the following complaints, use this section of the chapter to quickly focus your assessment.

Limb pain
Pain is perhaps the most common complaint involving the lower extremities. Most pain results from injury or inflammation, but it may also be caused by altered peripheral circulation or neurologic damage. (See 🖼 *Assessing Acute Leg Pain,* p. 312.)

NORMAL FINDINGS

WHAT TO EXPECT WHEN EXAMINING THE LOWER EXTREMITIES

Use this quick review to confirm normal findings when examining the lower extremities.

Inspection
- Symmetrical extremities
- Uniform skin color, light variation
- No swelling or varicosities
- No gross deformities

Palpation
- Cool to warm skin temperature
- Smooth skin with minimal moisture
- Equal, easily palpated femoral, popliteal, pedal, and posterior tibial pulses

- No edema or varicose veins
- Full range of motion (ROM)
- Symmetrical muscle tone
- Muscle strength at 5 on a scale of 1 to 5
- Deep tendon reflexes ++ bilaterally at knee and ankle
- Plantar reflex negative
- No clonus
- Superficial touch and pain sensations bilaterally
- Intact vibratory and position senses

If your patient complains of limb pain, investigate the symptom further by asking her the following questions:
- Where is the pain? Is it localized or generalized? Point to where you feel the pain. Is it deep or superficial pain? Does it radiate to another location, such as your back?
- How bad is the pain? Where is it on a scale of 0 to 10, with 0 being no pain and 10 being the worst pain possible? Are you able to perform your usual daily tasks? Can you walk without pain?
- In what setting does the pain occur? Does it occur only after walking long distances or going up and down stairs? Does it occur after repetitive movements? Only at night?
- When did the pain first begin? Is it a new problem, or have you had it before? Did it begin suddenly or gradually? Is it intermittent or continuous? How long does the pain last?
- Can you describe the pain in your own words (burning, stabbing, dull, throbbing)?
- Is the pain associated with any other problems, such as swelling, redness, or tingling?
- Does anything make the pain worse?
- Does anything make the pain better?

INTERPRETING ABNORMAL FINDINGS

ASSESSING ACUTE LEG PAIN

Determining if leg pain is acute or chronic will guide you in your assessment. Chronic pain persists for 3 months or more, whereas acute pain usually is more sudden in onset and associated with hyperactivity of the sympathetic nervous system (tachycardia, increased respiratory rate and blood pressure, dilated pupils). The etiology of acute limb pain is musculoskeletal, neurologic, or vascular. This chart reviews some commonly encountered causes of acute limb pain.

Type of pain	Typical findings	Associated characteristics	Probable cause
Musculoskeletal	• History of recent trauma • Refusal to bear weight or partial weight-bearing • Throbbing pain	• Obvious deformity • Swelling • Crepitus • Tenderness on palpation or movement • Ecchymoses • Paresthesias	• Fracture or dislocation
	• Usually involves only one joint • Sudden pain • Limited weight-bearing • Swelling • Erythema • Tenderness	• Fever • History of recent viral illness • Movement decreases pain (except with rheumatoid arthritis)	• Septic joint
Neurologic	• Shooting pain radiating down one or both legs following distribution of sciatic nerve • Often no complaint of back pain • Pain is electric, burning, aching • Associated with paresthesias	• Pain worsens with movement, such as walking, coughing, straining at stool • Positive straight-leg raising test • Decreased deep tendon reflexes • Local muscle weakness and atrophy	• Sciatica
Vascular	• Pain distal to the occlusion • Coldness • Numbness • Weakness • Skin pallor or cyanosis	• Diminished or absent pulses distally	• Acute arterial occlusion
	• Calf is common site • May or may not be painful	• Swelling of calf or ankle • Calf tenderness and erythema • Positive Homans' sign	• Deep vein thrombosis

Focusing your assessment

When examining a patient who complains of limb pain, focus your assessment as follows:

- Check to see if your patient can ambulate without difficulty and without assistance. Note whether she can bear weight on the affected leg. Also note whether her legs are symmetrical.
- Determine whether the patient has pain with ROM. Check to see if ROM is restricted because of the pain. Remember to compare each side against the other.

- Palpate the patient's pulses to see if they're equal and strong bilaterally. Compare the lower extremities for color, temperature, and amount and distribution of hair growth. Also look for areas of skin breakdown or ulceration, possibly from incompetent veins.
- Dorsiflex the appropriate foot, ankle, and calf area to see if the pain worsens. If your patient complains of lower leg pain with swelling and has risk factors for deep vein thrombosis (DVT), such as the use of oral contraceptives or prolonged immobility, check for Homans' sign. Dorsiflex the ankle while your patient's knee is slightly flexed. If she complains of pain, she may have DVT. Keep in mind, however, that a positive Homans' sign occurs in only 35% of patients who actually have DVT. It also can occur with a herniated lumbar disk.
- Check for sciatic pain. This involves placing your patient in a supine position on the examination table and passively raising her extended leg, flexing it at the hip. If she complains of posterior leg pain when it's elevated between 30 and 60 degrees, this suggests sciatic pain.

Possible causes
- *Soft tissue injury.* Pain can result from a fall or twisting injury, such as stepping the wrong way off a curb. The problem could affect muscles, tendons, or ligaments. Pain may be intense initially, improving with ice and rest. Gradual, progressive pain from activity or repetitive movements may also result from a sprain or strain. A sprain involves stretching or tearing a ligament; a strain involves stretching or tearing a muscle. An Achilles tear or a hamstring tear usually involves acute pain. Often, the patient can't bear weight.
- *Fracture.* Your patient almost certainly has a history of trauma or a fall that causes intense pain that's worse with movement. Your patient won't be able to bear weight on the painful extremity.
- *Tumor or metastasis.* This deep pain usually worsens at night.
- *Arterial embolism or thrombosis.* This sudden, severe pain is very localized. The affected limb will also become cold, pale, and pulseless.
- *Arterial or peripheral arterial disease.* Pain is gradual and intermittent in nature. If your patient has atherosclerotic disease in her peripheral arteries, she'll likely complain of calf pain from exercise (intermittent claudication). The pain abates with rest. In cases of severe disease, your patient will complain of resting leg pain.
- *Deep vein thrombosis.* Usually, this condition causes gradual leg pain. It worsens with walking and dorsiflexion of the foot, and it commonly is associated with swelling and erythema of the affected extremity.
- *Sciatic pain.* Commonly caused by a herniated lumbar disk, this pain feels electric to many patients and commonly is associated with a tingling or aching sensation that radiates down one or both legs. It worsens with activity and improves with rest. You can check for this condition with straight-leg testing.

- *Diabetic neuropathy*. This condition causes pain and paresthesias symmetrically in the feet and legs. Peripheral neuropathy is a syndrome involving sensory loss, muscle weakness and atrophy, pain, and vasomotor symptoms.
- *Peroneal nerve palsy*. This pain results from compression of the peroneal nerve against the lateral aspect of the head of the fibula. This cause of leg pain is common in bedridden patients and thin people who habitually cross their legs. If the problem is peroneal nerve compression, your patient will not be able to dorsiflex her great toe against resistance.

Joint pain or stiffness

Complaints of joint pain and stiffness are often used interchangeably. Stiffness is difficult to assess, but it refers to a perception of tightness or resistance to movement. If your patient complains of joint pain or stiffness, investigate the symptom further by asking her the following questions:

- Do you have other symptoms associated with the joint pain, such as swelling, tenderness, warmth, redness, or limited movement?
- Is the problem restricting any of your usual activities? Is walking difficult or painful? Can you use the stairs without pain? Do you have pain when rising from a sitting position?
- Does stiffness occur in the morning and, if so, how long does it last? (Stiffness associated with inflammatory arthritis usually lasts more than 60 minutes. Stiffness related to muscle soreness from strenuous exertion often peaks the second day after the exertion.)

Focusing your assessment

When examining a patient who complains of joint pain or stiffness, focus your assessment as follows:

- Inspect the joint, looking for erythema, swelling, or deformity.
- Check ROM for the lower extremities, comparing each side.
- Palpate the joint and surrounding tissues for tenderness while your patient flexes and extends the limb. Listen for crepitus, a crackling sound heard as the joints move.

Possible causes

- *Fracture or dislocation*. Consider the possibility of a hip fracture in an elderly patient who complains of hip pain after a fall. Fractures commonly involve the femur head or the pelvis. Dislocation of the hip joint is also common among the elderly.
- *Gout*. This inflammatory reaction to uric acid crystals in joints, bones, and subcutaneous structures causes a pain that usually begins suddenly. It's associated with swelling, erythema, and warmth, and it usually affects only one joint, most often the great toe. (See *Gout*.)

DISORDER CLOSE-UP

GOUT

A metabolic disorder characterized by elevated serum uric acid concentration and deposits of urate crystals in synovial fluid and surrounding joint tissues, gout causes joint pain, usually in the great toe, ankles, and midfoot. *Primary gout* occurs most often in men and postmenopausal women. *Secondary gout* usually affects elderly people.

The exact cause of gout is unknown, although primary gout is believed to involve an inborn error of purine metabolism or a decrease in renal uric acid excretion. Secondary gout, marked by hyperuricemia, can result from a disorder or medication.

Normally, uric acid production is balanced through excretion, with about two-thirds being excreted via the kidneys and the remainder in feces. When serum uric acid levels rise above 7 mg/dl, the serum is saturated, and monosodium urate crystals may form. These crystals tend to form in the body's peripheral tissues, where lower temperatures reduce the solubility of the uric acid.

Other factors that can precipitate crystal formation and tissue deposition include a decrease in extracellular fluid pH and reduced plasma protein-binding of urate crystals. Tissue trauma from a rapid change in uric acid levels also may lead to crystal deposits. Conversely, a rapid increase in uric acid may occur after tissue trauma and release of cellular components.

Unless treated, gout progresses in four stages: asymptomatic hyperuricemia, acute gouty arthritis (usually affecting a single joint), an intercritical period (an asymptomatic period that can last up to 10 years), and tophaceous or chronic gout. In this final stage, hyperuricemia continues untreated, with development of crystal deposits (tophi) in cartilage, synovial membranes, tendons, and soft tissues.

Health history
- Sedentary lifestyle
- History of hypertension
- History of renal calculi
- Complaints of sudden onset of pain, often in great toe, initially moderate but increasing in intensity
- Difficulty bearing even the weight of bed sheets on the affected area
- Chills

Characteristic findings
Expect your physical examination findings to vary among patients with gout, depending on the extent and severity of the disease. The information that follows will help you distinguish between expected and unexpected findings.

Inspection
- Swollen, dusky-red, or purple joint with limited movement
- Tophi, especially on outer ears, hands, and feet
- Ulceration of skin over tophi, with release of chalky white exudate or pus (in chronic stage)

Palpation
- Warmth and extreme tenderness over joint

Vital signs
- Fever
- Hypertension

Complications
- Renal calculi
- Atherosclerotic heart disease
- Cardiovascular lesions
- Cerebrovascular accident
- Coronary thrombosis
- Hypertension
- Infection, with tophi rupture and nerve entrapment

- *Septic joint.* This condition is characterized by fever and joint pain, swelling, redness, and warmth. It must be evaluated and treated quickly to prevent osteomyelitis, joint destruction, or both.
- *Rheumatoid arthritis.* A chronic systemic disease with articular inflammation, rheumatoid arthritis is characterized by morning stiffness lasting more than an hour each day, pain in at least two joint groups, symmetrical joint swelling, and subcutaneous nodules. The pain can be constant or intermittent.
- *Osteoarthritis.* The "wear-and-tear joint arthritis" is the most common form of joint disease, with progressive destruction and loss of joint cartilage. Weight-bearing joints of overweight patients are often involved. Prolonged occupational or sports stress can lead to osteoarthritis.

Swelling

Swelling is an excessive accumulation of interstitial fluid or edema. If your patient complains of swelling of the lower extremities, investigate the symptom further by asking her the following questions:

- Where is the swelling located? Does it affect both legs? Does it involve the entire leg or just a certain area? How far up the leg does the swelling go? (See 🗎 *Thrombophlebitis.*)
- Is the swelling slight? Or is it marked? If the swelling has occurred before, is it more severe or less?
- When does the swelling occur? Upon waking in the morning? Or at the end of the day? Is it constant or intermittent?
- When did you first notice the swelling? Was it gradual or sudden? Is it new or chronic? If intermittent, how long does it last?
- Do you have an imprint of a shoe or a sock line when you take your shoes and socks off (pitting edema)?
- Have you had surgery, or have you been injured recently? Do you have a history of heart or lung problems? Is the swelling associated with pain, warmth, or redness? Which medications do you take?
- Does anything make the swelling worse, such as sitting for long periods or eating salty foods?
- Does anything reduce the swelling, such as elevating your feet, using support hose, or putting ice on your feet?

Focusing your assessment

When examining a patient who complains of swelling, focus your assessment as follows:

- Inspect the skin for evidence of erythema, brawniness, skin breakdown, or ulceration.
- Palpate the swollen area for warmth and tenderness.
- Palpate for pitting or nonpitting edema.
- Note whether the swelling is unilateral or bilateral.

DISORDER CLOSE-UP

THROMBOPHLEBITIS

Inflammation of a vein associated with thrombus formation, thrombophlebitis can result from vessel wall trauma; hypercoagulability of the blood; infection; chemical irritation; postoperative venous stasis; prolonged sitting, standing, or immobilization; or long periods of intravenous catheterization.

Both deep and superficial veins can be affected by thrombophlebitis. Deep vein thrombophlebitis usually involves the deep veins of the legs, primarily the calf. Superficial vein thrombophlebitis typically involves the veins of the upper extremities and is commonly associated with trauma (for example, from insertion of catheters in the subclavian vein).

Three pathologic factors, known as Virchow's triad, are associated with thrombophlebitis: venous stasis, increased blood coagulability, and injury to the vessel wall. Two of these three factors must be present for thrombi to form in the vein.

Trauma to the endothelial venous lining brings subendothelial tissues in contact with platelets. These platelets aggregate, especially if the patient has venous stasis. Fibrin, leukocytes, and erythrocytes deposit into the platelet clump to cause a thrombus.

Initially, a thrombus floats within a vein. Within 7 to 10 days, it adheres to the vein wall, but a portion may still float in the lumen of the vessel. Pieces of the tail may break loose and travel through the circulation as emboli. Fibroblasts eventually invade the thrombus, scarring the vein wall and destroying the venous valves.

Health history
- Asymptomatic (early in the inflammatory process)
- Vague tightness or dull aching pain in affected extremity, especially on walking, increasing in severity
- Inability to walk without pain

- History of risk factors, including bed rest, use of intravenous catheters, immobilization, obesity, myocardial infarction, heart failure, multiple sclerosis, oral contraceptive use, pregnancy and childbirth, altered coagulability states, and surgery in patients older than age 40
- Tenderness over affected area
- General malaise

Characteristic findings
Expect your physical examination findings to vary among patients with thrombophlebitis, depending on the extent and severity of the disease. The information that follows will help you distinguish between expected and unexpected findings.

Inspection
- Redness, cyanosis, and swelling of the affected extremity
- Marked redness along the course of the vein (superficial thrombophlebitis)
- Increased size of affected extremity

Palpation
- Warm and tender to the touch
- Palpable cordlike structure (superficial thrombophlebitis)
- Positive cuff sign
- Possible positive Homans' sign
- Diminished or absent pedal pulse on affected extremity
- Slowed capillary refill

Vital signs
- Possible fever

Complications
- Pulmonary embolism
- Chronic venous insufficiency

- Measure the swollen areas, and record their sizes.
- If you find joint swelling, assess ROM for each affected joint.

Possible causes

- *Musculoskeletal problems.* Swelling from an injury, such as a fracture or sprain, commonly is associated with superficial bruising or hematomas. Swelling tends to occur a few hours after the initial injury. Localized joint swelling may indicate synovial inflammation, as in a septic joint or rheumatoid arthritis. Or you may notice an increase in synovial fluid around the joint after an injury.
- *Systemic sources of bilateral edema.* These conditions may include heart failure, which would be accompanied by shortness of breath; excessive renal retention of sodium and water, which may be accompanied by hypertension; and kidney failure, which most often would be accompanied by diminished urination or cirrhosis (you'll be able to palpate a firm, smooth liver with a blunt edge).
- *Local causes of bilateral edema.* This condition could stem from sitting or standing for long periods, pregnancy, or menopause. You may find unilateral edema if your patient has cellulitis, in which you would find local erythema and tenderness; osteomyelitis, a bacterial bone infection associated with pain and tenderness in the affected area; venous obstruction from a thrombus, in which you'd detect marked redness and a cordlike feeling along the course of the vein; or tumors that compress the vasculature.

Changes in sensation

This problem may involve anesthesia, paresthesias, or dysesthesias. Anesthesia (numbness) is a loss of sensation to a body part. Paresthesias are abnormal tactile sensations not produced by stimulation and usually described as tingling or prickling. Dysesthesias are distorted, typically unpleasant sensations in response to a stimulus. They commonly last longer than the stimulus itself. A burning sensation that occurs in response to a simple pinprick is an example of dysesthesia. If your patient complains of changes in sensation, investigate the symptom further by asking her the following questions:

- Where is the sensation? Is it in just one part of the leg, or does it involve the entire leg? Does it involve one or both legs?
- How intense is the sensation?
- When or where does it occur? Only when your legs are elevated? When bending over?
- When did this problem begin? Was its onset sudden or gradual? Is this a new or chronic problem?
- Can you describe the type of sensation? Is it associated with other problems, such as weakness or pain? If so, how significant? Any recent injury?

- What worsens this sensory change? Cold temperatures? Sitting for long periods? Does it seem to occur in response to another stimulation, such as a pinprick?
- Does rest or leg elevation make the sensation better?

Focusing your assessment

When examining a patient who complains of changes in sensation, focus your assessment as follows:

- Evaluate the sensory system, including your patient's perception of pain, temperature, position, vibration, and light touch.
- Assess muscle tone and strength by testing each major muscle group against resistance. This procedure checks not only the musculoskeletal system but also the neurologic system that innervates the muscles.
- Test the DTRs.
- Assess circulation to the extremity by palpating pulses, feeling for coolness, and inspecting for pallor and blanching.
- Assess your patient's respiratory patterns. Note any increased or rapid respiratory rate, especially if your patient appears anxious and looks as though she may be hyperventilating.
- Gently palpate the spinal column, feeling for protrusions or masses that could indicate a herniated vertebral disk or a tumor.
- Ask your patient to bend forward and touch her toes; then ask if this movement made the sensation better or worse. Also, while she's supine, raise her legs above heart level and see if this makes her symptoms worse.

Possible causes

- *Fracture, tumor, or swelling.* These conditions place pressure on a nerve or compress the nerve, resulting in anesthesia or paresthesias. Bending forward and flexing the spine may produce or aggravate these abnormal symptoms.
- *Spinal cord injury.* This condition commonly produces dysesthesias, or anesthesia below the level of the injury.
- *Occlusive vascular disease.* This condition produces a loss of sensation or a burning, prickling sensation in the extremities from diminished blood flow when the legs are elevated over the head. The extremities may pale and pulses diminish.
- *Neurologic disorder.* Vitamin B_6 deficiency or such neurologic disorders as multiple sclerosis and ALS can cause paresthesias. With ALS, your patient also may demonstrate increased DTRs and muscle weakness.
- *Hyperventilation.* This condition commonly causes a pins-and-needles sensation in the fingers and toes, along with a feeling of faintness.

Changes in skin color or temperature

Changes in skin color of the lower extremities, with or without temperature change, can suggest an inflammatory process or compromised vascular flow. If your patient complains of skin color or temperature change, investigate the symptom further by asking her the following questions:

- Where on your legs did you notice the change in color or temperature?
- Did you notice a marked change to a bluish or reddish color or a feeling of coldness?
- Have you been doing anything in particular when you've noticed the change, such as crossing your legs, standing for a long period, or exerting yourself?
- Does the change occur at any particular time of day?
- How would you describe the skin discoloration (pale, bluish, reddened)?
- Do you have any other symptoms associated with the change in color or temperature?
- Are you aware of anything that aggravates the problem, such as smoking?
- Are you aware of anything that relieves the problem?

Focusing your assessment

When examining a patient who experiences changes in skin color or temperature, focus your assessment as follows:

- Inspect the area for erythema, pallor, swelling, and deformity.
- Palpate the pulses of the lower extremities (femoral, popliteal, dorsalis pedis, posterior tibial) for equality and strength. Note if any are absent.
- Palpate for warmth and tenderness. If you find a localized area of erythema, measure and document it for future comparison. Also outline the area with a felt-tipped marking pen.

Possible causes

- *Anemia.* A common cause of pallor, this condition also causes fatigue.
- *Arterial insufficiency.* In this condition, your patient will have pain aggravated by exercise.
- *Respiratory conditions.* Chronic obstructive pulmonary disease and other respiratory conditions can cause generalized cyanosis—especially in the distal digits—from hypoxemia.
- *Heart failure or congenital heart disease.* These conditions produce generalized cyanosis from hypoxemia. They're usually associated with edema and shortness of breath on exertion.
- *Venous obstruction.* In this case, the area would be tender, edematous, and warm to the touch.
- *Arterial occlusion.* In this case, your patient would have pain and skin that is cold to the touch. (See *Responding to Acute Arterial Occlusion.*)

ACTION STAT

RESPONDING TO ACUTE ARTERIAL OCCLUSION

An acute arterial occlusion of the leg can result in loss of the affected limb if not recognized and treated immediately. Most patients with peripheral vascular disease have a chronic condition with symptoms that develop over years. However, if your patient has an acute arterial occlusion, she'll experience severe, unrelenting pain. Onset is sudden, and pain may involve the entire leg.

Occlusion of a major artery with acute loss of perfusion distal to it may result from a thrombus or an embolus that migrates to the point of occlusion. Diagnosis is based on a detailed examination, including history and Doppler studies. Prognosis varies. If the affected limb is in a confined space, such as with a cast, arterial occlusion can occur because of compartment syndrome. In this syndrome, tissue edema occludes arterial blood flow and presses on nearby nerves.

What to look for

Signs and symptoms of acute arterial occlusion vary, depending on the location of the obstruction. Typically, the skin of the affected extremity is cold. You can also remember signs and symptoms by using the five Ps:

- *P*ain that's diffuse and distal to the occlusion, not alleviated by position change
- *P*ulselessness
- *P*allor, followed by proximal mottling and distal cyanosis
- *P*aresthesias, with numbness, loss of light-touch sensation, and—in advanced ischemia—loss of pain or pressure sensation
- *P*aralysis, or motor deficits, that arise after sensory deficits in advanced ischemia

What to do immediately

If you suspect an arterial occlusion, notify the physician immediately. Anticipate these orders:

- Insert an intravenous line for thrombolytics and anticoagulants. Also, if your patient needs surgery, she'll need an intravenous catheter to administer fluids during the procedure.
- Prepare your patient for ultrasound studies, such as lower-extremity Doppler, to identify the extent and location of the blockage.
- Prepare your patient for surgery (such as femoral-popliteal bypass), percutaneous transluminal angioplasty of the affected artery, or thrombolytic therapy (such as recombinant tissue plasminogen activator or streptokinase).
- If compartment syndrome is the cause, prepare to take action to relieve pressure on the affected limb, such as cast removal or surgery.
- Maintain nothing by mouth status until you find out which of these interventions she'll need.

What to do next

- Administer analgesics, as prescribed, to relieve limb pain.
- Continue to monitor circulation to the extremity, including its color, temperature, and the presence and strength of distal pulses.
- Prevent injury to the extremity because healing will be impaired in the compromised limb.
- If your patient requires anticoagulation therapy, monitor the activated partial thromboplastin time if she's receiving heparin, or prothrombin time if she's taking warfarin sodium (Coumadin).
- Teach the patient how to check her peripheral pulses and look for signs of worsened circulation, such as pallor and coolness. Also teach her how to care for and protect the extremity.

- *Anxiety or cold environment.* In these conditions, the skin is usually cool to the touch.
- *Inflammation, infection, or recent trauma.* These conditions typically redden the skin. Bacterial infection can cause a septic joint. The joint will be erythematous, swollen, tender, and warm. Your patient will have a fever.
- *Cellulitis, first-degree (partial thickness) burns, and superficial thrombophlebitis.* In these cases, skin usually is warm to the touch and tender.
- *Gout or a flare-up of rheumatoid arthritis.* These conditions cause erythema around a joint.

Weakness or paralysis

If your patient complains of muscle weakness or decreased function related to paralysis, investigate the symptom further by asking her the following questions:
- Is the weakness in only one or both legs? Can you move the leg at all, or do you have no control over movements?
- When did the problem first begin? Is it a new or chronic problem? How often does it happen? Is it there all the time or just sometimes? Do you have other symptoms or weakness elsewhere?
- How bad is the weakness? Does it affect your independence?
- What makes the muscle weakness worse? What makes it better?
- Do you stumble frequently or trip when walking? Do you have difficulty rising from a chair?

Focusing your assessment

When examining a patient who complains of weakness or paralysis, focus your assessment as follows:
- Assess the musculoskeletal and neurologic systems any time a patient has a change in leg function.
- Assess your patient's ambulation status. Is her gait impaired?
- Look for muscle atrophy in the major muscle groups of her legs, comparing each side.
- Assess muscle tone and strength by testing each major muscle group against resistance. This procedure tests not only the musculoskeletal system but also the neurologic system that innervates the muscles. Absent or decreased muscle tone or strength may be caused by lower motor neuron disorders. Upper motor neuron disorders cause increased muscle tone and spasticity.
- Test DTRs. Absent or decreased DTRs occur with lower motor neuron disorders. Upper motor neuron disorders cause increased DTRs.

Possible causes

- *Fatigue.* When a patient complains of weakness in her extremities, she may, in fact, be fatigued and have decreased activity tolerance. True muscle weakness is different from fatigue and can be caused by injury or by central or peripheral nerve degeneration.
- *Hypokalemia or hypothyroidism.* Chemical changes that occur in these conditions can result in generalized muscle weakness.
- *Upper and lower motor neuron disorders.* Upper motor neuron disorders include cerebrovascular accident (CVA) or central nervous system (CNS) trauma. Lower motor neuron disorders include polio, ALS, and Guillain-Barré syndrome. With upper motor neuron disorders, increased or hyperactive DTRs accompany weakness. With lower motor neuron disorders, reflexes are diminished or absent.
- *Myopathies.* Caused by medications (such as corticosteroids) or diseases (such as muscular dystrophy), myopathies produce proximal muscle weakness (hips and thighs). Your patient will have difficulty rising from a seated position.
- *Neuropathies.* Seen in people with diabetes mellitus or lead poisoning, neuropathies cause weakness and loss of sensation in the feet and lower legs. Typically, your patient will trip or stumble while walking.
- *Paralysis.* An inability to voluntarily move a body part from loss of motor function, paralysis can occur in one, two, or all four limbs. Hemiplegia can be caused by a CVA or head injury. Paraplegia and quadriplegia can be caused by spinal cord injury.

Muscle spasm or cramping

If your patient complains of muscle spasm or cramping, investigate the symptom further by asking her the following questions:

- When did the spasm or cramping first begin? Is it a new or chronic problem? How often does it happen?
- How bad is the spasm or cramp? Does it affect your independence?
- When does the spasm or cramping occur? Does it occur only after strenuous activity or mostly at night? Is it constant or intermittent?
- What makes the muscle spasm worse? What makes it better?
- Do you take a diuretic, such as furosemide, or an immunosuppressive medication, such as cyclosporine?

Focusing your assessment

When examining a patient who complains of muscle spasm or cramping, focus your assessment as follows:

- Assess tone and strength by testing each major muscle group against resistance. This tests not only the musculoskeletal system but also the neurologic system that innervates the muscles.

- Test DTRs. Absent or decreased DTRs are observed in lower motor neuron disorders.
- Check your patient's serum electrolyte levels for imbalances.

Possible causes
- *Muscle spasticity.* This term refers to increased muscle tone (hypertonia) and exaggerated DTRs. Upper motor neuron disorders are associated with spasticity, as seen in CNS trauma or a CVA.
- *Muscle spasms.* These painful muscular contractions usually involve the calf or foot. Commonly, they result from fatigue in the muscle and abate with rest or stretching of the muscle.
- *Electrolyte imbalances.* Painful, nocturnal leg cramps can result from impaired peripheral circulation and such electrolyte imbalances as hypokalemia, especially when induced by diuretic use. Other medications, such as cyclosporine, have the side effect of leg cramps.

PUTTING IT ALL TOGETHER

For any nurse, accuracy represents the most important goal of physical assessment. Your patient—indeed, the entire health care team—relies on your skill and expertise to detect health problems and follow up with appropriate collaborative care. However, in this era of budget cuts and time demands, accuracy can't be your only assessment goal. Like it or not, you also must be fast.

If you've already applied the first nine chapters of *Expert 10-Minute Physical Examinations*, you're well on your way to ensuring accuracy in your physical examinations. This chapter presents guidelines for helping you stay focused and fast—10 minutes fast.

In addition to no-nonsense instructions on how to perform a quick head-to-toe assessment, this chapter outlines essential normal findings for each body area. Based on the special *Normal Findings* features that appear in earlier chapters, this information has been adapted to highlight the most crucial findings—findings you can investigate in just 10 minutes. Review them regularly to keep your assessments on target and on time.

Keep in mind, however, that the nature and complexity of a physical examination depends on your patient's condition at the time of your encounter. In other words, if your patient is acutely ill with a specific health problem, you'll probably be performing a series of focused physical examinations to track and evaluate his chief complaint. That's why throughout this book we've given you techniques for isolating your patient's chief complaint, performing a focused assessment, and pinpointing its probable cause.

On the other hand, let's say your patient doesn't have a pressing complaint, or you don't know his medical diagnosis. Even in this situation, you can perform a thorough assessment that includes all body systems. And if you follow the guidelines in this chapter, you can do it in about 10 minutes.

The thing to remember is that, above all else, fast and accurate assessment requires readiness and repetition. This review chapter will help you gain both speed and accuracy in your physical examinations. By learning how to better organize and prioritize examination steps, you can gather pertinent patient information quickly and identify abnormalities before they turn into crises.

FIRST THINGS FIRST

Remember that physical examination begins the moment you encounter a patient, whether during admission, a home or clinic visit, or during your shift. However, physical examination doesn't end with that single encounter. To provide quality, ongoing health care, you'll need to perform physical examinations at regular intervals to assess expected and unexpected changes in a patient's condition.

To set yourself up for successful assessment, you'll need to keep a few points in mind. First, always review the patient's health history for important medical, surgical, and family details before you start your examination.

Second, if your patient has a chief complaint, be sure you have enough information about it. Ask the patient to explain his complaint fully. Investigate whether the problem is ongoing and whether it changes in character or severity. Also ask about any new problems or symptoms that may have developed since the history was taken.

Third, think critically about the patient's chief complaint. Consider what might be causing it. Then, during the examination, look for related signs and symptoms that could confirm or disprove your suspicion. This focused approach will help you get to the root of your patient's problem more quickly.

Finally, make sure you have an appropriate environment and the proper equipment to perform your physical examination comfortably and completely. For example, check to see if the room is warm enough and the lighting sufficient for you to observe your patient clearly. Take steps to ensure your patient's privacy by closing the door, for example, or drawing the curtain. If visitors or other health care providers are in the room, either ask them to leave or delay your examination until another time, unless your patient wants them present for the examination.

To perform a 10-minute physical examination, make sure you have the following pieces of equipment within reach: a stethoscope, a thermometer, a sphygmomanometer, a penlight, cotton-tipped swabs, latex or vinyl gloves, a pupil gauge, a tongue blade, a scale (standing platform or bed), a reflex hammer, and a pulse oximeter.

Try to avoid waiting until the end of your examination to document your findings—even though waiting might seem like a time-saver. Instead, record your findings—both normal and abnormal—in note form as you go along. Doing so will keep you from forgetting important details that arise during your examination. Later, after the examination, you can enter the data onto a flow sheet or document your findings in your patient's medical record.

PERFORMING AN EXPERT 10-MINUTE EXAMINATION

In general, be aware of your patient's condition any time you're in his presence, whether or not you're engaged in a formal physical examination. In fact, you should assess your patient informally at every opportunity to catch changes or problems as early as possible.

In this informal assessment, consider your patient's condition and situation as you accomplish tasks that require you to be around him. Note whether anything seems awry. Look for obvious signs of distress or conditions that warrant immediate attention, such as bleeding or weakness.

If your patient is hospitalized, inspect all incisions and dressings for signs of bleeding, drainage, infection, dehiscence, and evisceration. Inspect the placement and function of drains and tubes, including postsurgical drainage or nasogastric tubes, and palpate IV insertion sites for infiltration or infection. Assess your patient's fluid balance by noting his intake and output (intake includes oral and IV sources; output includes urine, nasogastric substances, and postsurgical drainage). In addition, if your patient is connected to a monitoring device, evaluate the information it provides. Finally, if your patient has a cardiac or respiratory condition, check the arterial oxygen saturation levels.

When you're ready to turn to a formal assessment, you'll have to decide which areas of the patient's body you want to assess, based on his individual needs. No matter what his specific complaint, you may want to start with a general survey.

Taking a general survey
The goal of a general survey is to assess your patient's vital signs and general condition. Afterward, you'll be able to document a wide-ranging list of findings that offer a well-rounded view of your patient's condition. (See 📖 *What to Expect When Conducting a General Survey*, p. 328.)

NORMAL FINDINGS

WHAT TO EXPECT WHEN CONDUCTING A GENERAL SURVEY

Use this review to confirm normal findings when conducting a general survey.

- Facial expression free of distress. If the patient is relatively content, he may smile, make eye contact, and have relaxed facial muscles. (Remember facial expression reflects a patient's mood and physical condition.)
- Body temperature within the following ranges:
  Oral: 96.8° to 99.5° F (36° to 37.5° C)
  Rectal: 97.3° to 100.2° F (36.3° to 37.9° C)
  Tympanic (core): 97.2° to 100° F (36.2° to 37.8° C).
- Pulse rate between 60 and 100 beats per minute (bpm), with a regular rhythm, smooth upstroke and downstroke, and strong amplitude. Pulse rates less than 60 bpm are normal in athletes or people taking certain medications. Pulse rates greater than 100 bpm are normal when influenced by factors that stimulate the sympathetic nervous system.
- Respiratory rate between 12 and 20 bpm, with regular rhythm.
- Breathing quiet, easy, and effortless.
- Respiration producing pronounced abdominal movement and slight thoracic movement in a patient in the supine position. In a patient in the sitting position, thoracic movement is more pronounced.

- Systolic blood pressure ranging from 90 to 119 mm Hg.
- Diastolic blood pressure 60 to 80 mm Hg.
- Systolic blood pressure dropping by less than 20 mm Hg when the patient moves from a supine or sitting position.
- Diastolic blood pressure rising only slightly when the patient moves from a supine or sitting position.
- Blood pressure differing by no more than 10 mm Hg between the arms.
- Body movements smooth, easily controlled, and coordinated.
- Ambulation showing patient's ability to hold body and head erect, balance easily, and swing arms at his sides. Turns accomplished smoothly, with shoulders and hips level during each stride.
- Mechanisms intact for balance, coordination, and proprioception.
- Level of consciousness showing patient is awake, alert, and oriented. Patient should respond appropriately when addressed in normal tone of voice, participate in and pay attention during conversation.
- Speech fluid, articulate, and clear.

To perform a general survey, follow these steps:

- Measure vital signs, temperature, pulse, respirations, and blood pressure for signs of abnormality.
- Assess height, weight, and body build. Note a weight gain or loss of more than 2 pounds over 24 hours. Use a bed scale if your patient is bedridden or a chair scale if he's unsteady on his feet.
- Observe the patient's ability for self-care. Note personal hygiene and grooming. Also note the general condition of the patient's skin, hair, and nails. (See ⬦ *What to Expect When Examining the Skin, Hair, and Nails.*)

- Observe the patient's posture. Look for signs of abnormal posture in the comatose patient by checking for unnatural positions. Also look for signs of pain in an alert patient.
- Observe general body movements, and look for tics, tremors, rigidity, or flaccidity.
- Observe the patient's gait. Assess balance, coordination, and position sense.
- Assess level of consciousness, attention, orientation, and speech patterns.

Remember that you may need to alter your methods for this general examination, depending on your patient's condition. Ideally, you'll want him to stand and ambulate for important portions of the examination. However, if he's bedridden or comatose, you'll have to do your best to perform the examination while he's in bed.

Examining the head and neck

When examining your patient's head and neck, have him sit up, whether in a chair, on the side of the bed, or in the bed. When assessing jugular

NORMAL FINDINGS

WHAT TO EXPECT WHEN EXAMINING THE SKIN, HAIR, AND NAILS

Use this review to confirm normal findings when examining the skin, hair, and nails.

- Skin color even throughout the body, except in dark-skinned people, in whom it's lighter on the palms, soles, and nail beds.
- Skin texture smooth and soft, except for such joints as the elbows and knees.
- Skin warm and dry.
- Skin returning immediately to its normal position when pinched.
- Hair thin, fine, and usually light in color over all areas except the scalp, axillae, eyebrows, pubic areas, palms, and soles.
- Hair coarser, darker, and thicker on the scalp, axillae, eyebrows, and pubic areas. In males, facial hair coarse and thick.
- Hair texture and color that varies with race and age. Texture may be fine or coarse, straight or curly. Color is distributed evenly and ranges from light blond to black or gray.
- Hair distribution even, except in cases of male-pattern thinning or baldness.
- Nail plates smooth, round, and slightly convex, with angle of about 160 degrees between the nail and skin at the nail's base.
- Nail plates firmly attached to the nail beds.
- Nail bed firm upon palpation.
- Capillary refill time less than 4 seconds.
- Nail surface smooth, even, and hard, with smooth and rounded nail edges.
- Periungual skin unbroken, smooth, and flat.

venous pressure, however, position your patient in bed with his head elevated 45 degrees. For your patient's comfort, you may wish to delay this part of the examination until he's supine. (See 🖾 *What to Expect When Examining the Head and Neck.*)

Assess your patient's head and neck by following these steps:

• Inspect and palpate the skin of the scalp and face for integrity. Look for any lesions or scars.

NORMAL FINDINGS

WHAT TO EXPECT WHEN EXAMINING THE HEAD AND NECK

Use this review to confirm normal findings when examining the head and neck.

• Head round and symmetrical.
• Scalp flesh-colored, without scales, and covered with hair that's distributed evenly and is free from excess oils.
• Skin firm, smooth, intact on head and neck; color distributed evenly.
• Facial appearance symmetrical. Palpebral fissures and distances between the eyes and midline of nose are equal.
• Eyes symmetrical, including placement, shape, and motility.
• Eyelids free of drainage and edema, smooth and nontender to palpation. In elderly patients, ectropion or entropion can be a normal variant.
• Lashes free of granulations or scales.
• Lacrimal apparatus producing adequate tears, nontender and free of discharge.
• Conjunctiva clear and moist; sclera white and translucent; cornea smooth and transparent; iris flat and circular, with even bilateral pigmentation.
• Pupils round, equal in size and equally reactive to light and accommodation.

• Nasal mucosa flat and slightly redder than oral mucosa; nasal septum midline.
• Lips moist and free of cracks and fissures.
• Symmetrical movement of uvula, tongue, and soft palate; positive gag reflex.
• Auricles equal in height and size, symmetrically positioned, and able to move freely and painlessly. In the elderly patient, auricles may be more prominent and earlobes more pendulous.
• External auditory canal patent and free of nodules, cysts, and drainage. A small amount of cerumen is normal.
• Pulsation of the internal jugular vein visible and regular, changing with inspiration and expiration; no jugular distention.
• Lymph nodes either nonpalpable or small, soft, and nontender.
• Trachea midline without tugging.
• Carotid pulse regular, full, and smooth.

- Observe facial expressions for signs of distress or for the appearance of abnormal facies associated with disease. Observe the face for symmetry of structure and movement.
- Inspect the integrity of the mucous membranes of the nose and mouth.
- Inspect the placement and movement of the tongue, uvula, and soft palate. Check for the presence of a gag reflex.
- Inspect the neck for distention of the jugular vein, and estimate central venous pressure.
- Palpate for lymph node swelling in the preauricular and postauricular, submental and submandibular, and cervical chains located in and around the head and neck.
- Inspect and palpate the position and movement of the trachea.
- Auscultate for a carotid bruit and venous hum.
- Assess the symmetry and strength of neck and shoulder muscles.
- Inspect and palpate the eyes and associated structures for position, shape, and motility.
- Evaluate extraocular movements, observing for conjugate movement and any abnormal movements (such as nystagmus) in all six cardinal positions.
- Inspect pupil size, shape, and response to light and accommodation. After you use the penlight to test pupillary response, check the corneal reflections for bilateral symmetry.
- Inspect and palpate the external ear, noting skin color, texture, integrity, and any areas of tenderness. Note any drainage in the external ear canal.

Examining the chest and back

During most of the chest and back examination, your patient should be sitting on the side of the bed or sitting up in bed. However, when auscultating heart sounds, ask your patient to lean forward or assume a left lateral recumbent position. (See ▨ *What to Expect When Examining the Chest and Back*, p. 332.)

Assess your patient's chest and back by following these steps:
- Inspect skin integrity and color of the chest and back.
- Watch for the use of accessory muscles as your patient breathes.
- Assess anterior-posterior and lateral dimensions of the thorax to evaluate thoracic shape.
- Inspect the precordium for pulsations, and palpate the anterior chest for thrills. Locate the position and strength of the point of maximum impulse.
- Inspect the spinal column for curvature and obvious deformity.
- Evaluate respiratory excursion to observe equality of lung expansion.
- Auscultate the anterior chest for heart sounds.

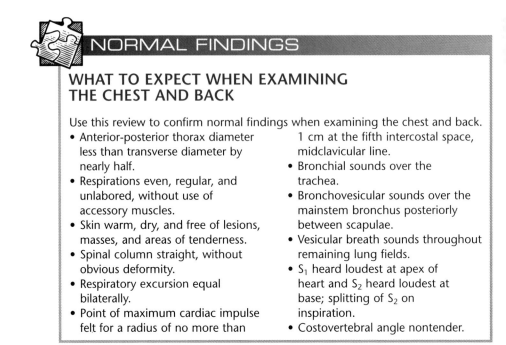

NORMAL FINDINGS

WHAT TO EXPECT WHEN EXAMINING THE CHEST AND BACK

Use this review to confirm normal findings when examining the chest and back.

- Anterior-posterior thorax diameter less than transverse diameter by nearly half.
- Respirations even, regular, and unlabored, without use of accessory muscles.
- Skin warm, dry, and free of lesions, masses, and areas of tenderness.
- Spinal column straight, without obvious deformity.
- Respiratory excursion equal bilaterally.
- Point of maximum cardiac impulse felt for a radius of no more than 1 cm at the fifth intercostal space, midclavicular line.
- Bronchial sounds over the trachea.
- Bronchovesicular sounds over the mainstem bronchus posteriorly between scapulae.
- Vesicular breath sounds throughout remaining lung fields.
- S_1 heard loudest at apex of heart and S_2 heard loudest at base; splitting of S_2 on inspiration.
- Costovertebral angle nontender.

- Auscultate the chest and back for the presence and quality of breath sounds.
- Palpate or use blunt percussion at the costovertebral angle to check for tenderness that may indicate pyelonephritis.

Examining the upper extremities

When examining the upper extremities, have your patient sit up. If necessary, however, he can be supine. (See 📋 *What to Expect When Examining the Upper Extremities.*)

Assess your patient's upper extremities by following these steps:

- Inspect the upper extremities for color and any obvious deformity, such as shortening of one arm, edema, disruption of skin integrity, or muscle atrophy.
- Palpate the upper extremities for temperature, moisture, and lesions.
- Palpate the radial, ulnar, and brachial pulses for rate, rhythm, and contour.
- Check the capillary refill of nail beds.
- Assess the range of motion (ROM) and bilateral strength of the patient's shoulders, upper arms, elbows, wrists, and hands. Palpate the joints, and listen for crepitation as the extremity flexes and extends.
- Palpate the infraclavicular and epitrochlear lymph nodes.
- Test deep tendon reflexes (DTRs), including the brachioradialis, biceps, and triceps.

NORMAL FINDINGS

WHAT TO EXPECT WHEN EXAMINING THE UPPER EXTREMITIES

Use this review to confirm normal findings when examining the upper extremities.

- Skin warm and smooth, with minimal moisture.
- Skin color matching rest of the body, except normal areas of pigmentation, such as freckles. Skin color may be darker than torso if upper extremities are routinely exposed to sunlight.
- Upper extremities with no edema or obvious deformity. Radial, ulnar, and brachial pulses easily palpated and bilaterally equal in strength and amplitude.
- Capillary refill brisk, less than 4 seconds.

- Full range of motion in all upper extremity joints without any pain.
- Upper extremities and shoulder muscles with symmetrical strength bilaterally.
- Handgrip strength equal bilaterally.
- Deep tendon reflexes—in brachioradialis, biceps, and triceps—measuring ++ bilaterally.
- Infraclavicular and epitrochlear lymph nodes either nonpalpable or small, soft, mobile, and nontender.

Examining the abdominal region

While you examine the patient's abdominal region, he should be lying down with his knees gently flexed to relax his abdominal muscles. (See 📑 *What to Expect When Examining the Abdominal Region,* p. 334.)

Assess your patient's abdominal region by following these steps:

- Inspect the abdominal skin and surface for discoloration, scars, striae (stretch marks), lesions, nodules, or dilated veins. Inspect the umbilicus, noting its color, contour, and location. Look for signs of inflammation or herniation.
- Note abdominal contour, symmetry, and movement. Have the patient take a deep breath and hold it while you look for bulges or masses. Do the same as the patient raises his head off the mattress.
- Using the diaphragm of your stethoscope, auscultate for the presence and quality of bowel sounds.
- Using the bell of your stethoscope, listen over the umbilicus (aorta) and the renal arteries for bruits.
- Palpate the abdomen for tenderness and masses. First palpate lightly over all four quadrants. Then palpate deeply, using one or both hands (bimanual palpation). If you suspect peritoneal irritation, check for rebound tenderness.

NORMAL FINDINGS

WHAT TO EXPECT WHEN EXAMINING THE ABDOMINAL REGION

Use this review to confirm normal findings when examining the abdominal region.

- Smooth, unbroken skin paler than other areas (if it hasn't been exposed to the sun). Fine, visible venous network. No lesions or nodules. You may see striae from pregnancy or weight gain; they're usually pink or blue but over time become silvery white.
- Symmetrical abdominal contour that's flat, rounded, or scaphoid (concave).
- Smooth, even movements during breathing. Abdominal movements

during breathing are typically seen in males; costal movements in females.
- Peristalsis not visible. Slight wavelike motion may be visible in thin patients.
- Aortic pulsations may be visible in thin patients.
- High-pitched bowel sounds at least every 15 seconds.
- Palpation that reveals no masses or tenderness.

Examining the lower extremities

When examining the lower extremities, have your patient sit up on the side of the bed or in a chair. (See *What to Expect When Examining the Lower Extremities*.)

Assess your patient's lower extremities by following these steps:
- Observe for any obvious deformity, such as shortening of one leg, asymmetrical alignment, edema, disruption of skin integrity, or muscle atrophy. Note the skin temperature and color, as well as the quantity and distribution of hair.
- Palpate the femoral, popliteal, posterior tibial, and dorsalis pedis pulses.
- Palpate the inguinal lymph nodes for size, mobility, and tenderness.
- Test the hip, knee, and ankle joints and their associated muscle groups for ROM and strength.
- Test superficial reflexes and DTRs, including the plantar (Babinski), patellar, and Achilles.

KNOWING WHEN TO SHIFT GEARS

In performing the complete 10-minute physical examination, keep in mind that you may have to shift gears at any time, particularly if you discover an alarming abnormal finding.

Suppose, for example, you find that your patient's blood pressure is unusually low, say 80/40 mm Hg, and he begins to complain of feeling

NORMAL FINDINGS

WHAT TO EXPECT WHEN EXAMINING THE LOWER EXTREMITIES

Use this review to confirm normal findings when examining the lower extremities.

- Skin warm and smooth, with minimal moisture.
- Skin color matching the rest of the body, except for normal areas of pigmentation, such as freckles. Skin color may be darker than the torso if the lower extremities are routinely exposed to sunlight.
- Leg hair distributed symmetrically.
- Lower extremities with no edema or obvious deformity.
- Range of motion full and painless in hip, knee, and ankle joints, as well as associated muscle groups.

- Dorsalis pedis, posterior tibial, popliteal, and femoral pulses present and bilaterally equal in strength and amplitude.
- Lower extremity muscles of equal strength bilaterally.
- Deep tendon reflexes (patellar and Achilles) ++ bilaterally. Normal response for the plantar (Babinski) reflex is downward, with inward curling of toes.
- Inguinal lymph nodes either nonpalpable or small, soft, mobile, and nontender.

light-headed. No matter what else you're assessing, you'll most likely want to focus your examination quickly on the possible causes of low blood pressure. You may want to examine your patient for signs of bleeding, dehydration, or cardiovascular compromise. Or, in some situations, your first step may be to call for help or notify the physician before proceeding with your examination.

You might also have to shift gears when it comes to your patient's comfort level. For example, if your patient is bedridden and has problems with mobility, you might want to assess his most accessible body parts (the front of his body) first before asking him to change positions. Whatever your approach, however, be sure it's systematic (head to toe and side to side), so you don't miss an important step.

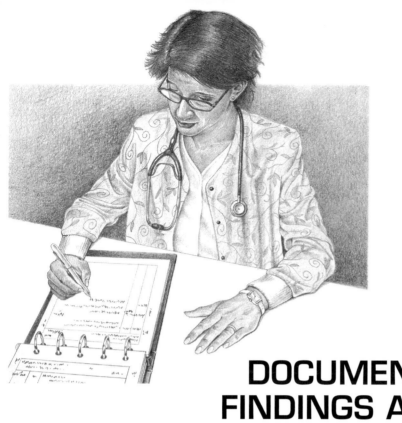

DOCUMENTING YOUR FINDINGS ACCURATELY

Rapid changes in the health care environment have placed greater importance on documenting care than ever before. How crucial is nursing documentation? As an information-sharing tool and a link between disciplines in a health care facility, accurate, thorough, and timely documentation of a patient's history and your physical examination findings becomes the road map that all members of the health care team rely on to guide the patient's treatment and follow her progress. Thorough, accurate documentation of the patient's physical, mental, and emotional condition is a fundamental nursing responsibility. Every time you document history and physical examination findings, interventions, or topics you've taught, you're helping to ensure the most effective treatment for your patient.

Documenting the initial assessment

From a legal standpoint, documentation is the best protection the patient, health care team, and health care organization have. If you fail to record your health history and physical examination findings, interventions, and teaching, you're not just depriving other team members of information they need to treat patients effectively. You're also putting yourself, your colleagues, and your employer in legal jeopardy. Remember—jurors rely heavily on what's documented in the medical records to determine if care was provided. Most malpractice cases that involve nurses arise from suspected failure to monitor a patient's condition or report changes in her clinical status—situations that wouldn't have arisen if the nurse had documented the patient's care properly.

Organizing your data

You no doubt recognize the importance of thoroughly documenting your health history and physical examination findings. But it's not always easy to make documentation a priority. Time constraints may make other patient care activities seem more important, especially during a crisis. When you consider the amount of information you must record, you may be tempted to push documentation to the bottom of your must-do list.

You can make documentation less burdensome by organizing the information into these logical categories:

• What the patient tells you—information you obtain directly from the patient (or from indirect sources, if the patient is incapacitated).
• What you assess—information you collect from health history and physical examination findings (vital sign measurement, inspection, palpation, percussion, and auscultation).
• What you do and teach—interventions you perform in response to health history and physical examination findings, as well as instructions you give the patient and family.

These categories serve as the framework for the entries that follow. Each one covers documentation for a specific clinical situation.

Document what the patient tells you

When obtaining the health history, gather information about the patient's

• Current symptoms (chief complaint).
• Past health status.
• Previous medical treatments.
• Responses to those treatments.

All these facts help the health care team identify successful interventions to incorporate into the treatment plan. Information you collect during the health history also serves as the basis of your teaching plan. By determining the patient's knowledge of her disorder, drugs, and health promotion measures, you can identify and prioritize appropriate teaching topics.

Identify the best information sources. Ideally, you should obtain information directly from the patient. In some situations—for instance, if your patient is unconscious—you'll need to interview family members, refer to the patient's medical records, and consult other health care team members to find out what you need to know. Be sure to document as many details as you can, leaving no gaps or uncertainties that a retrospective review might reveal. If you're unable to obtain part of the health history, document the reason, such as the inability to communicate with the patient and the absence of family members.

Quote the patient directly. Record the patient's exact words, placin quotes around them. This helps others clearly differentiate her words from yours.

If your patient has allergies, document her description of the allergic responses she has experienced. (What a patient reports as an allergy may be an expected or adverse effect of a drug.) Record information about her allergies in as many places as possible and according to your facility's policies and procedures. At the very least, it should appear on the initial history and physical examination findings form, the medication administration record, the nursing plan of care, the front of the patient's chart, and the patient's identification band.

Document what you assess

Next, document your findings from vital sign measurement, inspection, palpation, percussion, and auscultation. Describe abnormal findings in detail, paying special attention to those that relate to the patient's current condition. Also document findings related to symptoms the patient has denied. These pertinent negatives can be as useful as other data in determining the underlying problem.

Be objective and specific. Use objective language and avoid making judgments when documenting health history and physical examination data. For instance, if you write, "The patient's heart rate was only 60," this suggests that you think her heart rate is low.

Whenever possible, quantify your findings by citing specific numbers or ranges. Instead of "Mrs. Jones says she gets up a lot during the night to urinate," for example, write, "Mrs. Jones states she gets up 7 or 8 times during the night to urinate." Try to avoid phrases like "a little" and "a lot"—they're open to wide interpretation.

Be concrete. Describe only what you see, hear, feel, and smell during your history and physical examination. Don't document your interpretation of the patient's behavior. Instead of "Mary Smith was crying because of her depression," for example, write, "Mary Smith was crying during the physical examination." Also objectively document the patient's age, growth, physical abilities and limitations, and cognitive abilities. (See 🗐 *Documenting Growth and Developmental Information: What JCAHO Requires,* p. 340.)

Document what you do and teach

Your documentation should show that you took appropriate actions based on your health history and physical examination findings of the patient's condition. Try to record interventions as you perform them or soon afterward. Otherwise, you may forget to record important information. Note the time of each intervention to avoid the appearance that you took too long to intervene after assessing a significant finding.

LIFESPAN CONSIDERATIONS

DOCUMENTING GROWTH AND DEVELOPMENTAL INFORMATION: WHAT JCAHO REQUIRES

The Joint Commission on Accreditation of Healthcare Organizations (JCAHO) requires health care professionals to assess each hospitalized patient's physical, psychological, and social status. Also, JCAHO requires assessment of the patient's growth and development and the provision of age-appropriate care.

In most cases, you'll document growth and developmental needs as part of the admission assessment. The following examples show how you might document such needs for patients of various ages.

* *Male, age 70.* Mr. Harris talks about the recent loss of two close friends.
* *Female, age 58, who has sustained a hip fracture.* Ms. Robinson is concerned about her elderly uncle. She is the sole caregiver for the 88-year-old man and does not know how she'll care for him now that her injury prevents her from taking care of herself.
* *Male, age 17, who has paraplegia.* Billy describes his frustration with being dependent on his mother. He wants to attend a school on the West Coast and live in a dormitory.
* *Male, age 2, with respiratory syncytial virus.* Ryan cries for his mother and refuses to drink liquids.

Document the patient's response. Just because you've documented an intervention doesn't mean that your patient benefited from it. To indicate the effectiveness of an intervention, describe the patient's response—whether positive or negative. Be sure to evaluate her emotional response as well as her physical response.

Record referrals. Your documentation should indicate whether additional resources, such as home care, are needed, as well as any referrals you make to secure those resources. Record, too, your meetings with staff members from other disciplines who are involved in the patient's care. Also document the outcomes of discharge planning.

A patient's progress during your care and after discharge may depend on how well she understands her condition, treatment plan, and home care. When you document your teaching, clearly indicate your evaluation of her understanding of the instructions you've provided. If you think that she needs additional instructions, note this so that other health care team members can cover that topic in their teaching.

How documentation helps you evaluate the plan of care

All the information you obtain from the health history and physical examination along with the nursing interventions and the patient's response to those interventions contribute to the plan of care. Thorough documentation helps you evaluate the plan and revise it as needed.

DOCUMENTING PRIORITY HEALTH PROBLEMS

Document the patient's priority health problems as well as ongoing health history and physical examination findings of parameters related to these problems. If your patient has heart failure, for instance, be sure to document ongoing findings related to her heart, lungs, peripheral pulses, and fluid balance. (See *Key Priority Health Problems*.)

When your patient loses a peripheral pulse

Loss of a peripheral pulse may signal interruption of circulation—a potentially life-threatening event. If your assessment reveals this finding, you'll need to act rapidly. Besides reviewing your patient's medical history, you must quickly evaluate her current health status. You'll also need to notify the physician and record your findings accurately to ensure prompt, effective treatment.

Document what the patient tells you

Record an abbreviated version of the patient's medical history, especially noting a previous diagnosis of peripheral vascular disease, diabetes mellitus, heart disease, arterial occlusive disease, or other disorders that

KEY PRIORITY HEALTH PROBLEMS

When documenting patient care, you'll focus on what the patient tells you, what you assess, and what you do and teach. To help guide you through specific situations you may encounter in your daily practice, refer to the information that explains what to document when your patient

- Loses a peripheral pulse
- Has chest pain
- Has a myocardial infarction
- Has heart failure
- Has pneumonia
- Has an asthma attack
- Has a pulmonary embolism
- Has pulmonary edema
- Has pulmonary tuberculosis
- Has severe pain
- Is confused
- Has a seizure
- Has a cerebrovascular accident
- Has hypoglycemia
- Has hyperglycemia
- Has a pressure ulcer
- Has surgery

may predispose the patient to an arterial occlusion. If she reports chronic skin ulcers, injury, trauma, surgery, or wounds in the affected area, record that information. Pinpoint the exact location of the affected area, record the duration of the problem, and detail treatments the patient received for the condition.

Next, document reports of pain, weakness, numbness, tingling, and decreased sensation in the arm or leg that has lost the pulse. Determine if the patient's symptoms are relieved by rest, and note this in the medical record. Also document other symptoms, even if they seem unrelated to the absent pulse. Because decreased circulation in an arm or leg may reflect a systemic problem, you'll need to check for and document signs and symptoms of reduced cardiac output, such as hypotension, decreased level of consciousness (LOC), and chest pain.

Document what you assess

Although signs and symptoms vary with the cause of the absent peripheral pulse, you can expect these abnormal findings in the affected arm or leg:

- Weakness.
- Pain.
- Numbness.
- Tingling.
- Discolored nail beds or skin.
- Edema.
- Sluggish capillary refill.
- Cool skin.

Make sure you describe the affected arm or leg in detail, including its circumference, skin temperature and appearance, nail bed color, briskness of capillary refill, and the patient's ability to move the arm or leg.

Next, compare the affected arm or leg with the opposite one, and record your findings to help determine the circulatory status of the pulseless arm or leg. Measure the circumference of both arms or legs at two or more places. (See *Documenting Your Measurements.*)

Then, using a Doppler device if possible, auscultate for a pulse in the arm or leg. Record the presence or absence of a bruit. If you see an open area or a break in the skin, document its location, size, and color and carefully describe the lesion's edges. Also document the amount, color, and odor of drainage.

Next, record information that might help determine the cause of the pulse loss. To do this, measure the apical pulse and determine if a pulse deficit exists; assess LOC; measure blood pressure; evaluate urine output; and note dyspnea, chest or back pain, abdominal pain or distention, and nausea or vomiting. These assessments may help identify the cause of the lost pulse, such as shock, hemorrhage, or aneurysm.

DOCUMENTING YOUR MEASUREMENTS

If your patient loses her peripheral pulse, the circumference of the involved arm or leg may change. This may indicate whether her underlying condition is improving or worsening. To ensure accurate assessment over time, always measure the arm or leg at exactly the same location each time and thoroughly document the location you're using.

When possible, mark the patient's skin at the top and bottom edges of the measuring tape. If you're using such skin markings as a guide, note this in your documentation. For instance, you might write, "Right leg circumference: 30" midthigh, 20" midcalf, measured using skin markings."

If you can't mark the patient's skin, refer to an easy-to-find landmark to indicate where you took the measurement. For a thigh measurement, you might use the bend of the knee, as the following example shows: "Placed bottom edge of measuring tape on right anterior thigh, 6" above bend of knee."

You can also use a preprinted diagram to document measurement sites or to indicate skin abnormalities. To record a wound's location, for example, you can indicate its color and size in the margin. If the patient has multiple areas of skin breakdown, assign a number or letter to each area, and then reference the areas in the narrative section of your note. For instance, you may write, "Cultures taken from right leg wound A." You can also indicate changes in skin color or temperature on the human outline.

From Mosby. (1999). Surefire Documentation: How, What, and When Nurses Need to Document. St. Louis: Mosby.

Document what you do and teach

As you intervene during the patient's acute illness and her recovery, use the information below to guide your documentation and tailor the written plan of care to the patient's needs. Your documentation should also include the teaching you provide to help your patient prevent the underlying condition from recurring. Be sure to include the following, as needed:

- Ongoing monitoring of the affected arm or leg, along with vital signs.
- Removal of a constricting item, such as a bandage.

- Drugs and IV therapy.
- Proper positioning.
- Active or passive range-of-motion (ROM) exercises.
- Antiembolism stockings.
- Disease process.
- Diagnostic tests.
- Interventional procedures.
- Precautions and follow-up tests for anticoagulation.
- Activity.
- Proper positioning of the arm or leg.
- Avoidance of constrictive clothing, leg crossing, and staying in one position for prolonged periods.
- Smoking cessation.
- Proper nutrition.
- Signs and symptoms to report.
- Wound and skin care.
- Scheduled follow-up visits.

When your patient has chest pain

Because chest pain may indicate a myocardial infarction (MI) or another potentially fatal condition, always take this symptom seriously. Act quickly to perform a focused assessment and intervene promptly as indicated. Remember—documentation of your assessment findings must convey the essential information the health care team needs to guide treatment, especially when your patient's life is in danger.

Document what the patient tells you

When documenting your patient's chest pain, record her exact description of this symptom, placing quotes around her words. Ask her to rate pain severity on a scale of 0 to 10, with 0 indicating no pain and 10 indicating the worst pain imaginable.

Then have your patient point to the exact pain location; document her response. Ask if the pain radiates to other parts of her body, such as her jaws, shoulders, arms, or back. Document accompanying symptoms the patient reports, such as shortness of breath and nausea. Whenever possible, record her own words, not your interpretation of them.

Next, document the pain's duration. Ask when the pain started and whether it's steady or intermittent. Determine if the patient has had chest pain before. If she has, ask her to compare her current pain with that in previous episodes; carefully document her response.

Ask whether any factor (such as activity), triggered the chest pain. Find out if anything makes it better (such as rest or nitroglycerin) or worse (such as breathing deeply). Assess and document her emotional status, noting, for instance, if she is anxious or reports a feeling of impending doom.

Health history. Document pertinent health history information, such as a history of heart disease, hypertension, or hypercholesterolemia. Note other risk factors for heart disease, such as a family history of heart disease, advanced age, history of smoking, diabetes mellitus, obesity, and a sedentary or stressful lifestyle. Document the use of estrogen or oral contraceptives. Also record chronic diseases, hospitalizations, procedures, and surgeries the patient reports.

Obtain a drug history, recording the names, dosages, and administration times and routes for all drugs the patient uses. Record the time of her last dose of each. Document drug and other allergies the patient reports.

Document what you assess

Measure the patient's vital signs, especially noting tachycardia or bradycardia, an increased respiratory rate, and abnormally high or low blood pressure. Record your auscultation of heart sounds, including the presence of extra heart sounds or murmurs. If you hear abnormal sounds, note the stethoscope location, such as the fifth intercostal space, midclavicular line. Document whether the patient's heart rate is regular or irregular.

Then document patient actions (such as guarding and holding the chest) and behaviors (such as anxiety and restlessness) that suggest she's in pain. Note changes in her mental status, too, such as decreased LOC, disorientation, and confusion.

Next, evaluate the patient's respiratory rate and pattern. Record dyspnea, use of accessory breathing muscles, and jugular vein distention. Obtain and document the patient's pulse oximetry reading. Then assess her skin, recording such abnormalities as coolness, clamminess, pallor, and cyanosis.

Arrange for your patient to undergo a baseline 12-lead electrocardiogram (ECG). Then review it with the physician to detect abnormal rhythms and other changes. Place a copy of the tracing at the bedside for quick comparison during future ECG evaluations.

Document what you do and teach

As you intervene during the patient's acute illness and recovery, expect to implement and document the following general interventions. Because many interventions for a patient with chest pain depend on the underlying condition—for instance, if diagnostic tests reveal that your patient has had an MI—she may require additional interventions. As always, document your interventions and the patient's responses. Also, tailor the teaching plan to your patient's condition and treatment. Be sure to include the following, as needed:

- Diagnostic tests.
- Fluid intake and output.
- Oxygen therapy.
- Continuous cardiac monitoring.
- Drug and IV therapy.

- Activity.
- Emotional support.
- Transfer to the intensive care unit (ICU).
- Hemodynamic monitoring.
- Heart anatomy and physiology.
- Disease process.
- Interventional treatments.
- Signs and symptoms to report.
- Actions to take when chest pain occurs.
- Cardiac risk factor reduction.
- Nutrition.
- Activity.
- Resources for further information and support.

When your patient has a myocardial infarction

When caring for a patient who's experiencing an MI, accurate documentation can be as critical as rapid response. Your documentation can help ensure effective emergency treatment and tailor the plan of care to your patient's specific needs.

Document what the patient tells you

In this emergency, you probably won't have time to gather and document a complete health history. Once the crisis passes, be sure to question the patient or a family member or check medical records to obtain pertinent information.

To begin, determine if the patient has a history of atherosclerosis, coronary artery disease, or hyperlipoproteinemia. If she does, record the date the condition was diagnosed and its treatment, including drugs, activity guidelines, and dietary restrictions. If she smokes cigarettes or did so in the past, record the number of packs she smoked or smokes per day and the number of years she has smoked.

If she reports a history of hypertension and knows her most recent systolic and diastolic readings, document these readings to provide a baseline for comparison with current values. Record whether she complies with her hypertension treatment plan.

Find out if the patient has a history of diabetes mellitus. If so, record the date of diagnosis and the details of her treatment plan, including the type and dosage of the oral antidiabetic drug or insulin she takes. To help determine the effectiveness of diabetes treatment, document how often she monitors her blood glucose level at home, which methods she uses, and her most recent blood glucose level.

Then record the patient's reported activity level, including the types of activity and exercise she performs and the number of days per week she exercises. If she describes a sedentary lifestyle, record this. Document her weight and recent history of weight loss or gain.

If the patient has a family history of heart disease, note which family members are affected. You may want to use a genogram to record this information.

If the patient reports a previous MI, record the date and any complications. To aid your assessment of previous MI treatments and the patient's response, review the past medical record and document pertinent findings.

Next, document recent reports of crushing, substernal chest pain that radiates to the left arm, jaw, neck, or shoulder blades. Ask the patient to rate the pain's severity on a scale of 0 to 10, with 0 indicating no pain and 10 indicating the worst pain imaginable. Document her response, along with the time the pain started and factors that seem to improve or worsen it.

Ask if the patient recently had symptoms that typically precede or accompany an MI: indigestion or heartburn, more frequent angina attacks, feelings of impending doom, increased fatigue, and episodes of nausea, vomiting, or shortness of breath. Document her response fully. Discuss with the physician significant information you gather during the health history interview.

Document what you assess
Although signs and symptoms of MI vary among patients, you should assess for and document the following expected abnormal findings:
- Anxiety.
- Restlessness.
- Dyspnea.
- Tachypnea.
- Diaphoresis.
- Jugular vein distention.
- Cool, mottled skin.
- Diminished peripheral pulses.
- S_4 or S_3 (abnormal heart sounds).
- Paradoxical splitting of S_2.
- Systolic murmur.
- Pericardial friction rub.
- Low-grade fever.
- Tachycardia and hypertension (with an anterior MI).
- Bradycardia and hypotension (with an inferior MI).

Document what you do and teach
As you intervene during the patient's acute illness and recovery, document care and teaching related to these topics:
- Diagnostic tests.
- Fluid intake and output.
- Oxygen therapy.

- Continuous cardiac monitoring.
- Drug and IV therapy.
- Activity.
- Emotional support.
- Transfer to the ICU.
- Hemodynamic monitoring.
- Heart anatomy and physiology.
- Disease process.
- Interventional treatments.
- Signs and symptoms to report.
- Actions to take when chest pain occurs.
- Cardiac risk factor reduction.
- Nutrition.
- Smoking cessation.
- Cardiac rehabilitation.
- Resources for further information and support.

When your patient has heart failure

Successful management of heart failure focuses on three essential goals: maintaining fluid balance, controlling symptoms, and recognizing warning signs of complications. Your thorough documentation helps the health care team determine effective interventions and create a long-range treatment plan for your patient.

Document what the patient tells you

When obtaining your patient's health history, assess for and document signs, symptoms, and risk factors that could contribute to heart failure. If the patient has a history of heart failure, collect information about past treatments she has received, noting their effectiveness.

Ask the patient to relate her medical history, especially heart or circulatory diseases she has had. Along with this information, record the date of each diagnosis and treatment she received.

Document past or present signs and symptoms of heart failure she describes, and note whether she has new or worsening symptoms. In particular, ask about shortness of breath, edema, cough, tachycardia, chest pain, orthopnea, and fatigue. Record her responses in detail.

As necessary, ask the patient to elaborate on her symptoms. For example, if she says she gets tired from walking shorter and shorter distances, ask her to compare how far she can walk now before tiring compared to how far she could walk previously. Your documentation might read, "Patient states she previously could walk up to one block before feeling slightly short of breath. One week ago, she noted that she became short of breath after walking about 10 feet."

Next, elicit and record information about the patient's diet and recent dietary changes. Document your assessment of her sodium, fat, and cholesterol intake and her understanding of how an improper diet can contribute to heart disease. Note whether she has gained or lost weight recently and whether she weighs herself at the same time each day.

Ask about urination patterns, and document recent changes in urine output and frequency of urination. Also inquire about her daily fluid intake, and document her answer.

If the patient reports a history of hypertension, document this along with her most recent blood pressure reading, if known. Record the names and dosages of drugs she is using and her perception of the reason for using each one. Also document whether she complies with the prescribed drug regimen. Using her own words, record exactly how she uses her drugs. Finally, document recent changes in the amount of her daily activity, and determine if she's been under new or unusual stress.

Document what you assess

Perform and document a thorough patient assessment to establish a baseline. As treatment progresses, your documentation will help the health care team track the patient's condition.

Vital sign checks. Record the patient's pulse, respiratory rate, and blood pressure every 4 hours—more often if they're unstable. Document whom you notified and how you intervened for abnormal values and changes, especially tachycardia, tachypnea, and hypotension. When measuring vital signs, also document daily weights—a valuable indicator of fluid gain or loss for a patient with heart failure.

Respiratory system. Auscultate the patient's lungs every 1 to 2 hours. Document adventitious breath sounds and changes from the previous assessment—especially increased congestion and decreased air movement. Notify the physician of changes, and document that you did so.

Then evaluate for and record the use of accessory breathing muscles and signs and symptoms of decreased perfusion and hypoxia. Document the time dyspnea occurs and precipitating factors. Ask the patient if anything has improved the dyspnea in the past, and record her answer.

Cardiovascular system. Check for jugular vein distention. When documenting this finding, include the degree of distention. Document your assessment of heart sounds every 1 to 2 hours. Be sure to record abnormal sounds, especially S_3 or a prominent systolic murmur, which may indicate fluid overload.

Tissue perfusion. Record indicators of decreased tissue perfusion, especially pallor, diaphoresis, and cool, clammy skin. Also note confusion and decreased LOC, which may signal decreased cardiac output.

Fluid balance. Assess for and document signs and symptoms of fluid overload. If your patient has edema, note its location and whether it's pitting or nonpitting. Record the degree of pitting, if present. Document changes from the previous assessment.

Document what you do and teach

As you intervene to manage your patient's heart failure, document exactly what you did, when you did it, and the patient's response. This will help you identify effective interventions and refine your plan of care as needed. Also document all teaching you provide, along with measurable indicators of her understanding. Be sure your interventions, teaching, and documentation include the following topics:

- IV insertion.
- Drug and IV therapy.
- Oxygen therapy.
- Cardiac and hemodynamic monitoring.
- Heart anatomy, physiology, and disease process.
- Fluid intake and output.
- Daily weight.
- Nutrition, including dietary or fluid restrictions and referral to a dietitian.
- Signs and symptoms to report.
- Activity limitations.
- Diagnostic tests.
- Home monitoring, such as blood pressure measurement and Holter monitoring.

When your patient has pneumonia

Documentation for a patient with pneumonia can help her avoid complications, promote her progress toward self-care, and prevent recurrences. During the health history interview and physical examination, stay alert for risk factors or other conditions that make your patient vulnerable to the disease.

Document what your patient tells you

After documenting a complete health history, ask your patient to describe her symptoms. Then document them using her own words. Record the time of symptom onset, noting whether it was sudden or gradual. Ask about and record associated symptoms, such as fever, chills, cough, sputum production, weakness, fatigue, pain, and anorexia.

Risk factors. To further identify risk factors for pneumonia, note the patient's age and ask about a history of recent hospitalizations or surgery, chronic conditions, cardiopulmonary disease, immunosuppressive therapy, decreased LOC, and past bouts of pneumonia. Record complaints of difficulty eating, chewing, or swallowing, which predisposes the patient to developing aspiration pneumonia. Document whether she has received a pneumococcal vaccine. If she did, note the administration date.

Finally, record her report of allergies to drugs, foods, chemicals, and environmental elements, such as dust, pollen, and pets.

Pain. Document chest pain, headache, or other pain your patient reports. Using her own words, record the pain's characteristics, including intensity and duration. Note factors that she says make the pain better (such as splinting the chest while coughing and applying heat) or worse (such as coughing and breathing deeply).

Document what you assess

Assess and record the patient's vital sign measurements every 4 hours or more often if she's unstable. If you detect a fever, tachycardia, tachypnea, or hypotension, document this finding, notify the physician, and document your notification. Record all laboratory test results you obtain, such as arterial blood gas (ABG) levels.

Respiratory status. Record the respiratory rate and rhythm. Then auscultate for breath sounds, and document abnormalities, such as diminished breath sounds, wheezes, or crackles. Next, record percussion findings, such as areas of dullness, which may indicate consolidation. Also record other findings, including dyspnea, nasal flaring, use of accessory breathing muscles, and abnormal breathing patterns.

If the patient has a cough, document its frequency and its effectiveness in clearing secretions. If the cough is productive, describe the amount of sputum produced, frequency of sputum production, and sputum color, odor, and other characteristics.

Oxygenation. Record physical findings that reflect the patient's oxygenation, such as nail bed color and respiratory effort. Record pulse oximetry readings at the time of your initial assessment. Then obtain and document oximetry readings whenever the patient's condition changes or as required by the physician or facility policy. If the patient is receiving supplemental oxygen, note the amount of oxygen being administered at the time of the oximetry reading, along with the oxygen flow rate and delivery device. Do the same when recording ABG levels. Always record and report significant levels or important changes from previous ABG levels.

Next, document the patient's skin color, turgor, and temperature as well as capillary refill. Particularly note diaphoresis, pallor, and cyanosis, which may signal decreased oxygenation.

Finally, document your patient's LOC. Stay especially alert for confusion or disorientation—a sign of hypoxia or hypercapnia—and report this immediately.

Document what you do and teach

Record your interventions and teaching as you initiate them. This helps show that you provided timely and appropriate care, which may prove legally significant if the patient's care becomes an issue for litigation. Be sure to include the following, as needed:

- Frequent monitoring.
- Oxygen therapy.
- Pulse oximetry.
- Fluid intake and output.
- Drug and IV therapy.
- Diagnostic tests.
- Promoting coughing and deep breathing, performing chest physiotherapy, and suctioning.
- Nutrition.
- Activity.
- Disease process.
- Infection prevention.
- Signs and symptoms to report.
- Recommended preventive vaccines.
- Hydration.
- Resources for further information and support.

When your patient has an asthma attack

Potentially life-threatening, an acute asthma attack calls for prompt, accurate assessment and expert intervention—and complete documentation of those actions. To avoid future asthma attacks and help maintain an optimal activity level, the patient also needs effective teaching. Thorough documentation of your assessment, interventions, and teaching directs her plan of care during the acute episode. It can also help safeguard her long-term health.

Document what the patient tells you

Even after stabilizing a patient with an acute asthma attack, difficulty breathing and speaking may prevent her from supplying information. If she can nod or shake her head, ask essential yes-or-no questions, and record her responses. If she's accompanied by a family member or friend, obtain information from that person.

Then check the patient's medical record for data about a history of asthma or other respiratory problems, current drug use, and allergies. Be sure to note whether she uses oxygen, a nebulizer, or an inhaler at home, and document whether she's taking a steroid to treat asthma. If she is, record the dosage and the date she started taking it. Also find out if she takes peak-flow measurements at home. Ask about and document her best measurement.

Next, record data about the current asthma attack, including its onset, duration, and accompanying symptoms. Ask the patient or her companion how often she experiences asthma attacks and whether the current episode differs from previous attacks. Carefully document the answers.

Then identify and record recent exposure to irritants, such as smoke, allergens, and chemicals. Ask about symptoms of recent respiratory tract infections, such as fever and productive cough. Also document the treatments that have helped terminate previous asthma attacks.

Document what you assess

Record your findings from a rapid assessment. Include the following expected abnormal findings, if present, and any others you detect:
- Wheezing and dyspnea.
- Diminished or absent breath sounds.
- Difficulty speaking or performing activities (from dyspnea).
- Tachypnea.
- Use of accessory breathing muscles.
- Productive cough.
- Tachycardia.
- Hypotension.
- Anxiety and diaphoresis.
- Signs of decreased oxygenation, such as cyanosis.
- Change in LOC.

   If diagnostic test results are available, record pulse oximetry readings, ABG levels, and peak-flow measurements.

Document what you do and teach

To prevent the asthma attack from progressing, intervene rapidly, and record your actions as you take them. Expect to implement and document some or all of the following interventions and teaching points:
- Oxygen administration.
- Pulse oximetry.
- Nebulizer or inhaler administration.
- Drug and IV therapy.
- Diagnostic tests.
- Upright positioning.
- Breathing and relaxation techniques.
- Energy conservation.
- Emotional support.
- Respiratory system anatomy and physiology.
- Disease process.
- Peak-flow measurements.
- What to do if peak-flow measurements worsen or if an acute asthma attack occurs.
- Use of a prescribed metered-dose inhaler, dry powder inhaler, or nebulizer.
- Care of an inhaler and other respiratory equipment used at home.
- Signs and symptoms to report.
- Hygiene, and infection prevention.

- Allergen avoidance.
- Breathing techniques.
- Identifying and avoiding precipitating factors.
- Pacing activities with rest.
- Dietary and fluid recommendations.
- Stress management and relaxation techniques.
- Resources for further information and support.

When your patient has a pulmonary embolism

Without prompt assessment and treatment, pulmonary embolism can lead to serious complications and, possibly, death. If you suspect a pulmonary embolism, notify the physician at once, and take emergency steps to safeguard the patient's life. Then, as soon as possible, document the findings that led you to suspect pulmonary embolism.

When the patient's condition allows, review her history for factors that predispose her to this disorder. Then perform a thorough physical examination, focusing on her respiratory status and oxygenation. To show efficient nursing care and ensure clear communication with the rest of the health care team, document your interventions as you initiate them, along with the patient's response.

Document what the patient tells you

Record predisposing factors that the patient reports, such as a history of recent surgery, MI, heart failure, atrial fibrillation, venous insufficiency, thrombophlebitis, polycythemia vera, chronic illness, trauma, and immobilization after a fracture. Add other risk factors that you note, such as smoking, advanced age, and obesity. For a female patient, note recent pregnancy, childbirth, oral contraceptive use, and estrogen replacement therapy.

If your patient reports chest pain, ask her to describe it in detail, and record her answer in her own words. Include its precise location and time of onset. Record her rating of pain severity on a scale of 0 to 10, with 0 indicating no pain and 10 indicating the worst pain imaginable. Ask about and record factors that she says make the pain worse (such as breathing deeply and coughing) or better (such as lying still and splinting the chest while coughing). If she reports shortness of breath, document when she first noted this symptom. Also assess and record her anxiety level and if she reports a sense of impending doom.

Document what you assess

Focus your assessment and documentation on the patient's respiratory status and oxygenation. If you suspect that a blood disorder has contributed to the pulmonary embolism, check her most recent hemoglobin, erythrocyte, and thrombocyte values. Document that you notified the physician of abnormal values, along with the notification time and the physician's orders. Also, if you suspect the patient has deep vein thrombosis (DVT) that has embolized to the pulmonary vasculature, check her calves for evidence of erythema and edema, as well as the presence of Homans' sign.

Respiratory system. Document your assessment of the patient's respiratory status every 1 to 2 hours or as appropriate. Include the respiratory rate and rhythm, chest expansion characteristics (such as asymmetry), and any tachypnea, dyspnea, shallow breathing, or accessory muscle use.

Record the time of breath sound auscultation, noting such abnormalities as diminished breath sounds, wheezes, crackles, and friction rub. Document whether the patient has a cough. If the cough is productive, describe the amount of sputum produced and its characteristics.

Document what you do and teach

Act quickly to help your patient with a pulmonary embolism maintain adequate oxygenation and gas exchange. Try to document each intervention as you perform it, and then record the patient's response to your care and the teaching you provide. (See *Documenting by "AIR"*, p. 356) Be sure to cover the following areas:
- Oxygen therapy.
- Vital sign measurements and pulse oximetry readings.
- Drug and IV therapy.
- Proper positioning.
- Energy conservation.
- Comfort measures.
- Emotional support and anxiety relief.
- Respiratory system anatomy and physiology.
- Disease process.
- Signs and symptoms of respiratory insufficiency.
- Dietary restrictions.
- Bleeding precautions.
- Signs and symptoms to report.
- Diagnostic tests.
- Antiembolism stockings.

When your patient has pulmonary edema

Accurate documentation helps identify the cause of pulmonary edema and guides the health care team toward the most effective treatment. Pulmonary edema can rapidly progress to respiratory failure. By focusing your documentation on the key points described here, you can help your patient avert this acute emergency.

Document what the patient tells you

As necessary, gather information from the patient, family members, and existing medical records. In particular, document reports of chest pain. Using the patient's own words, record the pain's exact location, time of

DOCUMENTING BY "AIR"

Designed to avoid repetition of previously documented information, the AIR (Assessment, Intervention, Response) format promotes clear, concise recording of the patient's condition and nursing interventions—especially when used with flow sheets and the nursing plan of care. Using "AIR" allows you to document continual care. This can prove especially useful when the patient response you document doesn't reflect a final outcome. An explanation of AIR documentation follows:

A: Assessment

Summarize your assessment findings, including trends (worsening or improvement) and your impressions of the patient's problem. Organize the data into appropriate sections, using headings such as "Admission note" and "Discharge teaching."

I: Intervention

Describe your actions and those of other caregivers in response to assessment findings. Group information under the same headings you used in the "Assessment" section. You may want to include plans for additional monitoring or care.

R: Response

Document your patient's response to interventions, using the same headings you used for the other sections. Be aware that if the patient's response isn't expected for several hours or days after the intervention, another nurse may document it.

Oxygenation. To document the patient's oxygenation, record your assessment of her skin for circumoral cyanosis, pallor, coolness, clamminess, and diaphoresis. Also document pertinent negatives, such as absence of pallor. If the patient was admitted for thrombophlebitis, record your assessment of the affected leg, including its temperature and any edema, redness, or tenderness. Because impaired oxygenation can decrease the patient's level of consciousness (LOC), check for and record disorientation, confusion, and stupor.

Document the patient's pulse oximetry reading each time her condition changes. Write down the oxygen concentration she's receiving at the time of the reading. If she's not receiving oxygen, note that she's on room air. Record ABG levels each time a sample is drawn, and note the amount of oxygen she is receiving and any changes in her condition. Sample AIR documentation follows:

A: At 1240, patient had labored respirations of 24 breaths/minute. Breath sounds diminished in Ⓡbase. Skin cool and clammy. Fingernails cyanotic. ————————————————————————A. Casey, RN

I: At 1300, Dr. Williams notified of change in patient's clinical status and physical findings. Dr. Williams' verbal orders at that time included STAT ABGs and O₂ therapy to begin at 4 liters/minute. ABG sample obtained by respiratory therapist. Patient placed in semi-Fowler's position and nasal O₂ started at 4 liters/minute as prescribed. ——A. Casey, RN

R: At 1330, patient's respiratory rate 20 breaths/minute. Skin cool but no longer clammy. Nail beds show no cyanosis. Patient states he feels "much better." He appears comfortable while supine. ————————A. Casey, RN

From Mosby. (1999). *Surefire Documentation: How, What, and When Nurses Need to Document.* St. Louis: Mosby.

onset, duration, severity (on a scale of 0 to 10 with 0 indicating no pain and 10 indicating the worst pain imaginable), exacerbating factors (such as taking a deep breath), and alleviating factors (such as sitting upright).

Also check for and record preexisting cardiac or respiratory conditions that can precipitate pulmonary edema, past episodes of heart failure or acute respiratory distress syndrome, and a history of other predisposing factors, such as kidney or liver disease. Then record the names of drugs the patient reports taking and the allergies she describes.

Document what you assess
During the acute crisis, record the patient's vital sign measurements frequently and obtain her weight daily. Also thoroughly document the crucial findings described here.

Respiratory system and oxygenation. Document your frequent auscultation of the patient's breath sounds, including adventitious sounds (such as crackles and wheezes). Note dyspnea, labored breathing, and use of accessory breathing muscles. Also document whether the patient has a cough. If she does, check for sputum production and describe the amount, color, and odor of the sputum as well as other characteristics.

Then record significant skin findings, such as diaphoresis, abnormal temperature, clamminess, and cyanosis. Look for and document signs and symptoms of hypoxia, such as anxiety and restlessness. If the patient becomes short of breath during activity, record this fact. Indicate how much activity she can tolerate before becoming short of breath and how long it takes for her to recover a normal breathing pattern after rest. If she has difficulty lying flat, note this, too.

Finally, check for peripheral edema. Document its location, note any pitting, and record the degree of the pitting.

Cardiovascular system. Because pulmonary edema stresses the heart, document signs and symptoms of cardiac compromise. Record auscultation of heart sounds, noting decreased or abnormal sounds, such as an S_3. Then document the quality of the pulse, which may be bounding in pulmonary edema. Be sure to document that you assessed for jugular vein distention, too.

Document what you do and teach
To prevent your patient's condition from worsening, act quickly. Record your interventions as soon as possible after you implement them. Also document everything you teach. Keep these topics in mind as you intervene and teach:
- Airway, breathing, and circulation maintenance.
- Oxygen therapy.
- Continuous cardiac monitoring.

- Pulse oximetry.
- Diagnostic testing.
- Drug and IV therapy.
- Emotional support and anxiety relief.
- Proper positioning.
- Fluid balance.
- Fluid intake and output.
- Hemodynamic monitoring.
- Heart and respiratory system anatomy and physiology.
- Disease process.
- Dietary and fluid restrictions.
- Treatment procedures.
- Oxygen and energy conservation techniques.
- Signs and symptoms to report.

When your patient has pulmonary tuberculosis

Documenting your care for a patient with pulmonary tuberculosis (TB) can have far-reaching effects. Besides helping to ensure that your patient receives proper care, it can prevent the disease from being transmitted to others. By assessing and recording your patient's history, lifestyle, past treatments, and knowledge of TB and its transmission, you can evaluate her risk for developing active disease and infecting others. Your interventions and teaching plan can address these risks.

Document what the patient tells you

When obtaining your patient's medical history, be sure to elicit and record information about past pulmonary or infectious diseases and other respiratory conditions. If she has undergone a tuberculin skin test (intradermal injection of purified protein derivative [PPD]), record the test date and result. If she had a positive PPD reaction, document other tests she has undergone, such as chest X-rays and sputum tests, and their results. Find out if she has been treated for TB before. If she has, record the dates and duration of treatment, names of all prescribed drugs, and her compliance with treatment.

Then record current or recent symptoms your patient reports, including chronic cough, fever, chills, night sweats, bloody or purulent sputum, chest pain, weight loss, malaise, and anorexia.

Risk factors. Elicit and document your patient's risk factors for TB, such as a family history of the disease. Describe her living arrangements, especially if she lives in an institution, community residence, nursing home, or shelter. Note whether she has spent time in prison, in a shelter, in the military, or as a homeless person. Record other risk factors, such as a history of alcoholism, IV drug use, and positive human immunodeficiency virus status.

Document other risk factors you uncover, such as advanced age, a job in health care or day care, recent travel outside the country, or a condition that increases the risk of TB (such as malnutrition, chemotherapy, steroid or immunosuppressive therapy, chronic renal failure, other chronic disease, and recent loss of more than 10% of body weight).

Document what you assess

A patient who tests positive on a TB skin test doesn't necessarily have active TB. Your assessment can help determine her diagnosis and guide interventions.

When performing and documenting a complete nursing assessment, focus on the following expected abnormal findings:
- Cough.
- Fever.
- Hemoptysis or purulent sputum.
- Adventitious breath sounds.
- Dyspnea.
- Hoarseness.
- Tachycardia.
- Poor nutritional status.

Document what you do and teach

Documenting your interventions, teaching, and the patient's understanding is crucial in preventing pulmonary TB transmission. Make sure that your interventions, teaching, and documentation include the following topics:
- Isolation procedures, including a double-door isolation room with negative-pressure ventilation.
- Reporting to the local health authority and hospital infection control department.
- Prevention of disease transmission.
- Drug and IV therapy.
- Oxygen therapy.
- Pulse oximetry.
- Assistance with positioning, turning, coughing, and deep breathing.
- Suctioning, including proper care and disposal of suction equipment.
- Diagnostic tests.
- Drug compliance.
- Nutrition.
- Hygiene, and infection prevention, including hand-washing.
- Proper disposal of sputum and tissues.
- Follow-up testing.
- Signs and symptoms to report.
- Testing of family members and close contacts.

When your patient has severe pain

For a patient in severe pain, developing the plan of care hinges on careful assessment, appropriate interventions, and thorough evaluation of the patient's response. Documentation plays an important role in tailoring the plan to your patient's needs. It also communicates vital information to other health care team members so they can devise an effective pain-management plan.

Document what the patient tells you

Obtain and record a thorough health history from the patient. Include all possible sources of pain, such as chronic diseases, illnesses, and surgeries. Record her description of the circumstances when the pain first arose. Then elicit details about the pain, including its
- Onset.
- Location and radiation.
- Duration.
- Nature (such as sharp, dull, or stabbing).
- Severity rated on a 0 to 10 scale, with 0 indicating no pain and 10 indicating the worst pain imaginable.
- Exacerbating factors.
- Relieving factors.

Ask the patient if the pain prevents her from performing certain motions or activities, interferes with activities of daily living, or decreases her quality of life. Also record what she tells you about her usual activity level, sleep pattern, and appetite.

Next, document your patient's use of analgesics, including over-the-counter preparations. Quoting the patient directly, record her perception of whether these drugs are effective or cause adverse effects.

Then ask her to describe her use of alcohol and street drugs. Also find out if she uses nonprescription drugs or other substances to control her pain. Finally, ask her about allergies to drugs and other substances. Document all responses carefully.

Document what you assess

Record your findings from a thorough assessment. To avoid exacerbating the pain, be gentle when palpating, percussing, or auscultating the painful area.

First, document how well the patient can move the painful area, noting whether movement increases the pain. Describe weaknesses or functional limitations caused by the pain, and record diaphoresis or cool, clammy skin. Also record the patient's verbal response to pain, such as crying or shouting, and her nonverbal signs of pain, such as facial grimacing or guarding the painful area.

Next, measure and document the patient's vital signs. With severe pain, expect tachycardia, tachypnea, and hypertension. Assess whether the pain or analgesics have affected the patient's LOC or distorted her time perception. For instance, if she states, "My family left an hour ago" and you saw them leave 15 minutes earlier, document this alteration in time perception. Finally, record what you observe about her appetite.

Document what you do and teach

To evaluate the effectiveness of interventions and teaching, assess and record the patient's pain characteristics before and after each intervention, as well as her understanding of educational measures. As you document, be sure to cover these general areas:

- Drug administration.
- Comfort measures.
- Balance between activity and rest.
- External pain-relief measures, such as transcutaneous electrical nerve stimulation.
- Emotional support.
- Use of drugs for breakthrough pain, as indicated.
- Use of patient-controlled analgesia.
- Effective pain-control strategies, such as positioning, distraction, relaxation, guided imagery, and external measures.
- Signs and symptoms to report.
- Activity and rest guidelines.
- Factors that exacerbate pain.
- Realistic expectations.
- Ways to promote proper sleep patterns.
- Avoidance of alcohol and substance abuse.
- Stress management.
- Importance of follow-up care and complying with treatment.
- Resources for further information and support.

When your patient is confused

When documenting care for a confused patient, you must show that you assessed for physiologic causes of her confusion, evaluated her behavior carefully, and checked for exacerbating factors. You also must indicate that you took measures to help orient her and ensure her safety.

Document what the patient tells you

If your confused patient isn't a reliable information source, try to obtain data about her health history and current condition from family members, friends, and medical records. Check all three sources closely for clues to the cause of her confusion. Note information about chronic illnesses, hospitalizations, and surgeries as well as a history of neurologic problems, cerebrovascular accident (CVA), or transient ischemic attacks.

To discover if an adverse drug effect, drug interaction, or inappropriate dosage is causing the patient's confusion, record the names of all drugs she uses, along with their dosages and administration times and routes.

Next, determine and record the patient's alcohol consumption pattern. Document information about her living situation, including the names of people who normally are with her during the day and at night and the names of social contacts and sources of support.

To help evaluate the patient's sleep pattern, find out if she's exposed to natural light during the day. Such exposure aids time orientation and affects circadian rhythms. Disruption of circadian rhythms may reduce sleep, possibly causing confusion. Document how much sleep the patient usually gets, and describe her use of sedatives or other measures to promote sleep.

Also ask about sensory deficits, such as decreased visual acuity, hearing, and sensation. Describe corrective devices the patient uses, such as eyeglasses or a hearing aid, and record her perception of the effectiveness of these devices.

Document what you assess

Because confusion can take many behavioral forms and stem from various physical causes, you'll need to perform and document a complete patient assessment. Include the following information.

Onset and symptoms. If you notice that your patient becomes confused at certain times of day, document the behaviors, symptoms, and activities that occur at these times. Note whether the confusion has a gradual or sudden onset, and record the names, dosages, and administration times of drugs she received that day.

Determine if the patient experiences weakness when confused. Assess for and document bilateral hand grip and arm and leg strength. Note difficulty with coordinating fine and gross movements, and document speech abnormalities, such as garbled speech, word searching, aphasia, and difficulty articulating words. Also describe whether your patient is alert or lethargic. If she falls asleep frequently, record how long she can stay awake at one time and how easily you can arouse her from sleep.

Cognitive functions. Record your assessment of the patient's orientation to time, place, situation, and person. Using direct quotes, document her answers to questions you ask when evaluating her reality orientation. When recording her ability to understand what others say, use measurable behaviors. Don't simply rely on her statement that she understands. For instance, document whether she can repeat instructions, follow commands appropriately, and demonstrate procedures taught to her.

Also record your assessment of her short-term, midrange, and long-term memory. Start by asking her to repeat several words you tell her, then ask what she did yesterday, and, finally, question her about events that occurred many years ago.

Next, note whether the patient can focus on one activity for an extended period of time. In her own words, record inappropriate statements she makes; include a description of the circumstances. To make sure you didn't misinterpret her, ask her to explain her statement, and record her explanation.

If your patient exhibits abnormal behaviors or makes statements that suggest she's hallucinating, describe the specific behaviors and record her statements in her exact words. Document her emotional status, too, noting anxiety, irritability, or depression. If her behavior suggests she may harm herself or others, document this behavior and the measures you take to ensure safety, such as providing one-to-one supervision.

Sensory deficits. Document visual, hearing, or other sensory deficits you detect. Record exactly what the patient says and what you observe. For instance, you may write, "Patient states her hearing is adequate when wearing a hearing aid. She did not respond to her name when it was spoken in a normal volume from 2 feet away while she was wearing her hearing aid."

Document what you do and teach
Document interventions you take to keep your patient safe, decrease her confusion, and address its cause. Thorough documentation helps you detect factors that worsen or ease her confusion. Teaching a confused patient and her family helps ensure safe, appropriate care while she's hospitalized and after discharge. If your patient is so confused that you question whether she's capable of consenting to treatment, notify the physician. (See *Is Your Patient Competent?*, p. 364)

Depending on the cause of the patient's confusion, you may need to document the following interventions and teaching points:
• Frequent observation and orientation.
• Safety measures.
• Management of stimulation.
• Sensory and communication needs.
• Drug therapy.
• Laboratory test results.
• Potential hazards of taking nonprescription or herbal preparations without consulting the physician.
• Importance of avoiding potential substances of abuse, such as alcohol.
• Signs and symptoms to report.
• Ways to monitor the patient's condition.
• Follow-up tests.
• Nutrition.
• Importance of daily social contact and routine social activities.

IS YOUR PATIENT COMPETENT?

Legally, every adult is considered competent unless a judge finds otherwise in a formal hearing. A confused patient may be legally competent but unable to consent to treatment or otherwise participate in her treatment plan. If she can't understand the nature of her treatment, she's considered *clinically* incompetent (or incapacitated).

Determining clinical competency

In most facilities, the attending physician decides whether a patient is clinically competent. Nursing documentation of the patient's physical and psychosocial responses to therapy may play a major role in the physician's decision. To determine clinical competency, the physician typically evaluates whether the patient can

- Make definitive decisions
- Understand the information she's given
- Engage in rational decision-making and appreciate the possible outcomes of each option
- Make a reasonable decision about her treatment

Murky legal waters

If the patient falls short in any of the area just mentioned, above, the physician usually tries to obtain consent from the next-of-kin or the patient's appointed health care decision-maker. If the patient is legally competent, obtaining the consent of a surrogate may lead to a legal action for battery, based on unauthorized touching of the patient.

To clarify the issue, lawmakers are addressing the family's surrogate decision-making power. Typically, they favor granting such power if the family acts in good faith. Therefore, obtaining a surrogate's consent generally is considered safer than relying solely on the consent of a clinically incompetent patient.

Documenting care

If you care for a clinically incompetent patient, obtain the names of all family members and identify the next-of-kin, family-appointed spokesperson, or surrogate decision-maker to contact about treatment decisions. Also document conversations you have with these people. Record their names and telephone numbers in the medical record and your nursing documentation.

- Appropriate stimuli, such as a newspaper, radio, clock, calendar, and television.
- Avoidance of drastic changes, such as rearrangement of furniture.
- Keeping the home clean and clutter-free.
- Effective ways to manage agitation and irritability.
- Resources for further information and support.

When your patient has a seizure

Typically, a seizure is self-limited and poses no immediate threat to the patient's life. However, during a seizure, a patient may fall or aspirate gastric contents into the lungs. Also, status epilepticus (a series of uninterrupted seizures) may cause permanent brain damage or even death unless halted promptly by the administration of diazepam, phenobarbital, or another anticonvulsant. Your assessment and in-depth documentation of the patient's status and the actions you take to keep her safe can prove important to her diagnosis and treatment. For instance, your detailed record of her condition before, during, and after the seizure can help determine the seizure type and, possibly, its cause.

Document what the patient tells you

Ask your patient if she has experienced a seizure before, and determine if she has had other neurologic problems. Document her responses. Then record a history of diseases and conditions that increase the risk of seizures, such as hypoglycemia, head trauma, and alcohol or drug use.

If the patient has a history of seizures, document the date of the initial diagnosis and the current treatment plan, including prescribed drugs. Record the names, dosages, and administration frequency of anticonvulsants she's taking, along with the time of her last dose. If she reports a history of alcohol or drug use, document the substance, the time of her last use, and the amount she took. Next, explore factors associated with previous seizures, such as lack of sleep or emotional distress. Document them in the patient's medical record. Then, document nonspecific symptoms she reports just before the seizure, such as headache, mood changes, lethargy, muscle spasms, or jerking. Be sure to note the symptom's timing relative to the seizure. If the patient says she usually has an aura before a seizure, document her description of the aura in her exact words. For instance, she may describe a pungent smell, an unusual taste, nausea, indigestion, a rising or sinking feeling in her stomach, or a visual disturbance, such as seeing flashing lights.

Document what you assess

Besides offering valuable clues to the seizure type and its cause, accurate documentation of your patient's condition and behavior just before, during, and after the seizure provides baseline information that can help the health care team detect changes in her status. If you didn't witness the seizure, try to obtain information from someone who did.

Begin your documentation by describing events that preceded the seizure, such as an aura, outcry, or other behavior. Also record the following information:

- Time the seizure began.
- Time it ended.
- Length of clonic and tonic phases, if present.
- LOC before, during, and after the seizure.
- Neurologic status.
- Pupil responses and arm and leg strength after the seizure.
- Specific body parts affected by the seizure.
- Vital signs during the seizure (if they can be assessed without harming the patient).
- Vital signs after the seizure.
- Respiratory status, noting cyanosis and other signs of inadequate oxygenation.
- Urinary or bowel incontinence.

The patient may receive care before the seizure ends, such as drugs to halt the seizure and position changes to prevent injury. Recordthese interventions. Also document the name, dosage, and administration time and route of the anticonvulsant given, and note its effectiveness in resolving the seizure.

Assessment after the seizure. After the seizure ends, examine the patient for injuries sustained during the seizure, and assess her overall condition. Document your findings thoroughly. Depending on the seizure type and severity, she may display various behaviors immediately after the seizure. Besides documenting her LOC, check for and record other signs and symptoms that occur. Expected findings after a seizure include:
- Confusion.
- Emotional lability.
- Lethargy.
- Fatigue.
- Increased sensitivity to bright lights and noise.
- Amnesia related to the seizure.

Continue to observe and document the patient's condition until she returns to her baseline status.

Document what you do and teach

To promote continuity of care throughout your patient's stay, record the interventions and teaching you perform to maintain her safety before, during, and after the seizure. Include these items:
- The bed in a low position, near the nurse's station.
- Raised and padded side rails.
- Call button within easy reach.
- An emergency airway, supplemental oxygen, and suction equipment in the patient's room.
- Resuscitation equipment and an emergency drug tray nearby.
- Patient instruction to report an aura immediately.
- Patient positioning to one side to maintain an open airway and prevent aspiration.
- Removal of potentially dangerous objects from the area.
- Physician notification.
- Staying at the patient's side until the seizure ends, avoiding restraining the patient.
- Drug and IV therapy.
- Reorientation, reassurance, and reassessment of patient frequently (See *How Often Should You Reassess Your Patient?*).
- Diagnostic testing.
- Regular dental care to treat trauma to the teeth, gums, and mouth.
- Measures to help prevent seizures.
- Medical alert identification.
- Information about driver's license status.
- Resources for further information and support.

HOW OFTEN SHOULD YOU REASSESS YOUR PATIENT?

The Joint Commission on Accreditation of Healthcare Organizations (JCAHO) has developed the following recommendations for patient reassessment. Keep in mind that these recommendations represent the *minimum* requirements. However, your patient may need more frequent reassessment.

Patient	When to Reassess
Same-day surgery patient	On return from postanesthesia unit and immediately before discharge
Stable patient in medical-surgical unit	Every 24 hours
Patient with decreasing neurologic status	Every 15 minutes
Patient in labor	Every 15 minutes
Patient with active GI bleeding	Continuously, on a one-to-one basis
Suicidal patient	Continuously, on a one-to-one basis
Patient in rehabilitation	Every 1 to 2 weeks
Long-term care patient	Monthly

When your patient has a cerebrovascular accident

A patient who experiences a CVA (commonly called a stroke or brain attack) may be in immediate danger of airway obstruction and further brain damage. To help ensure prompt treatment and develop an effective nursing plan of care, you must document her condition thoroughly and record her responses to rapid interventions. Your documentation provides a crucial record of events throughout the course of the patient's illness.

Not all patients who have had a CVA require similar care. The history and assessment findings you'll document and the interventions you'll perform depend on the brain area affected and the cause of the CVA. The most common causes include thrombosis, embolus, and intracerebral hemorrhage. Although diagnostic tests help identify the precipitating condition, timely and effective management hinges on precise nursing observation and documentation.

Document what the patient tells you

During the health history interview, obtain information about the patient's medical history and symptoms just before and during the CVA. If your patient can't communicate, interview family members and check medical records for relevant information.

Medical history. Document a history of hypertension, cerebral aneurysm, or a bleeding disorder because these conditions can cause intracerebral hemorrhage. Also record a history of rheumatic heart disease, endocarditis, posttraumatic valvular disease, open heart surgery, and atrial fibrillation and other arrhythmias. These conditions suggest cerebral embolism as the cause of CVA. Then ask if the patient has a history of peripheral vascular disease, hyperlipidemia, heart disease, diabetes mellitus, transient ischemic attacks, and trauma. Record the information you obtain.

Next, document the names and dosages of prescription and over-the-counter drugs the patient has been taking. If she's taking an antihypertensive or anticoagulant, find out when she last took it and in what dosage; record the answer.

Your patient's lifestyle may provide clues to the cause of her CVA. Documenting this information also promotes more effective rehabilitation planning. Gather as much data as possible about the patient's smoking history, dietary sodium and fat intake, daily activity level, and drug history.

Symptoms. Record information about the patient's condition during the days and hours that led up to the CVA. Ask family members if the patient can't tell you herself. For example, document reports of headache, weakness, dizziness, confusion, memory disturbances, mood swings, tingling, numbness, poor muscle coordination, visual impairment (such as double vision), facial drooping, difficulty swallowing or talking, stiff neck, seizures, bowel or bladder incontinence, and bounding pulse.

Document what you assess
Besides aiding diagnosis and treatment, the data you collect and document during your physical assessment help ensure continuity of care by providing a baseline for later comparison. When documenting your assessment, focus especially on the patient's respiratory, neurologic, and cardiovascular systems.

Respiratory system. Quickly check your patient for a patent airway, and then take steps to maintain it. Measure her respiratory rate, pattern, and effort; evaluate her skin color; and review her pulse oximetry or ABG analysis results. Immediately notify the physician of abnormalities or changes in the patient's status. Then document your findings and your notification of the physician, including the time of notification.

Neurologic system. Accurate documentation of your patient's neurologic status can help caregivers track her progress or deterioration. Record your frequent assessments of her LOC. Remember, though, to document only specific and objective data, not interpretations of your findings. (See *Recording the Level of Consciousness: Objectivity Counts.*)

Because hemiplegia is a common sign of CVA, assess for and document weakness, numbness, and tingling in the arms or legs. Report these problems to the physician promptly. Also check for and record facial

RECORDING THE LEVEL OF CONSCIOUSNESS: OBJECTIVITY COUNTS

When documenting your patient's level of consciousness, include only specific, objective observations—not vague terms that one reader may interpret differently than another. For instance, if the patient is sitting up in bed talking with visitors, record this fact in detail. Don't state merely that she is "alert." If she is unresponsive with no reflexes, describe her that way rather than simply writing "comatose." For more hints, review the following documentation do's and don'ts:

Do write	Don't write
Awake and aware of environment. Interacting with visitors.	Alert
Oriented to her name, place, and today's date, including year.	Appears to know where she is
Sleeps when not stimulated. Easily aroused with verbal stimulation, and then is oriented to her name, place, and today's date.	Lethargic
Aroused with difficulty. Requires physical versus verbal stimulation. Nonsensical verbal responses.	Obtunded
Aroused only with painful stimuli. No verbal response.	Stuporous
Reflex activity only with painful stimulation. Cannot be aroused.	Semicomatose
No response or reflex reactions.	Comatose

drooping, loss of voluntary movement, changes in reflexes, and speech difficulties. When documenting these findings, describe the specific areas of the body affected and the severity of the abnormality.

Next, evaluate for aphasia (defective language function). Remember that aphasia may be receptive, expressive, or mixed. To detect receptive aphasia (inability to understand language), assess the patient's ability to follow simple commands. To detect expressive aphasia (inability to express or form words), ask her to identify an object or a person. Document your findings, which may suggest that she has a specific type of aphasia or mixed aphasia (both types).

Cardiovascular system and other findings. Evaluate and document your patient's cardiovascular system. Measure and record her blood pressure; typically, a CVA increases blood pressure, requiring frequent monitoring and an antihypertensive. If you administer an antihypertensive, document its effectiveness. Be sure to notify the physician if you detect a drop in blood pressure, which may promote brain tissue ischemia or death or indicate continued life-threatening bleeding. Document your notification, including its time, the physician's orders, and your actions.

Then assess for a positive Homans' sign. This sign may suggest DVT, a possible cause of the patient's CVA. Record your findings. Also monitor and document the patient's blood glucose level, which may increase as a result of steroid therapy used to reduce cerebral edema caused by the CVA.

Document what you do and teach

Document all actions you take to maintain the patient's respiratory status and vital signs, curb further cerebral ischemia and infarction, prevent injury, prevent or manage CVA complications, and help her communicate her needs. Also provide teaching to your patient and her family. Be sure to cover these general areas:

- Diagnostic tests.
- Drug and IV therapy.
- Artificial airway, if needed.
- Patient positioning to maintain a patent airway.
- Pulse oximetry.
- Oxygen therapy.
- Suctioning as needed.
- Endotracheal intubation and mechanical ventilation, if needed.
- Nothing by mouth (NPO) status, until swallowing ability is established.
- Fluid intake and output.
- Assistance for personal hygiene.
- Skin protection measures.
- Administration of gastric feedings, if ordered.
- Raised side rails and nearby placement of the call button.
- Toileting schedule and bowel program.
- Turning the patient frequently and using pressure-relief devices, such as a special mattress and heel protectors.
- Passive ROM exercises.
- Antiembolism stockings.
- Footboards, slings, splints, and braces.
- Help with communication.
- Referrals to a speech, occupational, or physical therapist.
- Disease process.
- Ways to reduce risk factors for CVA recurrence.
- Signs and symptoms to report.
- Safety measures and devices to use at home, such as a shower chair.
- Adaptive measures to use when performing activities of daily living.
- Use of ambulatory aids, if needed.
- Home exercise program.
- Telephone numbers for home health agencies.
- Resources for further information and support.

When your patient has hypoglycemia

Defined as a low blood glucose level, hypoglycemia can lead to coma, irreversible brain damage, and death unless treated promptly and effectively.

The condition occurs primarily in type 1 diabetic patients who don't eat enough food, who self-administer too much insulin, or who engage in unusual exertion. Other causes of hypoglycemia include cancer of the stomach, liver, or lung; adrenal gland hypofunction; malnutrition; liver dysfunction; alcoholism; and strenuous exercise.

To establish a foundation for the plan of care, focus your documentation on the patient's history of diabetes mellitus or other disorders, recent food and fluid intake, activity level, recent infections or emotional stress, and alcohol use. Be sure to document all physical assessment findings, laboratory test results, nursing interventions, and patient responses to interventions.

Document what the patient tells you

Most diabetic patients experience warning symptoms of hypoglycemia. Ask your patient to describe how she has been feeling for the past few hours, and record her response in her own words. If she noticed warning signs, try to determine—and then document—exactly when they began and how they progressed. Expect to document the following symptoms:

- Nervousness or shakiness.
- Dizziness or feeling faint.
- Numbness or tingling in the hands and feet.
- Weakness.
- Diaphoresis.
- Hunger or nausea.
- Headache.
- Palpitations.
- Double vision.

If the patient reports such symptoms, ask if she has had them before. If she has, find out if she knows what caused them. Record her responses in her exact words.

Document what you assess

Although the patient's symptoms are important, you'll also need to document objective signs of hypoglycemia. If you witnessed the hypoglycemic episode, record your observation of the following:

- Tremors.
- Personality changes, such as aggressiveness, stubbornness, negativity, or depression.
- Decreased LOC, such as confusion, difficulty speaking, delirium, seizures, or loss of consciousness.
- Poor coordination.
- Cold, clammy skin.
- Increased heart rate or a slow, bounding pulse.
- Increased respiratory rate.

Document what you do and teach

Hypoglycemia can rapidly progress to neurologic compromise, so you'll need to intervene immediately, and notify the physician. After verifying hypoglycemia, vary your interventions with the patient's LOC. Remember to take these general actions and to teach the following key points to prevent recurrence of hypoglycemia:

- Finger-stick glucose levels, using a portable blood glucose meter.
- Administration of 15 g of a simple oral carbohydrate (such as juice, candy, dextrose, or honey) if your patient is conscious and can swallow.
- Administration of an IV carbohydrate (such as dextrose) or subcutaneous, intramuscular, or IV glucagon, if your patient is unresponsive and can't swallow.
- IV access.
- Cause of hypoglycemia.
- Importance of maintaining a normal blood glucose level.
- Signs and symptoms to recognize and actions to take.
- Safety measures.
- Importance of carrying an oral carbohydrate at all times.
- Importance of eating regular meals and snacks, plus what to do if She's sick and unable to eat (sick-day rules).
- Importance of wearing medical alert identification.
- Importance of having regular medical checkups.

When your patient has hyperglycemia

Defined as a high blood glucose level, hyperglycemia seldom poses an immediate threat until the glucose level exceeds 240 mg/dl. With extreme blood glucose level elevation, the patient's condition may rapidly progress to ketoacidosis, a potentially fatal metabolic disorder.

Although commonly caused by diabetes mellitus, hyperglycemia also may stem from Cushing's syndrome (pituitary dysfunction), physical stress (such as trauma, burns, and surgery), and certain drugs (including corticosteroids and thiazide diuretics). In a diabetic patient, common causes of hyperglycemia include insufficient insulin dosage, dietary noncompliance, infection, and gastrointestinal illness.

To provide a basis for the nursing plan of care and the interdisciplinary treatment plan, first determine if your patient has been diagnosed with diabetes. Then explore and document other aspects of her health history, including recent food intake, infections, and physical injury.

Document what the patient tells you

Ask the patient how she has been feeling over the past few days, and record her response in her exact words. She may report these symptoms of hyperglycemia:

- Weakness.
- Unusual thirst.

- Frequent urination.
- Anorexia.
- Vomiting.
- Drowsiness.
- Abdominal pain.
- Headache.

Then find out if she has had hyperglycemia before. If so, record the symptoms she experienced at that time.

Document what you assess

Next, perform a physical examination. Expect to assess and document these signs and symptoms of hyperglycemia:
- Flushed cheeks.
- Dry skin and mouth.
- Acetone (sweet) breath odor.
- Kussmaul's respirations (fast, deep, labored breathing), especially if the blood glucose level exceeds 500 mg/dl.
- Weak, rapid pulse.
- Low blood pressure.
- Restlessness.
- Decreased LOC (possibly unresponsiveness).
- Electrolyte abnormalities, particularly potassium imbalance.
- Glucose and ketones in the urine.
- Signs of infection, such as a fever, increased pulse rate, or hot, dry skin that's flushed.

Document what you do and teach

Besides documenting your rapid interventions, record the patient's responses to these general interventions to show that you took appropriate actions to reverse hyperglycemia, and that she knows how to prevent further hyperglycemia:
- Insulin administration.
- Glucose monitoring.
- Fluid and electrolyte balance.
- Pathophysiology of the disorder.
- Mechanisms of hyperglycemia and ketoacidosis.
- Prescribed drugs, including their names, dosages, administration times and routes, adverse effects, and storage.
- Insulin administration, if indicated.
- Signs and symptoms of hypoglycemia and hyperglycemia, and actions to take if these conditions occur.
- Use of a blood glucose monitor.
- Importance of regular blood glucose monitoring.
- Effect of diet, infection, stress, and exercise on the glucose level.
- Dietary restrictions.

- Foot care.
- Importance of seeing the physician regularly and having regular eye examinations.
- Resources for further information and support.

When your patient has a pressure ulcer

Also called a pressure sore, decubitus ulcer, or bed sore, a pressure ulcer is an ulceration of the skin and underlying tissue. It results from prolonged pressure, primarily on a bony prominence, and reflects ischemic tissue hypoxia. A pressure ulcer may take a long time to heal and demands meticulous care by all health care providers.

When documenting your nursing care, include the patient's risk factors for developing a pressure ulcer, your assessment findings and interventions, and the patient's response. This information helps the health care team evaluate the treatment regimen's effectiveness as healing progresses.

Document what the patient tells you

To determine when the pressure ulcer developed and to detect contributing health care problems, obtain and document a thorough history from your patient and family members. Ask them to describe any changes in the ulcer's size, appearance, drainage, and odor. Document their description accurately.

Then record your patient's complete medical history. Especially note risk factors for pressure ulcers, such as diabetes mellitus, peripheral vascular disease, immunosuppression, smoking, and delayed healing. Collect and document data about the patient's dietary habits to determine whether she's meeting her nutritional needs. Determine if she has a history of incontinence, and document this information. Finally, ask about and record her usual daily routine, including her activity level. If she's bedridden, ask which positions she most often lies in.

Document what you assess

When documenting your initial assessment, be as specific as you can, especially when describing the pressure ulcer's size, stage, appearance, drainage, and odor. Remember—your record provides a baseline for evaluating healing and gauging treatment effectiveness.

Wound stage. Assess the stage of the pressure ulcer according to this guide:
- *Stage I.* Skin redness is unrelieved by removal of the pressure source.
- *Stage II.* Skin is chafed, cracked, blistered, or peeling, but the damage is superficial.
- *Stage III.* The full thickness of the skin and, possibly, subcutaneous (fatty) tissue is lost. Drainage, eschar, and necrotic tissue may be present.

- *Stage IV.* A deep, craterlike ulcer shows destruction of the full thickness of the skin and deeper tissues. Muscle and bone may be exposed and damaged.
- *Unable to stage.* Area covered with necrotic tissue; unable to stage precisely.

You may document wound appearance in a narrative format or by drawing a picture of the wound and labeling it appropriately. When describing wound characteristics, include these features:

- Precise location.
- Diameter in centimeters.
- Depth in centimeters.
- Amount, color, and location of granulation tissue (moist, pink tissue that represents new growth).
- Amount, color, and location of eschar (black or gray, scablike, crusty tissue covering the wound).
- Amount, color, and location of necrotic tissue (dry, black tissue that represents tissue death).
- Amount and description of drainage.
- Description of odor.
- Length and location of any undermining (cavity beneath the wound opening) or tunneling.
- Color and temperature of the surrounding skin.

Describe the amounts of granulation tissue, eschar, and necrotic tissue in percentages of total wound tissue. For instance, if granulation tissue accounts for about half of the pressure sore, record this as "50% granulation."

Nutritional and hydration status. Adequate nutrition and fluid intake are crucial for pressure ulcer healing. To assess your patient's nutritional and hydration status, evaluate and document her skin's general appearance and turgor. Also record the results of serum albumin and total protein assays.

Document what you do and teach

Your interventions for a patient with a pressure ulcer should focus on promoting healing and preventing further skin breakdown. Record each action you take and your patient's response. Also document interdisciplinary and collaborative consultations and interventions (See *Taking the Team Approach to Wound Care,* p. 376.) Your documentation for careful interventions and teaching should include these areas:

- Wound care.
- Pressure reduction.
- Frequent turning and repositioning.
- Good hygiene.
- Overhead trapeze to assist in repositioning.

TAKING THE TEAM APPROACH TO WOUND CARE

When developing a holistic plan of care for a patient with a pressure ulcer, expect to consult these health care team members. Document all pertinent communication with team members.

Dietitian	For strategies on optimizing the patient's nutrition
Occupational therapist	For advice on frequent repositioning to maximize pressure relief
Enterostomal therapist	To help assess the wound, form a plan of care, and evaluate the wound care regimen's effectiveness
Medical social worker	For referrals and resource information to ensure continuity of care after discharge
Plastic surgeon	To surgically repair, debride, and close certain wounds

- Pathophysiology of pressure ulcers.
- Wound care regimen.
- Signs and symptoms to report.
- Importance of good hygiene and skin care.
- Nutrition and fluid requirements to promote healing.
- Use of pressure-reduction or pressure-relief devices.
- Importance of frequent repositioning.

When your patient has surgery

With more same-day surgeries being performed and shorter hospital stays for major surgery, you may find it a challenge to gather and document all the necessary patient information in the time allotted. Yet, no matter how briefly you care for a patient, you must document all the care you provide. Besides serving as the basis for evaluating the plan of care, your documentation reflects the standard of care provided. This can prove important if the patient later sues you, other health care team members, or your health care facility.

Document what the patient tells you

Before surgery, document your patient's medical history. Ask her to describe previous health problems, treatments she received for them, and the effectiveness of those treatments. Then document the information she provides about previous surgeries and other medical procedures. Especially find out if she has experienced an allergic reaction to a food, drug, anesthetic, contrast medium, or dye. If she has never been anesthetized, ask if anyone in her family has experienced a reaction to an anesthetic.

Then determine if she has had a problem with bleeding, such as easy bruising, blood in the urine or stool, or difficulty stopping a cut from bleeding. Also document the use of warfarin or nonsteroidal anti-inflammatory agents. These factors indicate that the patient may have bleeding problems during and after surgery.

Next, have the patient tell you what she knows about the scheduled procedure, and document her response. If she'll go home shortly after surgery, record the type of transportation she'll use and the name of the person who'll accompany her. Also document whether someone will be at her home when she arrives or if she'll be alone that night.

Next, ask the patient when she last ate or drank and what drugs (if any) she has taken that day. Record her reply in her own words. Then question her about any recent symptoms she has had, especially if they seem unrelated to the reason for her upcoming surgery. In particular, document shortness of breath, chest pain, nausea, anxiety, and urinary difficulties.

Record the date of the patient's last bowel movement, and indicate whether she moves her bowels regularly. Also document her usual activity level and daily routine, which may be disrupted during her recovery.

Ask the patient if she has ever smoked. When documenting her answer, include the number of cigarettes per day she smokes or smoked. Also find out if she regularly drinks alcohol or uses recreational drugs, and record her response. Document her use of hearing aids, eyeglasses, and dentures. Finally, record the name of the patient's primary care physician.

During the postoperative period. After the patient returns from surgery, record reports of discomfort and other problems. Ask her to rate her pain's severity on a scale of 0 to 10, with 0 indicating no pain and 10 indicating the worst pain imaginable. Document her answer. Also record the following complaints:
- Urinary urgency with inability to void.
- Shortness of breath.
- Chest pain.
- Nausea.
- Leg pain or cramping.
- Anxiety or fear.

Document what you assess
Perform a physical examination before and after surgery, and document your findings.

Preoperative findings. Remember that your preoperative examination provides a baseline for later assessments. Notify the physician of abnormal findings, such as:
- Hypertension or hypotension.
- Tachycardia or bradycardia.
- Fever.
- Abnormal breath sounds.
- Irregular heart rate.

- Abdominal firmness or distention.
- Cold or discolored arms or legs.

Postoperative findings. Document your postoperative physical examination findings, and then compare them with preoperative findings. Measure and record the patient's vital signs every 5 to 15 minutes for the first hour after surgery and then hourly. Auscultate her lungs, noting the rate, rhythm, and depth of respirations; document these data carefully. Then palpate her peripheral pulses, recording the strength of each pulse. Assess for and document pain on ankle dorsiflexion (Homans' sign).

Next, record the amount of urine in the drainage bag, if present. Use this measurement as a baseline when assessing urine output over the next several hours. Then auscultate and palpate the patient's abdomen, recording abdominal tone and the type of bowel sounds.

Document the appearance of the dressing and the area around the incision, including the amount and color of drainage and skin discoloration. Assess the insertion site for tubes, drains, and catheters, and record their appearance.

Review the patient's latest blood chemistry and hematology results. Notify the physician of abnormal values, and document that you did so.

Document what you do and teach

Document all interventions you performed before and after surgery. In your preoperative documentation, include the steps you took to prepare the patient for surgery, including teaching. In your postoperative notes, record that you implemented all postoperative orders and helped the patient return to her baseline level of functioning. Make sure you cover the following areas in your documentation (see *Documenting Perioperative Care*):

- Completion of preoperative checklist.
- NPO status.
- Signed consent form.
- Correct identification band.
- Removal of personal clothing, jewelry, and prosthetics, such as dentures and contact lenses.
- Taping of wedding ring, if permitted.
- Itemized list of valuables.
- Postanesthesia care unit transfer information.
- Fluid intake and output.
- Diagnostic testing.
- Coughing and deep-breathing exercises.
- Splinting of incision.
- Pain control.
- Drug and IV therapy.
- Antiembolism stockings.
- Leg and foot exercises.

DOCUMENTING PERIOPERATIVE CARE

Before your patient is transferred from the postanesthesia care unit to the surgery suite, review your documentation to make sure it addresses all important aspects of her medical and recent history, the surgery she has just undergone, her postanesthesia care, and her current condition.

Medical and recent history

When documenting history information, be sure to include:
❑ The patient's medical and surgical history
❑ Events leading to current surgery
❑ Complications related to previous surgery or anesthesia (document this prominently at the front of the section)
❑ Drug or food allergies
❑ Current drugs
❑ Tobacco use

Surgery

Surgery documentation should cover:
❑ Type of procedure performed
❑ Time surgery began and ended
❑ Type of anesthesia used
❑ Duration of anesthesia
❑ Range of patient's vital signs during surgery
❑ Name, dosage, and administration time and route of each drug administered
❑ Fluid intake, output, and loss
❑ Use of devices to stop blood flow to a particular area, such as a tourniquet
❑ Type and location of drains, tubes, implants, and dressings left in place
❑ Patient's tolerance of the procedure
❑ Surgical complications

Postanesthesia period

During the postanesthesia period, you may document vital signs, assessment findings, and interventions on a postanesthesia flow sheet. No matter where you record the information, your documentation of the patient's postanesthesia course should include:
❑ Vital signs
❑ Level of consciousness (LOC)
❑ Skin color
❑ Name, dosage, and administration time and route of each analgesic or other drug given
❑ Patient's respiratory status, including the time of endotracheal tube removal, use of supplemental oxygen, if ordered, and arterial blood gas (ABG) levels or pulse oximetry readings
❑ Unusual events or complications, such as vomiting, hypothermia, arrhythmias, swollen tongue, or postspinal headache
❑ Interventions used to treat unusual events or complications documented earlier

Current condition

At the end of your postanesthesia documentation, document the patient's current condition. If the patient is being discharged to home (as with same-day surgery), be sure to document other pertinent findings, such as whether or not the patient can eat, walk, and urinate, as well as your patient's understanding of discharge instructions. Also, be sure to include:
❑ Vital signs
❑ LOC
❑ Interventions that will continue in the surgical unit

* Emotional support to the patient and family.
* Instructions for resuming previous drugs at home.
* Recommended activity level.
* Dietary recommendations or restrictions.
* Care of the incision and remaining drains.
* Signs and symptoms to report.
* Dates and times of follow-up medical appointments.

RISK OF FALLS ASSESSMENT TOOL

Use the following tool to help determine your patient's risk for fall. Remember that a score of 10 or more could indicate a high risk for fall and the need to initiate safety measures. Follow your institution's policies and procedures regarding the use of preventative measures.

Fall Assessment Scoring System	Points
I. Age 65-79 years (1) 80 & older (2)	
II. Mental Status Oriented at all times or comatose (0) Confusion at all times or agitated/uncooperative/anxious—moderate (2) Intermittent confusion or agitated/uncooperative/anxious—severe (4)	
III. Elimination Independent and continent (0) Catheter and/or ostomy (1) Elimination with assistance (3) Ambulatory with urge incontinence or episodes of incontinence (5)	
IV. History of Falling Within 6 Months No history (0) Has fallen one or two times (2) Multiple history of falling (5)	
V. Sensory Impairment Sensory impairment, such as blind, deaf, cataracts, not using corrective device (1)	
VI. Activity Ambulation/transfer without assistance (0) Ambulation/transfer with assistance of one person or an assistive device (2) Ambulation/transfer with assistance of two people (1)	
VII. Medications Narcotics ___ Diuretics ___ Tranquilizers ___ Chemotherapy ___ Sleeping aids ___ Antiseizure/antiepileptic ___ For the above medications, check how many the patient is currently taking at home or that the patient will be taking in the hospital. No medication (0) 1 medication (1) 2 or more medications (2) Add one more point if there has been a change in these medications or dosages in the past 5 days.	
A score of 10 or more indicates a high risk for falling, but if the patient does not meet a score of 10 and in the nurse's judgment is at risk for fall, initiate the high-risk fall protocol.	Total score:

Modified from MacAvoy, S., Skinner, T., & Hines, M. Clinical methods: falls risk assessment tool. *Applied Nursing Research.* 1996;9(4):213, 218.

NIH STROKE SCALE

B

N I H
STROKE
SCALE

Patient Identification __ __ - __ __ __ - __ __ __
Pt. Date of Birth __ __ / __ __ / __ __
Hospital _____ (__ __ - __ __)
Date of Exam __ __ / __ __ / __ __

Interval: ☐ Baseline ☐ 2 hours post treatment ☐ 24 hours post onset of symptoms ±20 minutes
☐ 7-10 days ☐ 3 months ☐ Other _____ (__ __)

Time: __ __ : __ __ ☐ am ☐ pm

Person Administering Scale _____

Administer stroke scale items in the order listed. Record performance in each category after each subscale exam. Do not go back and change scores. Follow directions provided for each exam technique. Scores should reflect what the patient does, not what the clinician thinks the patient can do. The clinician should record answers while administering the exam and work quickly. Except where indicated, the patient should not be coached (i.e., repeated requests to patient to make a special effort).

Instructions	Scale Definition	Score
1a. Level of Consciousness: The investigator must choose a response if a full evaluation is prevented by such obstacles as an endotracheal tube, language barrier, orotracheal trauma/bandages. A 3 is scored only if the patient makes no movement (other than reflexive posturing) in response to noxious stimulation.	0 = **Alert;** keenly responsive. 1 = **Not alert;** but arousable by minor stimulation to obey, answer, or respond. 2 = **Not alert;** requires repeated stimulation to attend, or is obtunded and requires strong or painful stimulation to make movements (not stereotyped). 3 = Responds only with reflex motor or autonomic effects or totally unresponsive, flaccid, and flexic.	_____
1b. LOC Questions: The patient is asked the month and his/her age. The answer must be correct – there is no partial credit for being close. Aphasic and stuporous patients who do not comprehend the questions will score 2. Patients unable to speak because of endotracheal intubation, orotracheal trauma, severe dysarthria from any cause, language barrier, or any other problem not secondary to aphasia are given a 1. It is important that only the initial answer be graded and that the examiner not "help" the patient with verbal or nonverbal cues.	0 = **Answers** both questions correctly. 1 = **Answers** one question correctly. 2 = **Answers** neither question correctly.	_____
1c. LOC Commands: The patient is asked to open and close the eyes and then to grip and release the nonparetic hand. Substitute another one-step command if the hands cannot be used. Credit is given if an unequivocal attempt is made but not completed due to weakness. If the patient does not respond to command, the task should be demonstrated to him or her (pantomime), and the result scored (i.e., follows none, one, or two commands). Patients with trauma, amputation, or other physical impediments should be given suitable one-step commands. Only the first attempt is scored.	0 = **Performs** both tasks correctly. 1 = **Performs** one task correctly. 2 = **Performs** neither task correctly.	_____

From National Institute of Neurological Disorders and Stroke, U.S. Department of Health and Human Service. www.ninds.nih.gov.

N I H
STROKE
SCALE

Patient Identification __ __ - __ __ __ - __ __ __

Pt. Date of Birth __ __ / __ __ / __ __

Hospital _____ (__ __ - __ __)

Date of Exam __ __ / __ __ / __ __

Interval: ☐ Baseline   ☐ 2 hours post treatment   ☐ 24 hours post onset of symptoms ±20 minutes
☐ 7-10 days   ☐ 3 months   ☐ Other _____ (__ __)

Instructions	Scale Definition	Score
2. Best Gaze: Only horizontal eye movements will be tested. Voluntary or reflexive (oculocephalic) eye movements will be scored, but caloric testing is not done. If the patient has a conjugate deviation of the eyes that can be overcome by voluntary or reflexive activity, the score will be 1. If a patient has an isolated peripheral nerve paresis (CN III, IV, or VI), score a 1. Gaze is testable in all aphasic patients. Patients with ocular trauma, bandages, preexisting blindness, or other disorder of visual acuity or fields should be tested with reflexive movements, and a choice made by the investigator. Establishing eye contact and then moving about the patient from side to side will occasionally clarify the presence of a partial gaze palsy.	0 = **Normal.** 1 = **Partial gaze palsy;** gaze is abnormal in one or both eyes, but forced deviation or total gaze paresis is not present. 2 = **Forced deviation,** or total gaze paresis not overcome by the oculocephalic maneuver.	_____
3. Visual: Visual fields (upper and lower quadrants) are tested by confrontation, using finger counting or visual threat, as appropriate. Patients may be encouraged, but if they look at the side of the moving fingers appropriately, this can be scored as normal. If there is unilateral blindness or enucleation, visual fields in the remaining eye are scored. Score 1 only if a clear-cut asymmetry, including quadrantanopia, is found. If patient is blind from any cause, score 3. Double simultaneous stimulation is performed at this point. If there is extinction, patient receives a 1, and the results are used to respond to item 11.	0 = **No visual loss.** 1 = **Partial hemianopia.** 2 = **Complete hemianopia.** 3 = **Bilateral hemianopia** (blind including cortical blindness).	_____
4. Facial Palsy: Ask – or use pantomime to encourage – the patient to show teeth or raise eyebrows and close eyes. Score symmetry of grimace in response to noxious stimuli in the poorly responsive or noncomprehending patient. If facial trauma/bandages, orotracheal tube, tape, or other physical barriers obscure the face, these should be removed to the extent possible.	0 = **Normal** symmetrical movements. 1 = **Minor paralysis** (flattened nasolabial fold, asymmetry on smiling). 2 = **Partial paralysis** (total or near-total paralysis of lower face). 3 = **Complete paralysis** of one or both sides (absence of facial movement in the upper and lower face).	_____
5. Motor Arm: The limb is placed in the appropriate position: extend the arms (palms down) 90 degrees (if sitting) or 45 degrees (if supine). Drift is scored if the arm falls before 10 seconds. The aphasic patient is encouraged using urgency in the voice and pantomime, but not noxious stimulation. Each limb is tested in turn, beginning with the nonparetic arm. Only in the case of amputation or joint fusion at the shoulder should the examiner record the score as untestable (UN), and clearly write the explanation for this choice.	0 = **No drift;** limb holds 90 (or 45) degrees for full 10 seconds. 1 = **Drift;** limb holds 90 (or 45) degrees, but drifts down before full 10 seconds; does not hit bed or other support. 2 = **Some effort against gravity;** limb cannot get to or maintain (if cued) 90 (or 45) degrees, drifts down to bed, but has some effort against gravity. 3 = **No effort against gravity;** limb falls. 4 = **No movement.** UN = **Amputation** or joint fusion, explain: _____ **5a. Left Arm** **5b. Right Arm**	_____ _____

N I H
STROKE
SCALE

Patient Identification __ __ - __ __ __ - __ __ __
Pt. Date of Birth __ __ / __ __ / __ __
Hospital _____ (__ __ - __ __)
Date of Exam __ __ / __ __ / __ __

Interval: ☐ Baseline   ☐ 2 hours post treatment   ☐ 24 hours post onset of symptoms ±20 minutes
☐ 7-10 days   ☐ 3 months   ☐ Other _____ (__ __)

Instructions	Scale Definition	Score
6. Motor Leg: The limb is placed in the appropriate position: hold the leg at 30 degrees (always tested supine). Drift is scored if the leg falls before 5 seconds. The aphasic patient is encouraged using urgency in the voice and pantomime, but not noxious stimulation. Each limb is tested in turn, beginning with the nonparetic leg. Only in the case of amputation or joint fusion at the hip should the examiner record the score as untestable (UN), and clearly write the explanation for this choice.	0 = **No drift;** leg holds 30-degree position for full 5 seconds. 1 = **Drift;** leg falls by the end of the 5-second period but does not hit bed. 2 = **Some effort against gravity;** leg falls to bed by 5 seconds, but has some effort against gravity. 3 = **No effort against gravity;** leg falls to bed immediately. 4 = **No movement.** UN = **Amputation** or joint fusion, explain: _____ **6a. Left Leg** **6b. Right Leg**	_____
7. Limb Ataxia: This item is aimed at finding evidence of a unilateral cerebellar lesion. Test with eyes open. In case of visual defect, ensure testing is done in intact visual field. The finger-nose-finger and heel-shin tests are performed on both sides, and ataxia is scored only if present out of proportion to weakness. Ataxia is absent in the patient who cannot understand or is paralyzed. Only in the case of amputation or joint fusion should the examiner record the score as untestable (UN), and clearly write the explanation for this choice. In case of blindness, test by having the patient touch nose from extended arm position.	0 = **Absent.** 1 = **Present in one limb.** 2 = **Present in two limbs.** UN = **Amputation** or joint fusion, explain: _____	_____
8. Sensory: Sensation or grimace to pinprick when tested, or withdrawal from noxious stimulus in the obtunded or aphasic patient. Only sensory loss attributed to stroke is scored as abnormal, and the examiner should test as many body areas (arms [not hands], legs, trunk, face) as needed to accurately check for hemisensory loss. A score of 2, "severe-to-total sensory loss," should only be given when a severe or total loss of sensation can be clearly demonstrated. Stuporous and aphasic patients will, therefore, probably score 1 or 0. The patient with brainstem stroke who has bilateral loss of sensation is scored 2. If the patient does not respond and is quadriplegic, score 2. Patients in a coma (item 1a = 3) are automatically given a 2 on this item.	0 = **Normal;** no sensory loss. 1 = **Mild-to-moderate sensory loss;** patient feels pinprick is less sharp or is dull on the affected side; or there is a loss of superficial pain with pinprick, but patient is aware of being touched. 2 = **Severe-to-total sensory loss;** patient is not aware of being touched in the face, arm, and leg.	_____

N I H
STROKE
SCALE

Patient Identification __ __ - __ __ __ - __ __ __
Pt. Date of Birth __ __ / __ __ / __ __
Hospital _____ (__ __ - __ __)
Date of Exam __ __ / __ __ / __ __

Interval: ☐ Baseline   ☐ 2 hours post treatment   ☐ 24 hours post onset of symptoms ±20 minutes
☐ 7-10 days   ☐ 3 months   ☐ Other _____ (__ __)

Instructions	Scale Definition	Score
9. Best Language: A great deal of information about comprehension will be obtained during the preceding sections of the examination. For this scale item, the patient is asked to describe what is happening in the attached picture, to name the items on the attached naming sheet and to read from the attached list of sentences. Comprehension is judged from responses here, as well as to all of the commands in the preceding general neurological exam. If visual loss interferes with the tests, ask the patient to identify objects placed in the hand, repeat, and produce speech. The intubated patient should be asked to write. The patient in a coma (item 1a = 3) will automatically score 3 on this item. The examiner must choose a score for the patient with stupor or limited cooperation, but a score of 3 should be used only if the patient is mute and follows no one-step commands.	0 = **No aphasia;** normal. 1 = **Mild-to-moderate aphasia;** some obvious loss of fluency or facility of comprehension, without significant limitation on ideas expressed or form of expression. Reduction of speech and/or comprehension, however, makes conversation about provided materials difficult or impossible. For example, in conversation about provided materials, examiner can identify picture or naming card content from patient's response. 2 = **Severe aphasia;** all communication is through fragmentary expression; great need for inference, questioning, and guessing by the listener. Range of information that can be exchanged is limited; listener carries burden of communication. Examiner cannot identify materials provided from patient response. 3 = **Mute, global aphasia;** no usable speech or auditory comprehension.	_____
10. Dysarthria: If patient is thought to be normal, an adequate sample of speech must be obtained by asking patient to read or repeat words from the attached list. If the patient has severe aphasia, the clarity of articulation of spontaneous speech can be rated. Only if the patient is intubated or has other physical barriers to producing speech should the examiner record the score as untestable (UN), and clearly write an explanation for this choice. Do not tell the patient why he or she is being tested.	0 = **Normal.** 1 = **Mild-to-moderate dysarthria;** patient slurs at least some words and, at worst, can be understood with some difficulty. 2 = **Severe dysarthria;** patient's speech is so slurred as to be unintelligible in the absence of or out of proportion to any dysphasia, or is mute/anarthric. UN = **Intubated** or other physical barrier, explain: _____	_____
11. Extinction and Inattention (formerly Neglect): Sufficient information to identify neglect may be obtained during the prior testing. If the patient has a severe visual loss preventing visual double simultaneous stimulation and the cutaneous stimuli are normal, the score is normal. If the patient has aphasia but does appear to attend to both sides, the score is normal. The presence of visual spatial neglect or anosagnosia may also be taken as evidence of abnormality. Since the abnormality is scored only if present, the item is never untestable.	0 = **No abnormality.** 1 = **Visual, tactile, auditory, spatial, or personal inattention** or extinction to bilateral simultaneous stimulation in one of the sensory modalities. 2 = **Profound hemi-inattention or extinction to more than one modality;** does not recognize own hand or orients to only one side of space.	_____

MINI-MENTAL STATE EXAMINATION

The Mini-Mental State Examination is a quick and easy objective test to gauge your patient's mental status. This standardized screening test gives a maximum score of 30. Patients who have altered mental states, such as depression, usually score between 24 and 30. Patients with dementia or delirium or other psychiatric disorders often score less than 20.

MAX SCORE	SCORE	QUESTION
		ORIENTATION
5		What is the (year)(season)(date)(day)(month)?
5		Where are we: (state)(county)(town)(hospital)(floor).
		REGISTRATION
3		Name three objects: Give 1 second to say each. Then ask the patient all three after you have said them. Give 1 point for each correct answer. Then repeat them until he learns all three. Count trials and record. Trials:
		ATTENTION AND CALCULATION
5		Serial 7's. (Count backward by 7's) 1 point for each correct. Stop after five answers. Alternatively, spell "world" backwards.
		RECALL
3		Ask for the three objects earlier. Give 1 point for each correct answer.
		LANGUAGE
9	Total:	Name a pencil and watch. (2 points) Repeat the following: "No ifs, ands, or buts." (1 point) Follow a 3-stage command: "Take a paper in your right hand, fold it in half, and put it on the floor." (3 points) Read and obey the following: CLOSE YOUR EYES. (1 point) Write a sentence. (1 point) Copy a design. (1 point)
		ASSESS LEVEL OF CONSCIOUSNESS ALONG A CONTINUUM: Alert Drowsy Stupor Coma

INSTRUCTIONS FOR ADMINISTRATION OF THE MINI-MENTAL STATE EXAMINATION

ORIENTATION

1. Ask for the date. Then ask specifically for parts omitted, for example, "Can you also tell me what season it is?" One point for each correct.
2. Ask in turn, "Can you tell me the name of this hospital?" (town, county, etc.). One point for each correct.

REGISTRATION

Ask the patient if you may test his memory. Then say the name of three unrelated objects clearly and slowly, about 1 second for each. After you have said three, ask him to repeat them. The first repetition determines his score (0 to 3), but keep saying them until he can repeat all three, up to six trials. If he does not eventually learn all three, recall cannot be meaningfully tested.

ATTENTION AND CALCULATION

Ask the patient to begin with 100 and count backwards by 7. Stop after five subtractions (93, 86, 79, 72, 65). Score the total number of correct answers.

If the patient cannot or will not perform this task, ask him how to spell the word "world" backwards. The score is the number of letters in correct order. For example, dlrow = 5 and dlorw = 3.

RECALL

Ask the patient if he can recall the three words you previously asked him to remember. Score 0 to 3.

LANGUAGE

Naming: Show the patient a wrist watch and ask him what it is. Repeat for pencil. Score 0 to 2.

Repetition: Ask the patient to repeat a sentence after you. Allow one trial. 0 or 1.

Three-Stage Command: Give the patient a piece of blank paper and repeat the command. Score 1 point for each part correctly executed.

Reading: On a blank piece of paper print the sentence, "Close your eyes," in letters large enough for the patient to see clearly. Ask him to repeat it and do what it says. Score 1 point only if he actually closes his eyes.

Writing: Give the patient a blank piece of paper and ask him to write a sentence for you. Do not dictate the sentence. It is to be written spontaneously. It must contain a subject and verb to be sensible. Correct grammar and punctuation are not necessary.

Copying: On a clean piece of paper, draw intersecting pentagons, each side about 1 inch, and ask him to copy it exactly as it is. All 10 angles must be present and 2 must intersect to score 1 point. Tremor and rotation are ignored.

Estimate the patient's level of sensorium along a continuum, from alert on the left to coma on the right.

COMPARING YOUR PATIENT'S WEIGHT
TO NATIONAL STANDARDS

D

The following table, compiled by the Metropolitan Life Insurance Company, is commonly used to compare a patient's weight to national standards. The weights are for adults ages 25 to 59 wearing clothing (3 lb. of clothes for women and 5 lb. for men). The weight ranges shown encompass all frame sizes. Heights are given without shoes.

Some studies suggest that these weights are nearly 10% lower than the average weight for the U.S. population. Therefore, you may also want to use other calculations, such as body mass index, when assessing your patient for being overweight or underweight.

METROPOLITAN WEIGHT AND HEIGHT TABLES

Women Weight (Pounds)		Height	Men Weight (Pounds)	
Average	Range		Average	Range
117	102-131	4'9"	-	-
119	103-143	4'10"	-	-
121	104-137	4'11"	-	-
123	106-140	5'0"	-	-
126	108-143	5'1"	139	128-150
129	111-147	5'2"	142	130-153
133	114-151	5'3"	144	132-156
136	117-155	5'4"	147	134-160
140	120-159	5'5"	150	136-164
143	123-163	5'6"	153	138-168
147	126-167	5'7"	156	140-172
150	129-170	5'8"	159	142-176
153	132-173	5'9"	162	144-180
156	135-176	5'10"	165	146-184
159	138-179	5'11"	169	149-188
-	-	6'0"	172	152-192
-	-	6'1"	176	155-197
-	-	6'2"	180	158-202
-	-	6'3"	185	162-207

Modified with permission from *1979 Build Study,* Society of Actuaries and Association of Life Insurance Medical Directors of America, 1980, Metropolitan Life Insurance Co.

LAB VALUES

NORMAL BLOOD TEST RESULTS

When you assess the results of your patient's blood tests, use the chart below to see if they fall within the normal range. Keep in mind that normal ranges vary somewhat depending on the laboratory used, so always compare the results to your institution's laboratory.

Blood test	Normal range	Container needed
Alanine aminotransferase (ALT, SGPT)	5 to 35 IU/L	Red top tube
Albumin	3.5 to 5 g/dl	Red top tube
Alkaline phosphatase	30 to 85 ImU/ml	Red top tube
Ammonia	15 to 110 mcg/dl	Green top tube
Amylase	56 to 190 IU/L	Red top tube
Arterial blood gases		Heparinized syringe
pH	7.35 to 7.45	
PCO_2	35 to 45 mm Hg	
HCO_3	21 to 28 mEq/L	
PO_2	80 to 100 mm Hg	
O_2 saturation	95% to 100%	
Aspartate aminotransferase (AST, SGOT)	8 to 20 units/L	Red top tube
Bilirubin (total)	0.1 to 1.0 mg/dl	Red top tube
Bilirubin (direct)	0.1 to 0.3 mg/dl	
Bilirubin (indirect)	0.2 to 0.8 mg/dl	
Bleeding time	1 to 9 min	N/A
Blood urea nitrogen (BUN)	10 to 20 mg/dl	Red top tube
C-reactive protein	Less than 0.8 mg/dl	Red top tube
Calcitonin	Less than or equal to 19 pg/ml (male) Less than or equal to 14 pg/ml (female)	Red or green top tube
Calcium (total)	9 to 10.5 mg/dl	Red top tube
Calcium (ionized)	4.5 to 5.6 mg/dl	
Carbon dioxide (venous)	23 to 30 mEq/L	Red or green top tube
Chloride	90 to 110 mEq/L	Red or green top tube
Cholesterol (total)	Less than 200 mg/dl	Red top tube
Creatine phosphokinase (CPK)	12 to 70 units/ml (male) 10 to 55 units/ml (female)	Red top tube
Isoenzyme MM	100%	
Isoenzyme MB	0	
Isoenzyme BB	0	
Creatinine (serum) /Creatinine clearance	0.6 to 1.2 mg/dl /90 to 139 ml/min (male) 0.5 to 1.1 mg/dl /80 to 125 ml/min (female)	Red top tube for blood
Erythrocyte sedimentation rate (ESR)	Up to 15 mm/hr (male) Up to 20 mm/hr (female)	Lavender top tube

Continued

Blood test	Normal range	Container needed
Ferritin	12 to 300 ng/ml (male) 10 to 150 ng/ml (female)	Red top tube
Fibrin degradation products (FDP)	Less than 10 mcg/ml	Blue top tube
Fibrinogen	200 to 400 mg/dl	Blue top tube
Folic acid	5 to 20 mcg/ml	Red top tube
Glucose (fasting)	70 to 115 mg/dl	Red or gray top tube
Glucose-2 hour post prandial	Less than 140 mg/dl (age 0 to 50) Less than 150 mg/dl (age 50 to 60) Less than 160 mg/dl (age 60 and older)	
Glucose tolerance test	Fasting: 70 to 115 mg/dl 1 hour: Less than 200 mg/dl 2 hours: 140 mg/dl 3 hours: 70 to 115 mg/dl 4 hours: 70 to 115 mg/dl	Gray top tube
Glycosylated hemoglobin	4% to 8%	Gray or lavender top tube
Hemoglobin	14 to 18 g/dl (male) 12 to 16 g/dl (female)	Lavender top tube
Hematocrit	42% to 52% (male) 37% to 47% (female)	Lavender top tube
High density lipoproteins (HDL)	40 to 60 mg/dl	Red top tube
Insulin	5 to 24 mcU/ml	Red top tube
Iron	60 to 90 mcg/dl	Red top tube
Iron binding capacity (TIBC)	25 to 420 mcg/dl	
Iron saturation (transferrin) Transferrin saturation	200 to 400 mg/dl 30% to 40%	
Lactic acid	0.6 to 1.8 mEq/L	Red top tube

Lactic dehydrogenase (LDH)
    LDH-1
    LDH-2
    LDH-3
    LDH-4
    LDH-5
	115 to 225 IU/L
	17% to 27%
	27% to 37%
	18% to 25%
	3% to 8%
	0 to 5%
		Red top tube

Lipase	0 to 110 units/L	Red top tube
Low density lipoproteins (LDL)	Less than 100 mg/dl (Optimal) 100 to 129 mg/dl (Near or above optimal) 130 to 159 mg/dl (Borderline high) 160 to 189 mg/dl (High) 190 mg/dl (Very high)	Red top tube
Magnesium	1.2 to 2.0 mEq/L	Red or green top tube
Osmolality	285 to 295 mOsm/kg H_2O	Red top tube
Parathyroid hormone (PTH)	Less than 2000 pg/ml	Red top tube
Partial thromboplastin time, activated (aPTT)	30 to 40 sec	Blue top tube
Phosphorus	3 to 4.5 mg/dl	Red top tube

Continued

Blood test	Normal range	Container needed
Platelet count	150,000 to 400,000/mm^3	Lavender top tube
Potassium	3.5 to 5.0 mEq/L	Red or green top tube
Protein, total	6.4 to 8.3 g/dl	Red top tube
Prothrombin time (PT)	11 to 12.5 sec	Blue top tube
Red blood cell count	4.7 to 6.1 million/mm^3 (male) 4.2 to 5.4 million/mm^3 (female)	Lavender top tube
Mean corpuscular volume (MCV)	80 to 95 mm^3	
Mean corpuscular hemoglobin (MCH)	27 to 31 pg/cell	
Mean corpuscular hemoglobin concentration (MCHC)	32 to 36 g/dl	
Red blood cell distribution (RDW)	11% to 14.5%	
Reticulocyte count	0.5% to 2%	
Sodium	136 to 145 mEq/L	Red top tube
Thyroid stimulating hormone (TSH)	2 to 10 mcU/ml	Red top tube
Thyroxine (T$_4$)	4 to 11 mcg/dl	
Triiodothyronine (T$_3$)	110 to 230 ng/dl	
Triiodothyronine (T$_3$) uptake	24% to 34%	
Triglycerides	150 mg/dl (Normal) 150 to 199 mg/dl (Borderline high) 200 to 499 mg/dl (High) 500 mg/dl or more (Very high)	Red top tube
Uric acid	2.1 to 8.5 mg/dl (male) 2.0 to 6.6 mg/dl (female)	Red top tube
White blood cell count	5000 to 10,000/mm^3	Lavender top tube
Basophils	0.5% to 1%	
Eosinophils	1% to 4%	
Lymphocytes	20% to 40%	
Monocytes	2% to 8%	
Neutrophils	55% to 70%	

STATURE-FOR-AGE AND WEIGHT-FOR-AGE PERCENTILES (GIRLS)

Mother's Stature _____ Father's Stature _____

Date	Age	Weight	Stature	BMI*

*To Calculate BMI: Weight (kg) ÷ Stature (cm) ÷ Stature (cm) x 10,000
or Weight (lb) ÷ Stature (in) ÷ Stature (in) x 703

AGE (YEARS)

STATURE

WEIGHT

Published May 30, 2000 (modified 11/21/00).
SOURCE: Developed by the National Center for Health Statistics in collaboration with
the National Center for Chronic Disease Prevention and Health Promotion (2000).
http://www.cdc.gov/growthcharts

CDC
SAFER · HEALTHIER · PEOPLE™

STATURE-FOR-AGE AND WEIGHT-FOR-AGE PERCENTILES (BOYS)

*To Calculate BMI: Weight (kg) ÷ Stature (cm) ÷ Stature (cm) x 10,000
or Weight (lb) ÷ Stature (in) ÷ Stature (in) x 703

Date	Age	Weight	Stature	BMI*

Mother's Stature _____ Father's Stature _____

AGE (YEARS)

STATURE

WEIGHT

Published May 30, 2000 (modified 11/21/00).

SOURCE: Developed by the National Center for Health Statistics in collaboration with
the National Center for Chronic Disease Prevention and Health Promotion (2000).
http://www.cdc.gov/growthcharts

CDC

SAFER · HEALTHIER · PEOPLE™

BRADEN SCALE FOR PREDICTING PRESSURE SORE RISK

Patient's Name _____ Evaluator's Name _____ Date of Assessment

SENSORY PERCEPTION Ability to respond meaningfully to pressure-related discomfort	**1. Completely Limited** Unresponsive (does not moan, flinch, or grasp) to painful stimuli, due to diminished level of consciousness or sedation. OR Limited ability to feel pain over most of body.	**2. Very Limited** Responds only to painful stimuli. Cannot communicate discomfort except by moaning or restlessness. OR has a sensory impairment which limits the ability to feel pain or discomfort over one-half of body.	**3. Slightly Limited** Responds to verbal commands, but cannot always communicate discomfort or the need to be turned. OR Has some sensory impair-ment, which limits ability to feel pain or discomfort in 1 or 2 extremities.	**4. No Impairment** Responds to verbal commands. Has no sensory deficit which would limit ability to feel or voice pain or discomfort.			
MOISTURE Degree to which skin is exposed to moisture	**1. Constantly Moist** Skin is kept moist almost constantly by perspiration, urine, etc. Dampness is detected every time patient is moved or turned.	**2. Very Moist** Skin is often, but not always moist. Linen must be changed at least once a shift.	**3. Occasionally Moist** Skin is occasionally moist, requiring an extra linen change approximately once a day.	**4. Rarely Moist** Skin is usually dry, linen only requires changing at routine intervals.			
ACTIVITY Degree of physical activity	**1. Bedfast** Confined to bed.	**2. Chairfast** Ability to walk severely limited OR nonexistent. Cannot bear own weight and/or must be assisted into chair or wheelchair.	**3. Walks Occasionally** Walks occasionally during day, but for very short distances, with or without assistance. Spends majority of each shift in bed or chair.	**4. Walks Frequently** Walks outside room at least twice a day and inside room at least once every 2 hours during waking hours.			
MOBILITY Ability to change and control body position	**1. Completely immobile** Does not make even slight changes in body or extremity position without assistance.	**2. Very Limited** Makes occasional slight changes in body or extremity position but unable to make frequent or significant changes independently.	**3. Slightly Limited** Makes frequent though slight changes in body or extremity position independently.	**4. No Limitation** Makes major and frequent changes in position without assistance.			
NUTRITION Usual food intake pattern	**1. Very Poor** Never eats a complete meal. Rarely eats more than one-third of any food offered. Eats 2 servings or less of protein (meat or dairy products) per day. Takes fluids poorly. Does not take a liquid dietary supplement. OR Is NPO and/or maintained on clear liquids or IVs for more than 5 days.	**2. Probably Inadequate** Rarely eats a complete meal and generally eats only about one-half of any food offered. Protein intake includes 3 servings of meat or dairy products per day. Occasionally will take a dietary supplement. OR Receives less than optimum amount of liquid diet or tube feeding.	**3. Adequate** Eats over half of most meals. Eats a total of 4 servings of protein (meat, dairy products) per day. Occasionally will refuse a meal, but will usually take a supplement when offered. OR Is on a tube feeding or TPN regimen, which probably meets most nutritional needs.	**4. Excellent** Eats most of every meal. Never refuses a meal. Usually eats a total of 4 or more servings of meat and dairy products. Occasionally eats between meals. Does not require supplementation.			
FRICTION & SHEAR	**1. Problem** Requires moderate to maximum assistance in moving. Complete lifting without sliding against sheets is impossible. Frequently slides down in bed or chair, requiring frequent repositioning with maximum assistance. Spasticity, contractures, or agitation leads to almost constant friction.	**2. Potential Problem** Moves feebly or requires minimum assistance. During a move skin probably slides to some extent against sheets, chair, restraints, or other devices. Maintains relatively good position in chair or bed most of the time but occasionally slides down.	**3. No Apparent Problem** Moves in bed and in chair independently and has sufficient muscle strength to lift up completely during move. Maintains good position in bed or chair.				
				Total Score			

IVs, Intravenous fluids; *NPO,* nothing by mouth; *TPN,* total parenteral nutrition.

BODY MASS INDEX-FOR-AGE PERCENTILES (GIRLS)

Date	Age	W	Stature	BMI*	Comments

*To Calculate BMI: Weight (kg) ÷ Stature (cm) ÷ Stature (cm) x 10,000
or Weight (lb) ÷ Stature (in) ÷ Stature (in) x 703

Published May 30, 2000 (modified 10/16/00).
SOURCE: Developed by the National Center for Health Statistics in collaboration with
the National Center for Chronic Disease Prevention and Health Promotion (2000).
http://www.cdc.gov/growthcharts

SAFER · HEALTHIER · PEOPLE™

BODY MASS INDEX-FOR-AGE PERCENTILES (BOYS)

Date	Age	Weight	Stature	BMI*	Comments

*To Calculate BMI: Weight (kg) ÷ Stature (cm) ÷ Stature (cm) x 10,000
or Weight (lb) ÷ Stature (in) ÷ Stature (in) x 703

BMI

AGE (YEARS)

kg/m²

kg/m²

Published May 30, 2000 (modified 10/16/00).
SOURCE: Developed by the National Center for Health Statistics in collaboration with
the National Center for Chronic Disease Prevention and Health Promotion (2000).
http://www.cdc.gov/growthcharts

SAFER · HEALTHIER · PEOPLE™

ASSESSING PAIN IN CHILDREN

K

Most pain scales are based on a numerical rating system, using a 0 to 10 scale for gauging the intensity of pain. But for young children, this system may be too complex to grasp. The Wong/Baker Faces Rating Scale is designed for children older than 3 years of age and can provide objective information about a child's pain experience. Starting at the left of the scale, the happy face represents little or no pain. As the scale progresses to the right, the face becomes progressively sadder and represents a greater intensity of pain.

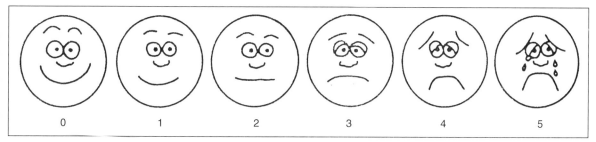

| 0 | 1 | 2 | 3 | 4 | 5 |

From Wong, D. L., Hockenberry-Eaton, M., Wilson, D., Winkelstein, M. L. & Schwartz, P. (2001). *Wong's Essentials of Pediatric Nursing* (6th ed.) p. 1301. St. Louis: Mosby.

Page numbers followed by b indicate boxes.